Heart Disease in Pregnancy

Second edition

EDITED BY

Celia Oakley, MD, FRCP, FESC, FACC
Professor (Emeritus) of Clinical Cardiology, Imperial College School of
Medicine at Hammersmith Hospital, London, UK

Carole A Warnes, MD, FRCP, FACC
Professor of Medicine, Mayo Clinic Consultant, Division of Cardiovascular
Diseases, Internal Medicine and Pediatric Cardiology, Mayo Clinic,
Rochester, Minnesota, USA

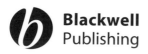
Blackwell
Publishing

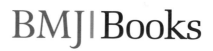
BMJ|Books

© 2007 by Blackwell Publishing
© 1997 BMJ Publishing Group
BMJ Books is an imprint of the BMJ Publishing Group Limited, used under licence

Blackwell Publishing, Inc., 350 Main Street, Malden, Massachusetts 02148-5020, USA
Blackwell Publishing Ltd, 9600 Garsington Road, Oxford OX4 2DQ, UK
Blackwell Publishing Asia Pty Ltd, 550 Swanston Street, Carlton, Victoria 3053, Australia

First published 1997
Second edition 2007

1   2007

Library of Congress Cataloging-in-Publication Data

Heart disease in pregnancy / edited by Celia Oakley, Carole A. Warnes. – 2nd ed. p. ; cm.
Includes bibliographical references and index.
ISBN-13: 978-1-4051-3488-0 (hardcover)
ISBN-10: 1-4051-3488-7 (hardcover)
1. Heart diseases in pregnancy.   I. Oakley, Celia.   II. Warnes, Carole A. [DNLM:
1. Pregnancy Complications, Cardiovascular. WQ 244 H436 2007]
RG580.H4H43 2007 618.3–dc22
2006024341
ISBN: 978-1-4051-3488-0

A catalogue record for this title is available from the British Library

Set in 9.5/12pt Meridien by SNP Best-set typesetter Ltd., Hong Kong
Printed and bound in Singapore by Fabulous Printers Pte Ltd.

Commissioning Editor: Mary Banks
Editorial Assistant: Victoria Pitman
Development Editor: Fiona Pattison
Production Controller: Debbie Wyer

For further information on Blackwell Publishing, visit our website:
http://www.blackwellpublishing.com

17806

Heart Disease in Pregnancy

Contents

Contributors

Dawn Adamson, MB, BS, MRCP, PhD
Specialist Registrar in Cardiology, Cardiology Department, Hammersmith Hospital, London, UK

Jorge R Alegria, MD
Fellow in Cardiovascular Diseases, Mayo Graduate School of Medicine, Rochester, Minnesota, USA

Philip N Baker, BMedSci, BM, BS, FRCOG, DM
Professor of Maternal and Fetal Health, Head of the Medical School, University of Manchester, UK

Giacomo G Boccuzzi, MD
Department of Invasive Cardiology and Coronary Care, Ospedale Humanitas, Milan, Italy

Felice L Bruno, MD, FICS, FACC
Associate Director, El Paso Southwestern Cardiovascular Associates, El Paso; Clinical Associate Professor of Surgery, Texas Technical University, El Paso, Texas, USA

Jack M Colman, MD, FRCPC
Staff Cardiologist and Co-director, Heart Diseases in Pregnancy Program, Toronto Congenital Cardiac Centre for Adults, Mount Sinai Hospital and Toronto General Hospital/UHN; and Associate Professor of Medicine, University of Toronto; Toronto Ontario, Canada

Heidi M Connolly, MD, FACC
Professor of Medicine, Mayo Clinic College of Medicine, Rochester, Minnesota, USA

Alexander Heazell, MBChB (Hons)
Clinical Research Fellow University of Manchester, UK

Graham RV Hughes, MD, FRCP
Lupus Research Unit, The Rayne Institute, St Thomas' Hospital, London; and The London Lupus Centre, London Bridge Hospital, London, UK

JMB Hughes, DM, FRCP
Professor Emeritus, Imperial College School of Medicine, London, UK

Lynne Hung, MD
Fellow in Cardiology, From Griffith Center, Division of Cardiovascular Medicine, Department of Medicine; and LAC USC Medical Center, Keck School of Medicine at University of Southern California, Los Angeles, California, USA

Bernard Iung, MD
Cardiology Department, Bichat Hospital, Paris, France

Munther A Khamashta, MD, FRCP, PhD
Senior Lecturer/Consultant Physician, Director, Lupus Research Unit, The Rayne Institute, St Thomas' Hospital, London, UK

David Lefroy, MD, FRCP
Senior Lecturer and Consultant Cardiologist, Cardiology Department, Hammersmith Hospital, London, UK

Michael D McGoon, MD
Professor of Medicine, Director, Pulmonary Hypertension Clinic, Mayo Clinic College of Medicine, Rochester, Minnesota, USA

Lilian J Meijboom, MD, PhD
Department of Radiology, Onze Lieve Vrouwe Ziekenhus, Amsterdam, The Netherlands

Barbara JM Mulder, MD, PhD
Professor of Cardiology, Cardiology Department, Academic Medical Center, Amsterdam, The Netherlands

Petros Nihoyannopoulos, MD, FRCP, FACC
Professor of Cardiology, Hammersmith Hospital, Imperial College School of Medicine, London, UK

Rick A Nishimura, MD
Judd and Mary Morris Leighton Professor of Cardiovascular Diseases, Mayo Clinic College of Medicine, Rochester, Minnesota, USA

Celia Oakley, MD, FRCP, FESC, FACC
Professor (Emeritus) of Clinical Cardiology, Hammersmith Hospital, London, UK

Joseph G Parambil, MD
Assistant Professor, Cleveland Clinic Lerner College of Medicine, Consultant, Department of Pulmonary and Clinical Care Medicine, Cleveland Clinic, Ohio, USA

Patricia Presbitero, MD
Director of Department of Invasive Cardiology and Coronary Care, Ospedale Humanitas, Milan, Italy

Shahbudin H Rahimtoola, MB, FRCP, MACP, MACC, DSc(Hon)
Professor University of Southern California G.C. Griffith Professor of Cardiology; Professor of Medicine Keck School of Medicine at USC; Griffith Center, Division of Cardiovascular Medicine, Department of Medicine; and *LAC USC Medical Center, Keck School of Medicine at University of Southern California, Los Angeles, California, USA*

Kirk D Ramin, MD
Associate Professor, Head, Division of Maternal Fetal Medicine, Department of Obstetrics and Gynecology, and Director, Maternal Fetal Medicine Fellowship Program, University of Minnesota, Minneapolis, USA

Guillermo Ruiz-Irastorza, MD, PhD
Consultant Physician, Professor of Medicine, Department of Internal Medicine, Hospital de Cruces, University of the Basque Country, Bizakaia, Spain

Claire L Shovlin, PhD, FRCP
Senior Lecturer, Cardiac Sciences, NHLI, Imperial College and Honorary Cansultant in Respiratory Medicine, Hammersmith Hospital, London, UK

Candice K Silversides, MD, FRCPC
Assistant Professor of Medicine (Cardiology), University of Toronto; Toronto Congenital Cardiac Centre for Adults; University of Toronto Cardiac Diseases in Pregnancy Program, Mount Sinai Hospital and Toronto General Hospital, Toronto, Ontario, Canada

Anita K Simonds, MD, FRCP
Consultant in Respiratory Medicine, Academic Department of Sleep and Breathing, Royal Brompton Hospital, London, UK

Philip J Steer, BSc, MB, BS, MD, FRCOG
Professor of Obstetrics and Gynaecology, Academic Department of Obstetrics and Gynaecology, Imperial College London, Faculty of Medicine, Chelsea and Westminster Hospital, London UK

James R Trimm, MD
Fellow in Cardiology, From Griffith Center, Division of Cardiovascular Medicine, Department of Medicine, LAC USC Medical Center, Keck School of Medicine at University of Southern California, Los Angeles, California, USA

Gurinder Vasdev, MD, FRCAnaes, FFARCSI
Assistant Professor of Anesthesia and Perinatology, Mayo Clinic College of Medicine, Rochester, Minnesota, USA

Carole A Warnes, MD, FRCP, FACC
Professor of Medicine, Mayo Clinic Consultant, Division of Cardiovascular Disease, Internal Medicine and Pediatric Cardiology, Mayo Clinic, Rochester, Minnesota, USA

Preface

The second edition, like the first one, is intended to provide practical guidance to clinicians looking after patients with heart disease, or who may be at risk of cardiac problems, in pregnancy and the puerperium. These will be hospital physicians and cardiologists, obstetricians, general practitioners and specialist nurses who provide direct care as well as the anaesthetists responsible for making delivery safe and the geneticists who answer the many questions posed by couples with a personal or family history of heart disease.

All of our contributors were chosen for the wealth of their personal clinical experience of pregnancy in a particular area of cardiovascular-respiratory disease. While modern cardiology has a broader evidence basis from clinical trials than any other speciality such evidence is singularly lacking for pregnancy in which practice is based at best on cohort studies, otherwise it relies on literature reviews, anecdote and personal experience. Clinical trials are sparse even in the area of hypertension and this will always be so because numbers are inevitably small and neither clinicians nor patients feel comfortable about randomisation into trials at this time. National registries may be a potential solution for the future.

Antenatal cardiac clinics and the practice of shared care with local cardiologists and general practitioners has expanded since the first edition, helped especially by the creation of regional centres for grown up congenital heart disease and combined clinics. Regional centres mean longer journeys but shared care reduces their frequency and brings patients access to local help when they need it. We hope you will find what you need in these pages.

Acknowledgments

We are grateful to all our contributors for responding to the call to write, for their enthusiastic participation and, mostly, on-time delivery. We thank Mary Banks, Veronica Pock and Fiona Pattison of Blackwells for guidance. I am grateful to my colleague Professor Petros Nihoyannopoulos for the echocardiograms shown in chapters 4, 14 and 17.

CHAPTER 1

Overview

Celia Oakley

It is nearly a decade since the first edition and, in the second edition, I am joined by my friend and colleague Professor Carole Warnes as co-editor. Together we have gathered our most wanted contributors from both sides of the Atlantic and from Europe.

Much has happened: exponential advances in the practice of cardiology and continued evolution of our case mix of pregnant patients with heart disease. The increasing success of neonatal surgery allows more and more infants with complex anomalies to reach adulthood, wanting normal lives with jobs and families. Except in developing countries, women with congenital heart disease now far outnumber those with rheumatic heart disease which used to be found in up to 1 per cent of all pregnant women. Career women postponing pregnancy account for larger numbers of older patients with hypertension and atheromatous coronary disease.

Heart disease is the third most common cause of maternal death and the leading non-obstetric cause. Some heart conditions, such as pulmonary embolism, arrhythmias, hypertension in pre-eclamptic toxemia and peripartum cardiomyopathy, develop as a complication of pregnancy in previously healthy women, but women with pre-existing heart disease may be predisposed to some of these complications and less able to cope with them.

Most women with heart disease who are in New York Heart Association class I or II before pregnancy accomplish pregnancy safely, but exceptions include patients with fixed left-sided obstruction such as mitral or aortic stenosis or those who have pulmonary vascular disease or fragile aortas. The risk is obviously high in women with NYHA class III or IV symptoms before pregnancy. Significant heart conditions are usually known about before pregnancy but there are important exceptions that paradoxically include just these high-risk conditions: pulmonary hypertension, mitral stenosis, some cardiomyopathies, the fragile aorta, atrial septal defect (ASD) and, nowadays, coronary artery disease as well.

Pregnant women do not want to travel and so they seek local care but most pregnant women have normal hearts, so local experience of heart disease is likely to be sparse. Women with known or suspected heart disease planning pregnancy, or pregnant women with unexplained shortness of breath, need to be referred for full diagnosis at a specialist center where the conduct of pregnancy can be planned. Antenatal care is then shared between the specialist center and the local cardiologist, obstetrician and GP. The site and mode of delivery can be planned according to individual need, with the local carers being confident that they know where and whom to call upon for advice if it is needed. The care of grown-up women with congenital heart disease, once consigned to adult cardiologists among whom few had relevant knowledge or interest, has improved through the appointment of appropriately trained cardiologists in the major cardiac units.

Echocardiography is the keystone of diagnosis and, along with an ECG, usually provides all that is needed for a clinical diagnosis; although the use of chest radiographs should be limited during pregnancy, they can provide useful information that is not otherwise easily obtained. An echocardiogram is always performed in the specialist center but so often, tragically, is not thought about by the generalist.

The use of drugs is avoided as much as possible during pregnancy, but they may be necessary and their possible effects on the fetus need to be known. Rhythm disturbances may first develop or become more frequent during pregnancy and cause considerable concern over the best choice of management. More reliance is placed on evidence from randomized trials in cardiology than in any other specialty, but there is no such evidence from which to guide management in pregnancy. Both clinicians and patients would probably be reluctant to join such trials and recruitment of adequate numbers would be difficult. Nearly all drugs prescribed in pregnancy have crept into common use without trial, and their use has been continued as long as their track record remained clean. Coumarin anticoagulants are the exception because, with no effective alternative, they continue to be recommended for patients with mechanical valves.

Previously undetected mitral stenosis is not uncommon in young immigrant women. It would be recognized immediately and treated promptly in their own countries, but tends to be missed in the west because it has become rare. Clinical competence is fast disappearing in favor of technology. Shortness of breath is too easily ascribed to the pregnancy or to asthma, and echocardiography requires at least a suspicion that there may be a cardiac cause. The radiation dose from a chest radiograph is only half as much as the natural background radiation received in the course of a year, and is about the same as that received during a flight across the Atlantic.

Patients with simple congenital cardiac defects do well but some more complex abnormalities may cause concern. Patients who have had holes closed or valves opened will sometimes have residual problems. Those who have survived heroic surgery during infancy for the palliation of complex defects need detailed assessment. Some of these patients face trouble in pregnancy. Aortic valve stenosis, previously mild in childhood, may have become more severe but the patient has been lost to follow-up until a pregnancy. Other patients who have considered themselves cured may have been left with substantial, but undiagnosed and progressive, pulmonary hypertension. Ebstein's anomaly, Eisenmenger syndrome or corrected transposition may be recognized for the first time at an antenatal clinic. Women with valved conduits, univentricular circulations or interatrial (or arterial) switches for transposition all want to live normal lives and have families. A rich variety is seen. These patients seek advice about the risks of future pregnancy and they want to know the genetic risks to a potential child.

Optimum management requires correct appraisal of the probable ability of the abnormal heart to make the necessary adaptations to the major hemodynamic and respiratory changes that take place during pregnancy, labour and delivery. It is important to predict potential trouble in advance both for the mother and for the baby, and so reduce any likely adverse influences on the developing fetus, whose risks may be both environmental and genetic. Percutaneous intervention with appropriate shielding can be performed when necessary.

The increases in blood volume, stroke output and heart rate (particularly if stroke volume cannot be increased) may not be well tolerated. The relaxation of smooth muscle, which allows accommodation of the increased blood volume, and the profound fall in systemic vascular resistance are beneficial to patients with regurgitant valve disease or left-to-right shunts because the abnormal flows tend to diminish Patients with impaired left ventricular function may benefit from the fall in afterload but this may be offset by an increase in preload. When the left atrial pressure is raised, it will rise further during pregnancy because of the increase in intrathoracic blood volume. Reflex tachycardia, when stroke volume fails to rise appropriately, betrays a lack of circulatory reserve. This may not matter when left ventricular filling is rapid but may precipitate pulmonary edema when it is slow in patients with left ventricular inflow or outflow obstruction and increase myocardial ischaemia, and failure in patients with aortic stenosis, hypertrophic cardiomyopathy or pulmonary hypertension.

The fall in systemic vascular resistance causes right-to-left shunts to increase during pregnancy, with more shortness of breath, more cyanosis and a rise in packed cell volume. Fetal perfusion suffers with risk of miscarriage, prematurity and dysmaturity. When cyanosis is associated with pulmonary stenosis the mother may tolerate pregnancy (with risk of venous thrombosis and paradoxical embolism), but if she has pulmonary hypertension (Eisenmenger syndrome) the risk is mortal.

The highest maternal mortality from heart disease is in patients with pulmonary hypertension, whether idiopathic, or associated with other disease or with reversed central shunt in Eisenmenger syndrome. New drugs (no track record) offer some amelioration in milder disease but patients with Eisenmenger syndrome are usually unresponsive. The maternal mortality rate may be as high as 50%, the result of tilting the finely balanced systemic and pulmonary vascular resistances upon which survival and well-being depend. A fall in systemic resistance, associated perhaps with a vagally induced systemic depressor reflex or increase in pulmonary vascular resistance, may cause the right ventricle to empty most of its output into the aorta, with consequent plummeting of arterial oxygen saturation and ventricular fibrillation. In patients with pulmonary hypertension unassociated with septal defects, the stroke output may be low and fixed. Any systemic vasodilatation may lead to a fall in blood pressure, right ventricular ischaemia, loss of output and sudden death. Most deaths occur in the puerperium either suddenly or associated with a seemingly immutable increase in pulmonary vascular resistance, which is unresponsive to all efforts to bring about vasodilatation.

In the peripartum and postpartum periods, maternal heart failure may develop with seemingly explosive suddenness in peripartum cardiomyopathy or coronary dissection may cause sudden myocardial infarction. Thromboembolism is a hazard after cesarean section and in women with restricted cardiac outputs or cyanotic heart disease.

The management of delivery, whether natural or cesarean under general or regional anesthesia, is crucial to the survival of both mother and baby in women with heart disease. The obstetric anesthetist is an important member of the team and there should be early discussion of the mode of delivery among cardiologist, obstetrician and anesthetist. Although epidural analgesia or anesthesia is well tolerated by patients with abundant circulatory reserve, vasodilatation can cause a redistribution of blood volume away from the thorax, resulting in a fall in filling pressure and cardiac output that needs to be compensated by fluid loading. This has to be finely judged when systemic and pulmonary venous filling pressures are critical. If the stroke output cannot be raised, the slight fall in blood pressure that usually accompanies epidural anesthesia may become profound. Vasodilatation increases fetal as well as maternal hypoxemia in patients with right-to-left shunts and, in those with outflow obstruction vasodilatation may lead to failure of distal perfusion.

In general, normal delivery has been favored for women with heart disease. This dates from a time when the most common maternal disease was mitral stenosis. Patients were kept in bed during the latter part of pregnancy and, with the inferior vena cava compressed by the gravid uterus and intrapulmonary pressures thus minimized, they came to term without the need for beta-blocking drugs to prevent tachycardia. The progress of labour was apparently expedited by the inotropic effects of digitalis on the contracting uterus, and a little postpartum blood loss helped as well.

Good arguments can be made for more frequent use of cesarean delivery for certain cardiac patients. Heart disease tends to get worse, so the first pregnancy may be the only pregnancy. In addition to protecting the child, it safeguards patients with fragile circulatory reserve by eliminating maternal physical effort and expediting the birth process. In cyanosed women the effort of normal delivery increases right-to-left shunting. cesarean section gives babies who are usually premature and small for dates their best chance of survival. cesarean delivery under epidural anesthesia minimizes aortic wall stress in women with Marfan syndrome and is obligatory to prevent skull compression if the baby is anticoagulated by maternal warfarin in patients with mechanical valves.

The clinical geneticist plays an increasing part as more becomes known about the inheritance of cardiovascular defects and cardiomyopathies. Antenatal diagnosis by fetal echocardiography or sometimes by fetal sampling offers early diagnosis or reassurance.

Optimum management of pregnancy in women with heart disease is a team effort. Patients are best seen in joint antenatal cardiac clinics where their progress can be monitored and the delivery strategy planned.

We hope that readers will find practical help from the wealth of clinical experience built into this second edition. If we seem to concentrate on potential disaster it is to help to avert it. Most patients with heart disease do well.

CHAPTER 2

Physiological changes in pregnancy

Candice K Silversides, Jack M Colman

Physiological changes during pregnancy facilitate the adaptation of the cardiovascular system to the increased metabolic needs of the mother, thus enabling adequate delivery of oxygenated blood to peripheral tissues and the fetus. Changes occur in circulating blood volume (affecting preload), peripheral vascular compliance and resistance (affecting afterload), myocardial function and contractility, heart rate, and sometimes heart rhythm and the neurohormonal system (Table 2.1). Women without heart disease adapt well and adverse cardiac events are rare. In some women, heart disease may first be detected during pregnancy when inadequate adaptation exposes previously unrecognized limitations of cardiac reserve. In the presence of important maternal structural heart disease, increased cardiovascular demands of pregnancy can result in cardiac decompensation, arrhythmias, and, rarely, maternal death. This chapter examines the physiologic changes of pregnancy as they occur in the antepartum period, at the time of labour and delivery (peripartum), and in the postpartum period.

Changes in the antepartum period

An increase in blood volume and heart rate as well as a reduction in systemic vascular resistance bring about the increase in cardiac output necessary to sustain pregnancy.

Circulating blood volume

An increase in blood volume has been documented in a number of studies; however, there is variability among studies with regard to the magnitude and timing of this increase. The increased blood volume delivered to the ventricle during pregnancy increases the preload (the distending force on the ventricular wall) and can be estimated by examining ventricular diastolic volume and pressure.

Blood volume begins to increase in week 6 of gestation and by the end of pregnancy it will have reached approximately 50% more than in the pre-pregnant state (Figure 2.1).[1,2] Individuals differ considerably; one study demonstrated individual increases from 20% to 100% above pre-pregnant

Table 2.1 Hemodynamic changes during pregnancy, peripartum and post partum

	Pregnancy	Peripartum	Post partum
Blood volume	↑	↑	↓
Systolic blood pressure	↓	↑	↑
Diastolic blood pressure	↓	↑	↑
Systemic vascular resistance	↓	↑	↑
Heart rate	↑	↑	↓
Stroke volume	↑	↑	↓
Cardiac output	↑	↑	↓

Hemodynamic changes are discussed in more detail in the text.

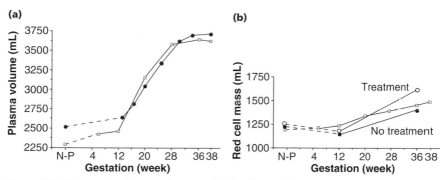

Figure 2.1 Changes in plasma volume and red cell mass during pregnancy. N-P, not pregnant. (Plasma volume data reproduced from Lind[1] and Pirani et al.[2] Red cell mass reproduced from Lind[1] and Taylor and Lind.[5]) (b) The treatment group (white circles) included women treated with folic acid and iron. Women in the no-treatment group (black circles) were not given any supplements.

blood volume.[3] All studies have shown that blood volume progressively increases, at least until mid-pregnancy; some studies have found that it plateaus in the third trimester,[4,5] whereas others suggest that it increases continuously until term.[6] The increase in blood volume is more pronounced in twin pregnancies.[7] Red cell mass increases as much as 40% above pre-pregnancy levels.[2,5] The plasma volume increase is proportionally greater than the increase in red blood cell mass, and the resulting hemodilution explains the so-called 'physiological anemia of pregnancy'. Reduced plasma volume expansion has been associated with low birthweight and intrauterine growth retardation.[8]

In normal pregnancies, there is an increase in the left ventricular end-diastolic volume (assessed echocardiographically), which can be noted by 10 weeks' gestation and peaks during the third trimester. There are also increases in the left atrial, right atrial and right ventricular diastolic dimensions (Table 2.2).[9]

Preload is influenced by maternal position: the supine position results in compression of the inferior vena cava and consequent obstruction of venous return and decreased cardiac output. The effect is more profound in twin

Table 2.2 Cardiac chamber dimensions (measured by echocardiography) during pregnancy and post partum in pregnant women ($n = 18$)

Chamber	Weeks 8–12	Weeks 20–24	Weeks 30–34	Weeks 36–40	Puerperium	Control
LVd (mm)	41.1 ± 3.1	42.7 ± 2.2	43.0 ± 1.7	43.6 ± 2.5	41.8 ± 1.8	40.1 ± 3.0
LA (mm)	29.6 ± 2.1	31.5 ± 2.4	33.1 ± 2.4	32.8 ± 3.0	29.9 ± 3.1	27.9 ± 2.4
RVd (mm)	30.1 ± 2.0	31.9 ± 2.1	35.5 ± 3.2	35.5 ± 2.3	31.1 ± 2.1	28.5 ± 3.0
RA (mm)	42.8 ± 2.3	47.4 ± 2.4	50.8 ± 2.7	50.9 ± 2.8	46.6 ± 3.3	43.7 ± 4.4

LVd, left ventricular diastolic dimension; LA, left atrial dimension; RVd, right ventricular diastolic dimension; RA, right atrial dimension.

Values represent the mean value ± standard deviation (SD).

Reproduced from Campos.[38]

compared with singleton pregnancies. A paravertebral collateral circulation can develop that allows blood to bypass the obstructed inferior vena cava.

A number of mechanisms are postulated for the hypervolemia of pregnancy. Estrogen increases renin levels and causes sodium retention and an increase in total body water. Other hormones, such as prolactin, placental lactogen, prostaglandins and growth hormone, are increased during pregnancy and may contribute to fluid retention.

Despite increasing blood volume and atrial and ventricular distension, cardiac filling pressures (central venous pressure and pulmonary capillary wedge pressure) have not been shown to be higher in women at term compared with women 11–13 weeks' postpartum (Table 2.3).[10] The ability of a normal heart to adapt to chronic volume overload probably prevents pressures from increasing in women without heart disease.

Women with dilated cardiomyopathy, obstructive valve lesions such as mitral stenosis or pulmonary hypertension may not be able to adapt to the increased blood volume. In such patients, increased preload can result in decompensation. In contrast, in patients with hypertrophic obstructive cardiomyopathy, increased preload and larger ventricular dimensions may diminish the degree of left ventricular outflow tract obstruction, improving the hemodynamics during pregnancy.

Peripheral vascular compliance and resistance

Afterload is the force against which the ventricular muscle contracts; typically it is reduced during pregnancy. In the absence of outflow tract obstruction, systemic ventricular afterload can be approximated by either measuring the arterial systolic pressure or calculating the systemic vascular resistance.

During pregnancy, there is a fall in systemic (peripheral) vascular resistance beginning in week 5 of gestation with a nadir between weeks 20 and 32. After week 32 of gestation, the systemic vascular resistance slowly increases until term. There is a corresponding initial decrease in the systemic arterial pressure, which begins in the first trimester and reaches its nadir at mid-pregnancy.[11,12] Thereafter, systemic pressure begins to increase again and ultimately reaches or

Table 2.3 Hemodynamic changes at term and post partum (measured by cardiac catheterization)

Measurement	Post partum (mean ± SD)	At term (mean ± SD)	Percentage change	P
Cardiac output (L/min)	4.3 ± 0.9	6.2 ± 1.0	44	0.0003
Heart rate (beats/min)	71 ± 10	83 ± 1.0	17	0.015
Mean arterial pressure (mmHg)	86.4 ± 7.5	90.3 ± 5.8	4.5	0.210
Systemic vascular resistance (dyn cm/s^{-5})	1530 ± 520	1210 ± 266	−21	0.100
Pulmonary vascular resistance (dyn cm/s^{-5})	119 ± 47	78 ± 22	−34	0.022
Central venous pressure (mmHg)	3.7 ± 2.6	3.6 ± 2.5	−2.7	0.931
Pulmonary capillary wedge pressure (mmHg)	6.2 ± 2.1	7.5 ± 1.8	19	0.187
Left ventricular stroke work index (g m/m^{-2})	41 ± 8	48 ± 6	17	0.040

Reproduced from Clark et al.[10]

SD, standard deviation.

exceeds the pre-pregnancy level. The overall fall in systemic vascular resistance is a result of changes in resistance and flow in multiple vascular beds. During pregnancy, blood flow increases in the low impedance uteroplacental circulation, reaching up to 500 mL/min at term, measured in the supine position, and even higher in the left lateral decubitus position.[13] Placental flow increases until week 25 of gestation and then remains unchanged. In addition there is a fall in resistance caused by increased levels of peripheral vasodilators, in particular prostacyclin (PGI_2).

Renal blood flow increases during pregnancy, peaking in the third trimester at about 60–80% above pre-pregnancy levels. This coincides with a 50% increase in the glomerular filtration rate.[14] Changes in renal blood flow are primarily caused by renal vasodilatation and are also altered by positional changes. Supine recumbency and sitting result in lower glomerular filtration rates. The blood flow to the hands and feet increases during pregnancy, with an increase in cutaneous flow that results in warm erythematous extremities. Nasal congestion results from increased flow to the nasal mucosa. Mammary blood flow increases, causing breast engorgement, dilatation of superficial veins and a continuous murmur known as the mammary souffle. No changes have been shown to occur in cerebral or hepatic blood flow. Coronary blood flow has not been studied in pregnancy.

Not only is the inferior vena cava compressed in the supine position, but the uterus may obstruct the abdominal aorta and the iliac arteries.[15] This compression is relieved by shifting to the left lateral decubitus position. The decreased cardiac output that occurs in the supine position is usually compensated by an increase in supine systemic vascular resistance. The 'supine hypotensive syndrome of pregnancy' occurs when there is inferior vena caval obstruction, possibly further exacerbated by an underdeveloped paravertebal collateral system, and insufficient increase in the systemic vascular resistance or heart rate.

Generally a decrease in afterload will not exacerbate cardiac dysfunction; in fact, the decreased afterload in women with regurgitant valve lesions helps to attenuate the severity of the regurgitation. However, in specific situations, decreases in afterload can be detrimental, e.g. in women with Eisenmenger syndrome and also in other types of cyanotic heart disease, a decrease in afterload facilitates an increase in right-to-left intracardiac shunting, leading to increased cyanosis and hypoxemia. As another example, changes in renal blood flow impacting on drug excretion and changes in the volume of distribution of drugs together explain in large part the need for modified drug dosing during pregnancy.

Anatomical changes during pregnancy

The physiological changes in preload and afterload are accompanied by remodeling of the ventricles and atria. All four cardiac chambers increase in size from the first trimester to the end of the third trimester. The dimensions decrease to baseline levels in the postpartum period (see Table 2.2). Left ventricular remodeling also manifests as increases in left ventricular wall thickness and mass.[16–20] Structural changes also occur at the level of the valve annulus: increases in mitral, tricuspid and pulmonic annular diameters lead to increasing degrees of mitral, tricuspid and pulmonic regurgitation. Small pericardial effusions are frequently found, which usually resolve after delivery.[21]

Increases in atrial size may contribute to atrial arrhythmias during pregnancy. Other changes, such as small pericardial effusion, may have little clinical significance. Although the prognostic significance of changes such as ventricular remodeling are well described in non-pregnant women, their magnitude and direction, and their long-term prognostic significance, have not yet been well studied in pregnant women with structural heart disease.

Myocardial function and contractility

Both systolic and diastolic function contribute to overall cardiac performance. Contractility is the ability of the heart to generate force and shorten, and is usually approximated by surrogate assessments of systolic myocardial function such as cardiac output (index), velocity of circumferential fiber shortening and ejection fraction. Left ventricular diastolic function, which influences the ability of the heart to fill effectively, is assessed most commonly by examining echocardiographic Doppler-filling patterns.

Cardiac output has been the most extensively studied measure of cardiac performance during pregnancy and is dependent on heart rate and stroke volume, both of which increase during pregnancy (Figure 2.3). Cardiac output increases by about 30–50%,[10,11,16,17,22] with the first increase noted as early as week 5 of gestation and reaching a peak at approximately the end of the second trimester

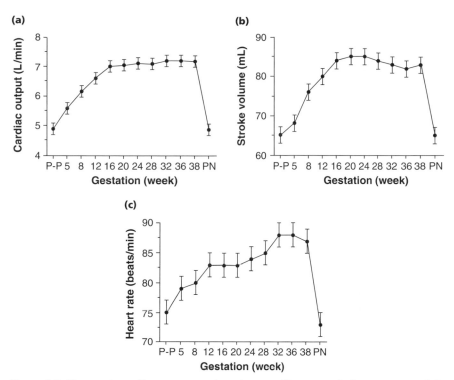

Figure 2.2 Changes in cardiac output, stroke volume and heart rate during pregnancy. P-P, prior to pregnancy; PN, postnatal – 6 months after delivery. (Adapted from Robson et al.[11])

according to some (see Figure 2.2)[11] and later in the third trimester, according to others.[23] Thereafter, cardiac output remains unchanged till term, or decreases slightly near term. Although most of the increase in cardiac output results from increase in stroke volume, increased heart rate also contributes; this becomes more important later in the pregnancy when the stroke volume plateaus while the heart rate continues to rise.[11,24] Although less information is available about the cardiac response to pregnancy of women with heart disease, Ueland et al. showed that pregnant women with underlying cardiac disease have lower cardiac output than pregnant women with normal cardiac function.[25]

Studies vary with regard to the effect of pregnancy on left ventricular ejection fraction. Some studies have demonstrated increases in ejection fraction,[11] whereas others have shown no significant change.[17,26,27] Ejection fraction is sensitive to changes in both preload and afterload, and differences in study results may be related to differences in loading conditions. In one study, an afterload-adjusted and preload-insensitive index of contractility (afterload-adjusted velocity of circumferential fiber shortening) decreased during pregnancy and returned to normal 2–4 weeks postpartum.[27]

Diastolic function has been studied less than systolic function during pregnancy. Using echocardiography, the ratio of early to late diastolic flow velocity

(*E*/*A* ratio) has been shown to be lower during the third trimester compared with post partum.[28] The mechanism and significance of this finding are not known.

As a result of increased fetal and maternal tissue mass and cardiac and respiratory work, maternal peak oxygen consumption can increase by 20–30% at term.[29] Whereas most of the increase in cardiac output occurs early, the increase in oxygen consumption occurs progressively throughout the pregnancy.

The increased demands and stresses of pregnancy may be detrimental to women with limited cardiac reserve. Women who are unable to increase cardiac output or who require elevated filling pressures to do so may develop evidence of right- or left-sided heart failure. Fixed stenotic valvular lesions, such as aortic stenosis, may limit the ability of the heart to provide the increased cardiac output necessary, resulting in adverse maternal and fetal events. For women with coronary disease, increased cardiac work during pregnancy, and hence increased myocardial oxygen consumption, may trigger ischaemia. In women with Marfan syndrome the increased cardiac output and hypervolemia of pregnancy, as well as the changing hormonal milieu, contribute to the observed increase in risk of aortic dissection.

Heart rate and rhythm

Mean heart rate usually increases by 10–20 beats over the course of pregnancy, peaking in the late second trimester or early third trimester (see Figure 2.3), although there is wide individual variation. Most women remain in sinus rhythm during pregnancy; however, premature atrial and ventricular complexes may become more frequent. The frequency of new-onset supraventricular arrhythmias and even ventricular tachycardia has been shown to increase during preg-

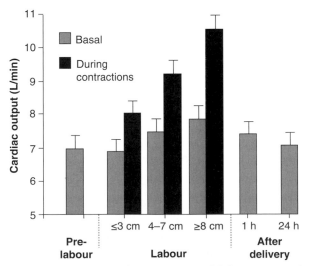

Figure 2.3 Changes in cardiac output during labour and delivery. (Reproduced from Robson et al.[37])

nancy. Furthermore, pregnancy may increase the frequency of supraventricular and ventricular arrhythmias in women with a prior history of such arrhythmias. Women with a history of arrhythmias before pregnancy are at increased risk for adverse cardiac events during pregnancy.

Neurohormonal factors

An alternative method of exploring the hemodynamic changes is to examine the neurohormonal response to pregnancy. Nitric oxide and the prostaglandins are vasodilators that may be responsible for the observed drop in peripheral resistance and for changes in uterine and renal blood flow. These hemodynamic changes initiate additional baroreceptor-mediated neurohormonal events, including activation of the renin–angiotensin–aldosterone and sympathetic nervous systems, and release of natriuretic peptides.

The renin–angiotensin system regulates salt and water hemostasis in the body. There is an increase in both renin and angiotensin levels during pregnancy.[30] This paradoxical increase in renin secretion occurs despite the normal expansion of extracelluar volume during pregnancy.

Activation of the sympathetic nervous system typically occurs in response to a decrease in peripheral vascular resistance and arterial pressure. Conversely, plasma volume expansion suppresses catecholamine levels. During pregnancy, both opposing influences are active and the findings in the literature vary with regard to the extent and nature of net sympathetic activation during normal pregnancy and in patients with hypertensive disorders of pregnancy.[31,32]

The natriuretic peptides are involved in integration of cardiovascular and renal function. Atrial natriuretic peptide (ANP) and brain natriuretic peptide (BNP) are released in response to volume overload states. Release of ANP and BNP occurs in response to atrial and ventricular distension, respectively. In healthy pregnant women, ANP and BNP levels increase during the course of pregnancy.[33] Among pregnant women with pre-eclampsia, increased levels of ANP and BNP are related to changes in left ventricular mass and left ventricular volume.[34]

Overactivity of the autonomic nervous and the renin–angiotensin systems, and impairment in production or activity of vasodilators such as nitric oxide and PGI_2, have all been implicated in the pathogenesis of pre-eclampsia. Plasma catecholamine and neurohormone levels have not been examined in pregnant women with structural cardiac disease, and the role and behavior of these systems in pregnant women who develop cardiac decompensation are unknown.

Respiratory changes

Minute ventilation increases during pregnancy because of increases in tidal volume; the respiratory rate does not change. The increase in minute ventilation is greater than the increase in oxygen consumption and this results in both hyperventilation and an increased ventilatory equivalent for oxygen (the ventilation in liters required for each 100 mL of oxygen consumed). Subjective awareness of increased ventilation is one explanation for the sensation of dyspnea in pregnant women without cardiopulmonary limitation. Functional residual capacity decreases and, along with the increased oxygen consumption described earlier, results in less oxygen reserve. Exercise can further deplete this reserve in women with little ability to compensate.

Changes in the peripartum period

Pain, anxiety and uterine contractions all alter the hemodynamics at the time of labour and delivery. Increases in cardiac output, tachycardia and hypertension may stress the marginally compensated woman with heart disease and also lead to decompensation.

During the first stage of labour uterine contractions can increase central blood volume by as much as 500 mL, a so-called 'autotransfusion'.[35] On average, vaginal delivery results in the loss of 10% and cesarean delivery in 29% of total blood volume, although there is wide individual variation in the magnitude of blood loss.[36] Placental separation does not usually cause any significant change to the circulation. The basal blood pressure increases during labour and further increases with each uterine contraction; this is thought to result partly from the increasing cardiac output. In addition, compression of the lower limb vessels may redistribute blood to the upper limbs and add to upper body hypertension. Heart rate increases during labour secondary to increased circulating catecholamines. Reports vary with regard to the effect of uterine contractions on heart rate; some investigators have demonstrated increasing heart rate and others no significant change or a decrease.

Heart rate changes are variable among individuals, dependent on position and attenuated by anesthesia. Basal cardiac output increases during labour by about 10%.[37] The increased cardiac output is the result of increased heart rate and stroke volume. There is an additional 7–15% increase in cardiac output with each uterine contraction (see Figure 2.3). The increase in cardiac output is more pronounced during the second stage of labour and in the left lateral decubitus position compared with the supine position. Early after delivery, cardiac output may continue to increase to as much as 80% above pre-labour values, as a result of the relief of inferior vena cava compression and autotransfusion from the placenta. Cardiac output returns to pre-labour levels about 1 hour post partum. Immediately post partum, cardiac output can continue to increase and women need to be monitored closely during this time period. Appropriate anesthesia and careful monitoring can help to prevent serious adverse events.

Anesthesia and analgesia can significantly alter the hemodynamics during the peripartum period, e.g. epidural anesthesia can help to alleviate pain and anxiety, thereby reducing increases in heart rate, blood pressure and oxygen consumption. However, epidural anesthesia may cause significant hypotension as a result of venous pooling and decreased venous return. Compared with pudendal or paracervical anesthesia, caudal anesthesia results in less increase in cardiac output during labour, and thus limits the absolute increase in cardiac output at the time of delivery. Induction of general anesthesia can exacerbate hypertension and tachycardia. Anesthetic issues are discussed in more detail in Chapter 20.

Women at high risk during labour and delivery include women unable to accommodate to increases in preload, such as those with mitral stenosis, and women unable to accommodate to the increased cardiac output, such as those with dilated cardiomyopathy. Women with Marfan syndrome are at risk for aortic dissection especially if there are significant blood pressure elevations.

Changes in the postpartum period

Hemodynamic parameters slowly return to baseline values, but full resolution may take as long as 6 months after delivery. Thus, hemodynamic studies that used early postpartum values as surrogates for pre-pregnancy baseline values, when the latter were unavailable, may underestimate the actual changes that occur during pregnancy.

The blood volume decreases by 10% within the first 3 days after delivery. The hemoglobin level and the hematocrit increase progressively for the first 2 weeks after delivery and stabilize thereafter. Systolic and diastolic blood pressures remain unchanged from late pregnancy values until about 12 weeks post partum, after which they increase. Within 2 weeks post partum, systemic vascular resistance increases by 30%.[18] After the initial tachycardia associated with labour and delivery, a bradycardia often develops in the early puerperium. The heart rate slowly returns to baseline levels over the next 2 weeks. There is an immediate increase in cardiac output after delivery (within the first hour) by as much as 80%.[35] After this there is a decrease over the next 24 weeks.[18] Similarly, stroke volume decreases for the first 24 weeks after delivery. Most studies have demonstrated regression towards a baseline of left atrial and left ventricular dimensions and left ventricular mass by 24 weeks post partum (Table 2.3).[38] The left ventricular ejection fraction and rate of circumferential fiber shortening decrease following pregnancy. There has been concern that the anatomical changes in left ventricular mass and the function associated with pregnancy may not all ultimately return to pre-pregnancy values.[18]

Conclusion

During pregnancy and post partum, changes occur in the circulating blood volume, peripheral vascular compliance and resistance, myocardial function, heart rate and the neurohormonal system. These changes allow the cardiovascular system to meet the increased metabolic demands of pregnancy. Although these changes have been examined in normal pregnancies, less well understood is how these changes may differ in women with structural heart disease compared with women without heart disease and the mechanisms responsible for the differences that may exist.

References

1 Lind T. Hematologic system. Maternal physiology. *Washington: CREOG* 1985;**25**:7–40.
2 Pirani BB, Campbell DM, MacGillivray I. Plasma volume in normal first pregnancy. *J Obstet Gynaecol Br Commonw* 1973;**80**:884–7.
3 Pritchard JA, Rowland RC. Blood volume changes in pregnancy and the puerperium. III. Whole body and large vessel hematocrits in pregnant and nonpregnant women. *Am J Obstet Gynecol* 1964;**88**:391–5.
4 Rovinsky JJ, Jaffin H. Cardiovascular hemodynamics in pregnancy. I. Blood and plasma volumes in multiple pregnancy. *Am J Obstet Gynecol* 1965;**93**:1–15.
5 Taylor DJ, Lind T. Red cell mass during and after normal pregnancy. *Br J Obstet Gynaecol* 1979;**86**:364–70.
6 Lund CJ, Donovan JC. Blood volume during pregnancy. Significance of plasma and red cell volumes. *Am J Obstet Gynecol* 1967;**98**:394–403.
7 Thomsen JK, Fogh-Andersen N, Jaszczak P. Atrial natriuretic peptide, blood volume, aldosterone, and sodium excretion during twin pregnancy. *Acta Obstet Gynecol Scand* 1994;**73**:14–20.
8 Salas SP, Rosso P, Espinoza R, Robert JA, Valdes G, Donoso E. Maternal plasma volume expansion and hormonal changes in women with idiopathic fetal growth retardation. *Obstet Gynecol* 1993;**81**:1029–33.
9 Campos O. Doppler echocardiography during pregnancy: physiological and abnormal findings. *Echocardiography* 1996;**13**:135–46.
10 Clark SL, Cotton DB, Lee W, et al. Central hemodynamic assessment of normal term pregnancy. *Am J Obstet Gynecol* 1989;**161**:1439–42.
11 Robson SC, Hunter S, Boys RJ, Dunlop W. Serial study of factors influencing changes in cardiac output during human pregnancy. *Am J Physiol* 1989;**256**:H1060–5.
12 Duvekot JJ, Cheriex EC, Pieters FA, Menheere PP, Peeters LH. Early pregnancy changes in hemodynamics and volume homeostasis are consecutive adjustments triggered by a primary fall in systemic vascular tone. *Am J Obstet Gynecol* 1993;**169**: 1382–92.
13 Jurkovic D, Jauniaux E, Kurjak A, Hustin J, Campbell S, Nicolaides KH. Transvaginal color Doppler assessment of the uteroplacental circulation in early pregnancy. *Obstet Gynecol* 1991;**77**:365–9.
14 Davison JM. Kidney function in pregnant women. *Am J Kidney Dis* 1987:**9**: 248–52.
15 Bieniarz J, Yoshida T, Romero-Salinas G, Curuchet E, Caldeyro-Barcia R, Crottogini JJ. Aortocaval compression by the uterus in late human pregnancy. IV. Circulatory homeostasis by preferential perfusion of the placenta. *Am J Obstet Gynecol* 1969;**103**:19–31.
16 Rubler S, Damani PM, Pinto ER. Cardiac size and performance during pregnancy estimated with echocardiography. *Am J Cardiol* 1977;**40**:534–40.
17 Katz R, Karliner JS, Resnik R. Effects of a natural volume overload state (pregnancy) on left ventricular performance in normal human subjects. *Circulation* 1978;**58**: 434–41.
18 Robson SC, Hunter S, Moore M, Dunlop W. Haemodynamic changes during the puerperium: a Doppler and M-mode echocardiographic study. *Br J Obstet Gynaecol* 1987;**94**:1028–39.
19 Vered Z, Poler SM, Gibson P, Wlody D, Perez JE. Noninvasive detection of the morphologic and hemodynamic changes during normal pregnancy. *Clin Cardiol* 1991;**14**:327–34.

20 Mone SM, Sanders SP, Colan SD. Control mechanisms for physiological hypertrophy of pregnancy. *Circulation* 1996;**94**:667–72.
21 Abduljabbar HS, Marzouki KM, Zawawi TH, Khan AS. Pericardial effusion in normal pregnant women. *Acta Obstet Gynecol Scand* 1991;**70**:291–4.
22 Ueland K, Novy MJ, Peterson EN, Metcalfe J. Maternal cardiovascular dynamics. IV. The influence of gestational age on the maternal cardiovascular response to posture and exercise. *Am J Obstet Gynecol* 1969;**104**:856–64.
23 Bader RA, Bader ME, Rose DF, Braunwald E. Hemodynamics at rest and during exercise in normal pregnancy as studies by cardiac catheterization. *J Clin Invest* 1955;**34**:1524–36.
24 Mabie WC, DiSessa TG, Crocker LG, Sibai BM, Arheart KL. A longitudinal study of cardiac output in normal human pregnancy. *Am J Obstet Gynecol* 1994;**170**:849–56.
25 Ueland K, Novy MJ, Metcalfe J. Hemodynamic responses of patients with heart disease to pregnancy and exercise. *Am J Obstet Gynecol* 1972;**113**:47–59.
26 Mashini IS, Albazzaz SJ, Fadel HE, et al. Serial noninvasive evaluation of cardiovascular hemodynamics during pregnancy. *Am J Obstet Gynecol* 1987;**156**:1208–13.
27 Geva T, Mauer MB, Striker L, Kirshon B, Pivarnik JM. Effects of physiologic load of pregnancy on left ventricular contractility and remodeling. *Am Heart J* 1997;**133**: 53–9.
28 Sadaniantz A, Kocheril AG, Emaus SP, Garber CE, Parisi AF. Cardiovascular changes in pregnancy evaluated by two-dimensional and Doppler echocardiography. *J Am Soc Echocardiogr* 1992;**5**:253–8.
29 Elkus R, Popovich J Jr. Respiratory physiology in pregnancy. *Clin Chest Med* 1992;**13**:555–65.
30 August P, Lenz T, Ales KL, et al. Longitudinal study of the renin–angiotensin–aldosterone system in hypertensive pregnant women: deviations related to the development of superimposed preeclampsia. *Am J Obstet Gynecol* 1990;**163**:1612–21.
31 Natrajan PG, McGarrigle HH, Lawrence DM, Lachelin GC. Plasma noradrenaline and adrenaline levels in normal pregnancy and in pregnancy-induced hypertension. *Br J Obstet Gynaecol* 1982;**89**:1041–5.
32 Davey DA, Macnab MF. Plasma adrenaline, noradrenaline and dopamine in pregnancy hypertension. *Br J Obstet Gynaecol* 1981;**88**:611–18.
33 Yoshimura T, Yoshimura M, Yasue H, et al. Plasma concentration of atrial natriuretic peptide and brain natriuretic peptide during normal human pregnancy and the postpartum period. *J Endocrinol* 1994;**140**:393–7.
34 Borghi C, Esposti DD, Immordino V, et al. Relationship of systemic hemodynamics, left ventricular structure and function, and plasma natriuretic peptide concentrations during pregnancy complicated by preeclampsia. *Am J Obstet Gynecol* 2000;**183**: 140–7.
35 Ueland K, Hansen JM. Maternal cardiovascular dynamics. 3. Labour and delivery under local and caudal analgesia. *Am J Obstet Gynecol* 1969;**103**:8–18.
36 Ueland K. Maternal cardiovascular dynamics. VII. Intrapartum blood volume changes. *Am J Obstet Gynecol* 1976;**126**:671–7.
37 Robson SC, Dunlop W, Boys RJ, Hunter S. Cardiac output during labour. *Br Med J (Clin Res Ed)* 1987;**295**:1169–72.
38 Campos O. Doppler echocardiography during pregnancy. *Echocardiography* 1996;**13**: 135–146.

CHAPTER 3

Cardiovascular examination in pregnancy and the approach to diagnosis of cardiac disorder

Petros Nihoyannopoulos

Pregnancy is a physiological phenomenon during which there are major cardiovascular changes affecting the loading conditions of the heart. The mechanisms of the various cardiopulmonary adaptations during pregnancy are discussed in detail in Chapter 2. Briefly, during the first trimester there is a steep increase in plasma volume, which causes dilution and anemia. The stroke volume and, to a lesser extent, the heart rate increase and the cardiac output increases progressively. This increase is around 40–50% above the pre-pregnancy level and is maintained throughout pregnancy. There is an accompanying decrease in vascular resistance, and diastolic and mean blood pressure. In cyanotic or potentially cyanotic congenital heart disease, the drop in peripheral vascular resistance encourages right-to-left shunting, leading to increasing cyanosis, and a rise in hematocrit with increased risk of thrombosis and paradoxical embolism.

Although the normal heart tolerates the added load easily, abnormal hearts may not. When trouble occurs it usually begins early, often by the end of the first trimester. These considerations are of pivotal importance if the physician is to advise the woman correctly and not simply retreat with the easy option of advising against pregnancy or encouraging early termination.

Examination

History

Many disorders are apparent from the personal and family history, particularly cardiomyopathies, Marfan syndrome and congenital heart disease. It is important to ask specifically for possible sudden deaths in the family, which could potentially put this pregnant woman at a higher risk. There may be previous knowledge of a cardiac murmur, which may or may not be linked to a specific valve disease. The outcome of any previous pregnancies will be noted with particular attention to hypertension, pre-eclampsia, pulmonary edema or peripartum cardiomyopathy. Previous unsuccessful pregnancies ending in termination or stillbirth may signify maternal disease such as anti-phospholipid antibody syndrome causing recurrent mid-trimester termination. Fetal abnormality may have been related to maternal medication such as anti-epileptic drugs or it may reflect a genetic disorder.

Systemic blood pressure

Pregnancy hypertension has been the largest cause of maternal death in England and Wales over the last 30 years, and continues to be so, and cerebrovascular accident is the most common mode of death.[1] In systemic hypertension, the risks to the mother are largely related to the level of blood pressure and development of stroke or heart failure, whereas the risk to the fetus is from failure of placental function. The ability of the placenta to exchange nutrients and gases with the fetus is dependent on blood flow. In systemic hypertension, blood flow to the placenta is reduced. When the blood pressure is above 170/110 mmHg, cerebral blood flow autoregulation is lost, the maternal risks are greatly increased and treatment should be prompt.

The blood pressure tends to fall in the first part of pregnancy, mainly as a result of the fall in peripheral vascular resistance, but then it gradually rises to equal or exceed pre-pregnancy levels in the last 6 weeks. Blood pressure should be measured with the woman seated or lying on her left side because, if a woman lies supine, the blood pressure may be misleadingly reduced. Even profound hypotension can occur in late pregnancy from mechanical obstruction of the inferior vena cava by the gravid uterus.

The measurement of blood pressure is confounded by non-standardized methodology. In the non-pregnant patient the fifth Korotkoff sound is usually noted, because it corresponds best to the intra-arterial measurement. In pregnancy the fourth Korotkoff sound has been recommended in the USA as more reproducible because audible sounds may continue down to zero.[2] Recently, de Swiet et al. have made a compelling plea for recording diastolic pressure at the fifth Korotkoff sound as in the non-pregnant state. In a carefully conducted study, they found that observers could always identify the fifth sound whereas interobserver variation of the level of the fourth sound was much greater.[3]

Protein excretion increases during pregnancy from a maximum of 18 mg in 24 hours in the non-pregnant woman to over 300 mg total protein with albumin, representing roughly 55% of this. A total protein excretion of over 300 mg is considered to be abnormal.[4] Women who develop pregnancy induced hypertension in the second trimester may show steadily worsening hypertension accompanied by the development of proteinuria, thrombocytopenia, and failing renal and hepatic function, which define pre-eclampsia. It is crucial to follow the blood pressure using a standardized method and to look for proteinuria, particularly in women with a family history of hypertension or pre-eclampsia (see Chapter 18).

Physical signs

Adaptive mechanisms bring variation into the cardiovascular examination that may mimic heart disease. The palms flush, the extremities are warm, the soft tissues become more tense, the digital vessels throb, there may be capillary pulsation, and the pulse is full, bounding and often collapsing. The heart rate is slightly faster and there may be slight peripheral edema.[5]

The jugular veins look distended from about week 20 of pregnancy. The venous pressure may be raised with prominent 'a' and 'v' waves and brisk 'x' and 'y' descents because of hypervolemia and vasodilatation. The increase in blood volume causes the heart to be mildly overloaded and may lead to an overestimation of valve regurgitation. The increased intra-abdominal pressure caused by the gravid uterus indirectly leads to an increased intrathoracic pressure, which in turn raises the jugular venous pressure but not the right ventricular filling pressure. This is important to differentiate from heart failure and to avoid the potentially harmful administration of diuretics.

Normal pregnancy in a woman without heart disease is commonly accompanied by tachycardia, palpitations, and increased numbers of premature atrial or ventricular beats, sometimes multiple. It is important to recognize these usually benign symptoms.

During pregnancy the apical impulse is slightly displaced to the left and is more abrupt and lively. It signifies an overfilled ventricle working against a low resistance as a result of peripheral vasodilatation. Pathological volume-loaded conditions such as aortic or mitral regurgitation, or left-to-right shunting should be distinguished (Table 3.1).

The mitral closure sound may be slightly increased in intensity. A loud third sound confirms rapid ventricular filling and is found in up to 90% of pregnant women. There is no change in the character of the second heart sound during the first 30 weeks of pregnancy, but later on pulmonary closure may be slightly increased with persistent expiratory splitting.[6]

A systolic aortic or pulmonary flow murmur is heard in 90% of pregnant women. A cervical venous hum, best heard over the supraclavicular fossa, is common in children, and is also found in pregnancy. The mammary souffle (murmur), either systolic or continuous, is heard maximally at the second left

Table 3.1 Normal clinical findings that can mimic heart disease in pregnancy

- Raised jugular venous pressure (prominent 'a' and 'v' waves, brisk 'x' and 'y' descents)
- Volume-loaded left ventricle; full, sharp and collapsing pulse
- Warm extremities
- Peripheral edema
- Palpitations
- Tachycardia
- Premature atrial/ventricular beats
- Increased intensity of mitral closure sound
- Third heart sound
- Systolic murmur
- Continuous murmur from venous hum, mammary soufflé

or right intercostal space during late pregnancy in some women. This is easily differentiated from a persistent arterial duct by applying gentle pressure, which makes the mammary souffle disappear.

Special investigations

Electrocardiography

Electrocardiographic (ECG) changes can be related to a gradual change in the position of the heart. The ECG often shows a gradual shift of the QRS axis to the left in the frontal plane with a small Q wave, and inverted T wave in lead III as a result of rotation.

The heart rate may be increased by 10–15%. Re-entrant supraventricular tachycardia is a relatively common benign arrhythmia. Conversely, persistent sinus tachycardia, atrial flutter, atrial fibrillation or ventricular tachycardia suggests underlying heart disease and should prompt further investigation. The appearance of ventricular tachycardia in late pregnancy or in the puerperium should arouse suspicion of peripartum cardiomyopathy.[7]

Chest radiograph

The most common normal finding in pregnancy is slight prominence of the pulmonary conus and simulation of left atrial enlargement in the lateral views.[8] These changes are predominantly the result of hyperlordosis and may in some instances suggest mitral stenosis.[9] Progressive elevation of the diaphragm leads to a more horizontal position of the heart and an increase in the cardiothoracic ratio. An increased intrathoracic blood volume and heavy breast shadows may raise suspicion of left-to-right shunting from an atrial septal defect or pulmonary venous congestion caused by mitral stenosis.

A chest radiograph should be considered in any pregnant patient with new onset of dyspnea. Failure to do so has led to mistaken diagnosis of chest infection or adult respiratory distress syndrome and to missing mitral stenosis.[10] The general physician, intensive care consultant or obstetrician does not resort to echocardiography unless he or she suspects heart disease. This practice is, however, steadily changing and more and more pregnant women will have an echocardiographic examination requested as soon as an 'unusual' physical sign is present. As echocardiography causes no radiation, it has become the preferred screening method to assess the state of the heart, largely replacing the chest radiograph.

Echocardiography

Modern echocardiography with its sophisticated Doppler and transcsophageal arsenal is well suited to rapid diagnosis in pregnant women with known or suspected cardiac disorders. The performance and visual interpretation of echocardiographic studies can be achieved speedily and has a crucial impact on management. It is particularly important during pregnancy when the physical signs may be misleading with potential hazard to both mother and fetus. The

Table 3.2 Echocardiographic challenges during pregnancy

- Normal study
- Mitral stenosis
- Aortic stenosis
- Simple congenital heart disease (atrial septal defect or ASD, ventricular septal defect or VSD)
- Complex congenital heart disease
- Deterioration of ventricular function
- Assessment of prosthetic valves

recent introduction of hand-held echocardiographic machines makes bedside diagnosis easier and quicker.

Referral is often triggered by the detection of a systolic murmur by the obstetrician (Table 3.2). Occasionally, the distinction between normality and abnormality may be subtle and an expert interpretation should be sought before the final report. Doctors and technicians involved in the performance and interpretation of echocardiographic studies should be accredited by their national authority and fully acquainted with artifacts or variation of normal structures that are often seen in normal echocardiographic examinations. In most pregnancies echocardiography will reassure the mother-to-be who can then continue to enjoy her pregnancy.

A progressively increasing awareness in pregnant women during the third trimester is the presence of breathlessness. Although breathlessness may be a common symptom during pregnancy, this may be difficult to distinguish from breathlessness related to the onset of peripartum cardiomyopathy. New onset of intraventricular conduction delay or left bundle-branch block on the ECG, together with an 'unusual' breathlessness, should constitute an absolute indication for an early echocardiographic examination to assess left ventricular function. The test can easily be repeated as often as necessary so that progression or stability of ventricular function can be ascertained.

Valve disease

Most commonly echocardiography is requested for assessment of a patient with known valve disease. As a result of the hyperkinetic circulation and increased stroke output, systolic and diastolic velocities across native or prosthetic valves rise, leading to an apparent 'increase' in systolic or diastolic gradients, which should not be misinterpreted as indicative of increased disease severity. Similarly, in regurgitant lesions, the physiological increase in volume, which occurs during pregnancy, may render a minor valvar leak more impressive. Multivalvar regurgitation (affecting all except the aortic valve) is a common finding on Doppler echocardiography during pregnancy and should not be reported as abnormal if the regurgitation is slight and the valves look structurally normal.[11] Obviously the existence of a previous echocardiographic examination to serve as a comparison would facilitate this process, but the chance of this happening is rather unusual.

Despite the decline in rheumatic heart disease, one reason for echocardiography during pregnancy is to assess the severity of mitral stenosis in a pregnant woman or to establish the reason for breathlessness or pulmonary edema. Mitral stenosis may be difficult to diagnose clinically with uncontrolled tachycardia or the onset of atrial fibrillation, which prevents accurate measurement of the pressure half-time of mitral valve filling from the continuous Doppler display. Indeed, uncontrolled atrial fibrillation or, more often, sinus tachycardia is often the cause of pulmonary edema even when mitral stenosis is only moderate. If the heart rate cannot be slowed by carotid massage[12] planimetry of the mitral orifice area at the tips of the leaflets is the best alternative using a frame-by-frame method. Care should be taken to measure the smallest possible area at the leaflet tips from short-axis projections with optimal gain settings. An alternative would be to first slow the heart rate using beta blockers and then to measure the pressure half-time and gradient by Doppler.

Another echocardiographic task during pregnancy is assessment of the severity of aortic stenosis. The morphological features of the aortic valve can readily be described but the velocities and the derived pressure gradients across the valve are higher than in the non-pregnant state because of the increased stroke volume. This may lead to over-assessment of severity.[13] In such circumstances calculation of the effective aortic valve area by Doppler is an absolute necessity.

The reduced systemic resistance in pregnancy may precipitate effort-induced syncope if stroke volume fails to increase. Even then, pregnancy can be continued with bed rest and beta blockers in most patients until the baby is viable. Serial echocardiographic studies greatly help in decision-making in those difficult patients. Intervention is needed if left ventricular systolic function deteriorates or congestive heart failure develops. Balloon dilatation of the valve may provide temporary palliation if the valve is pliable and non-calcified, although this technique is now less often used in adults because of the poorly sustained benefits. Otherwise aortic valve replacement should be preceded by cesarean delivery of the baby if viable.[14]

Valve regurgitation is generally well tolerated during pregnancy, primarily because of the afterload reduction and increased heart rate. As a result, it is common for the calculated regurgitant volume and regurgitant fraction to be reduced.

Congenital heart disease

The decreasing incidence of rheumatic heart disease and advances in medical and surgical treatment have resulted in an increase in both the relative and absolute incidence of congenital cardiac disorders seen in pregnancy.[15] Their assessment can be one of the most challenging tasks for the echocardiographer.

Patients with unoperated congenital heart defects are usually acyanotic and the defects include pulmonary stenosis, persistent ductus arteriosus, coarctation of the aorta, atrial and ventricular septal defects, aortic valve disease secondary to some form of bicuspid aortic valve and Ebstein's anomaly. Pregnancy increases the risk of aortic dissection complicating coarctation and should be considered if such a patient develops chest pain. Interestingly, the incidence of toxemia is lower in coarctation-related hypertension than in primary systemic hypertension.[16] Although patients with tetralogy of Fallot tolerate pregnancy well, patients with pulmonary hypertension do not.[14] Pulmonary vascular disease may deteriorate during pregnancy with possible fatal outcome and the decreased arterial oxygen content in Eisenmenger syndrome leads to poor fetal growth or spontaneous abortion.

The advantage of echocardiography lies in its ability to perform serial studies in the assessment of intracardiac flow disturbances and left and right ventricular function. Most patients with simple defects will see their pregnancy through with no complications and the role of echocardiography is simply documentary, although sometimes rare complex or potentially dangerous abnormalities are first recognized on antenatal echocardiographic screening. These include corrected transposition and coronary anomalies.

The second category of patients with congenital heart disease includes those who have had previous surgery. If the operation were 'corrective', pregnancy would usually proceed normally but would sometimes be complicated by arrhythmia, usually benign, and endocarditis. Patients who have undergone palliative surgery may be at risk of heart failure or thromboembolism as well as infection and arrhythmia. Patients with Mustard or Senning repairs, Rastelli valve-bearing conduits or Fontan univentricular circulations can have successful pregnancies (see Chapter 5). Echocardiography and transesophageal imaging in these conditions permits detailed description of the surgical procedure and helps both in initial assessment of risk and in serial documentation of progress. Cardiac magnetic resonance imaging (MRI) may be complementary in these complex corrections, particularly in defining surgical shunts.

Cardiomyopathies

In women with cardiomyopathies, echocardiography has an important role in assessing left ventricular function. Cardiomyopathy may be first diagnosed during pregnancy. The left ventricle in hypertrophic cardiomyopathy seems to fill better during pregnancy and to accommodate the physiological increase in blood volume, without undue rise in filling pressure in most cases. Pressure gradients may be high but usually do not affect outcome. Coexisting mitral regurgitation can readily be detected. Generally, hypertrophic cardiomyopathy is well tolerated during pregnancy.

When discovered late in pregnancy, dilated cardiomyopathy may be regarded as peripartum because of its temporal relationship with pregnancy, but when detected earlier in pregnancy the condition is likely to have been pre-existing. Echocardiography shows a hypokinetic left ventricle that may or may not be dilated. In peripartum cardiomyopathy ventricular function may gradually improve within 6 months to a year of delivery. In an echocardiographic study of left ventricular function in 10 women with peripartum cardiomyopathy, the severity of left ventricular dysfunction did not predict outcome.[17] Over the first month after delivery, five of seven patients (71%) increased their ejection fraction and at 4 months left ventricular size and mass index decreased with further

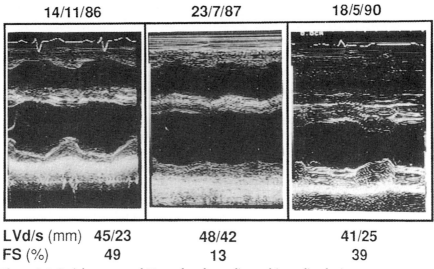

14/11/86   23/7/87   18/5/90

LVd/s (mm)   45/23   48/42   41/25
FS (%)   49   13   39

Figure 3.1 Serial parasternal M-mode echocardiographic studies during pregnancy (first panel), 3 months after delivery (middle panel) and 3 years later (third panel). The middle panel shows right ventricular hypertrophy and transient substantial left and right ventricular dysfunction. The fractional shortening dropped from 49% during pregnancy to 13% after delivery and subsequently recovered at 39%. (Reproduced with permission from Perloff.[16])

improvement in ejection fraction. Despite this improvement, the ejection fraction became normal in only 57% of women. Interestingly, two of these patients had subsequent normal pregnancies.[17] One of the patients with Eisenmenger ventricular septal defect (VSD) developed peripartum cardiomyopathy.[18] Echocardiography during pregnancy had shown excellent left and right ventricular function throughout. Repeat serial echocardiography after delivery showed sudden deterioration in ventricular function. Complete recovery of ventricular function occurred within 2 years with no advance in the pulmonary vascular disease (Figure 3.1).

Women with Marfan syndrome are always a worry in pregnancy. The family history is important and serial measurement of aortic root diameter are important particularly in patients with either a family history of aortic rupture or evidence of aortic root widening (see Chapter 10).

Transesophageal echocardiography

Multiplane transducers have made transesophageal echocardiography the ultimate echocardiographic method in the assessment of adults with complex congenital heart disease, thromboembolic episodes and infective endocarditis, particularly in patients previously operated on or with prosthetic valves. Transesophageal echocardiography is safe during pregnancy.[19] Oxygen saturations should be monitored when midazolam is used for premedication, particularly in patients with chronic obstructive airway disease or in cyanotic patients, because of the risks of hypoxia to the fetus. Antibiotic prophylaxis is not given because there is no evidence, even in high-risk patients with prosthetic valves, that transesophageal echocardiography has caused endocarditis.[19]

Some patients with severe mitral stenosis may require balloon valvotomy, which is successful in suitable valves identified by echocardiography. The procedure can be monitored by transesophageal echocardiography in the catheter laboratory to reduce the amount of radiation to the fetus.

Imaging the heart from the esophagus using multiplane transducers has many advantages over precordial imaging in adults with complex congenital heart disease. One should adopt a sequential approach to the diagnosis of congenital heart lesions. The atrial situs (by defining the atrial appendages), the venous connection and the detailed morphology of the atrial chambers and septum can easily be defined, in contrast to transthoracic windows when these posterior structures tend to be poorly imaged. The transesophageal probe lies in contiguity with the posterior wall of the left atrium and is in an excellent position to image the morphology and sites of drainage of the pulmonary veins and venae cavae. Previous surgery may have been undertaken many years earlier and the details may not be available. Transesophageal echocardiography therefore has a descriptive role as well as being diagnostic when possible sources of embolism, vegetation or abscesses are being sought.

Assessment of the function of a Fontan circulation by transesophageal imaging allows direct visualization of atriopulmonary and cavopulmonary connections, together with pulsed Doppler estimation of velocity profiles through the connections. Direct visualization of Glenn or Blalock anastomoses, precise measurement of atrial shunting, and identification or exclusion of obstruction to pulmonary arterial or venous blood flow can all be achieved.

Patients who have undergone Senning or Mustard procedures can be difficult to assess by transthoracic imaging alone. From the transesophageal approach, caval obstruction or obstruction within the midportion of the systemic venous atrium, the sites of baffle leakage or obstruction to the drainage of individual pulmonary veins can easily be identified.

Stress testing

Coronary artery disease is rare during pregnancy but may be seen in women with familial hypercholesterolemia, particularly the rare homozygotes, or in patients with lupus erythematosus or anti-phospholipid syndrome.

Treadmill exercise testing is useful in the pre-pregnancy assessment of patients, particularly in symptom-free patients with aortic stenosis, looking for evidence of subendocardial ischemia that can be provoked or a fall in blood pressure as an indication of probable risk. More formal measurement of cardiopulmonary exercise tolerance may be used before giving advice about fitness for pregnancy in borderline patients.

Stress echocardiography, with either exercise or dobutamine infusion, may add to the diagnostic specificity of treadmill exercise testing in detecting the

Table 3.3 Routine checklist of fetal echocardiography

- Heart one-third of the fetal thorax
- Two atria of equal size
- Two ventricles of equal size contracting briskly
- Two equal size atrioventricular valves
- Patent foramen ovale
- Intact ventricular septum

presence and extent of ischemia in high-risk patients with possible coronary artery disease.

Fetal echocardiography

Over the past 20 years fetal echocardiography has undergone major developments. The heart can usually be visualized at 16–18 weeks' gestation[20,21] and abnormalities can be detected as early as 18–20 weeks.[22,23] The single most valuable view is the four-chamber view centered on the atrioventricular junction. It gives the opportunity to assess the number and relative sizes of the ventricles and atria as well as the atrioventricular valves, and can be obtained in 95% of pregnancies.[22–24] The following features should be sought (Table 3.3):

- The heart should occupy no more than one-third of the fetal thorax
- There should be two atria of equal size
- There should be two ventricles of equal size that contract equally briskly
- The two atrioventricular valves should meet the atrial and ventricular septa at the crux
- The foramen ovale should be present
- The ventricular septum must be intact.

Fetal echocardiography should be performed by operators with skills based on experience of pathology rather than just on the performance of a large number of 'normal' scans. Transvaginal fetal echocardiography facilitates early visualization of the fetal heart.

Recognition of cardiovascular pathology is of great importance to adjust any medication appropriately and to plan the delivery and mode of anesthesia. There are a few cardiac conditions, such as Eisenmenger syndrome and primary pulmonary hypertension, that indicate the need for early interruption of pregnancy because of high maternal risk.

References

1 Turnbull A, Tindall VR, Beard RW et al. Report on confidential enquiries into maternal deaths in England and Wales 1982–1984. *Rep Health Soc Subj Lond* 1989;**34**:1–166.
2 MacGillivray I, Rose G, Row B. Blood pressure survey in pregnancy. *Clin Sci* 1969;**37**:395–9.

3 Shennon A, Gupta M, Halligan A, Taylor DJ, de Swiet M. Lack of reproducibility in pregnancy of Korotkoff phase IV as measured by mercury sphygmomanometry. *Lancet* 1996;**347**:139–42.

4 Hughes EC. *Obstetrics–Gynecological Terminology*. Philadelphia: Davis, 1972: pp 422–3.

5 Wood P. *Diseases of the Heart and Circulation*, 2nd edn. London: Eyre & Spottiswoode, 1956: pp 902–9.

6 Cutforth R, MacDonald CB. Heart sounds and murmurs in pregnancy. *Am Heart J* 1966;**71**:741–7.

7 Perloff JK. *The Cardiomyopathies*. Philadelphia: WB Saunders, 1988.

8 Szekely P, Snaith L. *Heart Disease and Pregnancy*. Edinburgh: Churchill Livingstone, 1974.

9 Turner AF. The chest radiograph in pregnancy. *Clin Obstet Gynecol* 1975;**18**:65–74.

10 Morley CA, Lim BA. The risks of delay in diagnosis of breathlessness in pregnancy. *BMJ* 1995;**311**:183–4.

11 Campos O, Andrade JL, Bocanegra J et al. Physiological multivalvular regurgitation during pregnancy: a longitudinal Doppler echocardiographic study. *Int J Cardiol* 1993;**40**:265–72.

12 Torrecilla EG, Garcia-Fernandez MA, Dan Roman DJ, Alberca MT, Delea JL. Usefulness of carotid sinus massage in the quantification of mitral stenosis in sinus rhythm by Doppler pressure half time. *Am J Cardiol* 1994;**73**:817–21.

13 Burwash IG, Forbes AD, Sadahiro M et al. Echocardiographic volume flow and stenoses severity measures with changing flow rate in aortic stenosis. *Am J Physiol* 1993;**265**:H1734–43.

14 Oakley CM. Pregnancy in heart disease. In: Jackson G (ed.), *Difficult Cardiology*. London: Martin Dunitz, 1990: pp 1–18.

15 Perloff JK. Pregnancy and congenital heart disease. *J Am Coll Cardiol* 1991;**18**:340–2.

16 Perloff JK. *Clinical Recognition of Congenital Heart Disease*. Philadelphia: WB Saunders, 1987.

17 Cole P, Cook F, Plappent T, Salzman D, Shilton M St J. Longitudinal changes in left ventricular architecture and function in peripartum cardiomyopathy. *Am J Cardiol* 1987;**60**:871–6.

18 Oakley CM, Nihoyannopoulos P. Peripartum cardiomyopathy with recovery in a patient with coincidental Eisenmenger ventricular septal defect. *Br Heart J* 1992;**67**:190–2.

19 Saltissi S, de Belder MA, Nihoyannopoulos P. Setting up a transoesophageal echocardiography service. *Br Heart J* 1994;**71**(suppl):15–9.

20 Allan LD, Tynan MJ, Cambell S, Wilkinson JL, Anderson RH. Echocardiographic and anatomical correlates in the fetus. *Br Heart J* 1980;**44**:444–51.

21 Wyllie J, Wren C, Hunter S. Screening for fetal cardiac malformations. *Br Heart J* 1994;**71**(suppl):20–7.

22 Allan LD, Chita SK, Sharland GK, Fegg NLK, Anderson RH, Crawford DC. The accuracy of fetal echocardiography in the diagnosis of congenital heart disease. *Int J Cardiol* 1989;**25**:279–88.

23 Allan LD, Crawford DC, Chita SK, Tynan MJ. Prenatal screening for congenital heart disease. *BMJ* 1986;**292**:1717–19.

24 Copel JA, Pila G, Green J, Hobbins JC, Kleinman CS. Fetal echocardiographic screening for congenital heart disease: the importance of the four chamber view. *Am J Obstet Gynecol* 1987;**57**:48–55.

CHAPTER 4

Acyanotic congenital heart disease

Celia Oakley, Heidi M Connolly

Both the relative incidence and the absolute numbers of pregnant women with congenital heart disease have risen. This is because rheumatic heart disease in young adults is rare in developed countries and more children with complex congenital heart disease are surviving into the reproductive age after surgery in infancy or childhood.[1–4] Congenital heart disease is not infrequently discovered first during pregnancy, particularly now that structural heart disease can be differentiated by echocardiography whenever there is clinical doubt. Many congenital cardiac defects are compatible with survival to adult life. Most of the simple acyanotic defects cause no trouble during pregnancy, but women from medically unmonitored communities with previously unsuspected major cardiac defects may be seen first in pregnancy.

Most infants and children in developed countries are examined regularly and simple cardiac defects are usually corrected at a young age. Only correction of a patent arterial duct can be regarded as a complete 'cure'. Problems in pregnancy may occur after repair for congenital heart disease (Table 4.1).

Arrhythmias may develop after closure of secundum atrial septal defect (ASD), especially when either there is residual atrial enlargement or the repair was performed later in life. Pulmonary vascular disease may progress after closure of non-restrictive ventricular septal defects (VSDs) and such patients are at risk because they may consider themselves normal and have been lost to follow-up. Survivors of heroic but palliative surgery for complex congenital heart disease need to be considered for cardiovascular reserve, possibly outgrown grafts or prosthetic values, presence of pulmonary hypertension, arrhythmia, and conduction defects, before proceeding with pregnancy.

Optimal management of the pregnant patient with congenital heart disease includes accurate diagnosis, and the correct prediction of the hemodynamic consequences of both the pregnancy on the cardiac disorder and the cardiac disorder on the baby's development.

A comprehensive pre-pregnancy assessment is recommended for all patients with a history of operated or unoperated congenital heart disease. Maternal prognosis during pregnancy may be determined by a cardiovascular risk index suggested in a prospective multicentre study on the outcome of pregnancy in women with cardiovascular disease.[5]

Four risk factor categories were identified, and included:

1 Prior history of congestive heart failure, transient ischemic attack, stroke or arrhythmia
2 Baseline NYHA (New York Heart Association) class > II or the presence of cyanosis
3 Left heart obstruction
4 Reduced systemic ventricular function.

When none of the risk factors was present, the risk of a cardiovascular complication during pregnancy was less than 5% (there were no patients with severe pulmonary hypertension in the study). The presence of one of the above risk factor categories suggested a risk of a cardiovascular complication during pregnancy of over 20% and, when more than one risk factor category was present, the risk of a cardiovascular complication during pregnancy was over 60%. Fetal mortality was also related to maternal functional class.

Pre-conceptual counseling with explanation of the genetic risks is recommended. Fetal echocardiographic evaluation is also suggested in selected cases to determine the presence of congenital heart disease in the fetus. The comprehensive pre-pregnancy evaluation and monitoring during pregnancy are best provided by a team made up of a cardiologist, obstetrician and obstetric anesthetist.

Table 4.1 Congenital heart disease and pregnancy

Well tolerated:
• Uncomplicated atrial septal defect
• Restrictive ventricular septal defect
• Small persistent ductus arteriosus
• Mild Ebstein's anomaly
• Mild or moderate pulmonary stenosis
• Mild or moderate aortic stenosis
• Corrected transposition without other significant defects

Moderate risk:
• Coarctation of the aorta – previously repaired without obstruction or sequelae
• Pulmonary stenosis with central right-to-left shunt
• Mild or moderate pulmonary hypertension with left-to-right shunt

High maternal (and fetal) risk:
• Severe pulmonary hypertension with reversed central shunt (Eisenmenger syndrome)
• Severe pulmonary hypertension without residual shunt
• Mechanical prosthetic values
• Severe aortic stenosis
• Severe coarctation
• Severe symptomatic pulmonary stenosis:
• Marked cyanosis

Atrial septal defect

Secundum ASDs in the region of the fossa ovalis and the rarer sinus venosus defects sited at the junction of the superior vena cava behave similarly and are

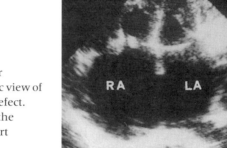

Figure 4.1 Apical four-chamber transthoracic echocardiographic view of a large secundum atrial septal defect. The caudal and ventral parts of the septum are intact. The right heart chambers are dilated.

considered together. ASD is by far the most common congenital cardiac defect to escape recognition until adult life and is two or three times more common in women than in men. It is not uncommon for an ASD to be detected during pregnancy (Figure 4.1) when the pulmonary flow murmur becomes louder and echocardiography is undertaken.

Most patients with ASDs tolerate pregnancy without difficulty in the absence of atrial arrhythmias or pulmonary hypertension. The effect of the increased cardiac output during pregnancy on the volume-loaded right ventricle in patients with left-to-right shunts may be counterbalanced by the decrease in peripheral vascular resistance.[6] A large left-to-right intracardiac shunt rarely causes congestive heart failure during pregnancy.

A frailty of ASD that it is useful to know is poor tolerance of acute blood loss. If this occurs, systemic vasoconstriction, coupled with a reduction in systemic venous return to the right atrium, can cause massive diversion of blood from the left to the right atrium. This can occur after a postpartum hemorrhage. The onset of atrial flutter or fibrillation is uncommon but, if it occurs, it should be treated by either direct current or medical cardioversion, depending on the severity of symptoms at presentation. Anticoagulation is recommended for 4 weeks after medical or electrical cardioversion or if atrial fibrillation persists.

Paradoxical embolism is a rare complication of ASD.[7,8] A small right-to-left shunt can be shown by intravenous contrast echocardiography in most ASDs but the much larger flow of blood left to right probably checks entry of particulate matter into the systemic circulation. Occasionally, however, stroke may be the presenting symptom during pregnancy. Empirical treatment with aspirin may help prevent thrombus and docs no harm to the fetus. Patients with ASD should receive venous thrombosis prophylaxis for prolonged immobility.

Patency of the foramen ovale (PFO) is found in about a quarter of adults with otherwise normal hearts so hardly qualifies as congenital heart disease (or as *acyanotic* congenital heart disease as any shunting is right to left) but paradoxical embolism through it has been increasingly recognised as a cause for stroke and a potential hazard in divers. PFO may be shown by injection of echo contrast (transesophageal imaging is superior) during Valsalva (or by transcranial Doppler) after unexplained stroke and also in patients with atypical, infrequent, migraine.[9,10]

Pulmonary embolism needs to be sought after unexpected stroke if a PFO is present (Chapter 17). Percutaneous closure should be considered if a PFO is held responsible for neurological events.[11,12]

A raised pulmonary vascular resistance is a relatively rare late complication and the pulmonary artery pressure is rarely raised in young women with ASD. A pulmonary artery systolic pressure of over 50 mmHg was found in only 7% of ASD patients in the third decade.[12,16] Primary pulmonary hypertension is sometimes associated with an anatomical secundum ASD in young women with undilated right heart chambers who have never developed left-to-right shunts because they have retained a high pulmonary vascular resistance from birth. In these patients the physical signs, behavior and prognosis are similar to those of primary pulmonary hypertension. The atrial communication provides a vent for the right ventricle and allows maintenance of systemic output through right-to-left shunting, although at the expense of reduced systemic arterial oxygen content. The risk of syncope and sudden death appears to be less and the prognosis somewhat better than in pulmonary hypertension without septal defect, but pregnancy carries a high risk (see Chapter 6) and should be strongly discouraged in any patient with severe pulmonary hypertension.

Patients with secundum ASD do not need antibiotic prophylaxis to cover dental treatment or delivery unless there is coexistent valvular disease.

Most ASDS are sporadic with a recurrence risk of about 2.5% in the offspring of patients with secundum ASD.[14] There are two types of familial ASDs, both inherited in an autosomal dominant pattern. The more common condition involves secundum ASD and atrioventricular conduction delay. The second familial type of ASD is Holt–Oram syndrome; careful inspection and occasionally radiological examination of the upper limbs of the proband are helpful on this account. This autosomal dominant condition is characterized by dysplasia of the upper limbs and ASD. Upper-extremity deformity is usually bilateral but may be asymmetrical. The atrial involvement ranges from an intact atrial septum to a large secundum ASD.

Elective surgical or device closure of a large ASD should be considered before pregnancy whenever possible.

Atrioventricular canal defects (endocardial cushion defects)

Atrioventricular canal defects, whether partial or complete, are usually diagnosed and treated surgically during infancy or childhood.

Partial atrioventricular defects with interatrial shunts and normal right ventricular pressures (ostium primum defects) are occasionally first diagnosed in young women and behave much like secundum ASDs during pregnancy, unless mitral regurgitation is considerable and complicated by pulmonary hypertension. Mitral, and less commonly tricuspid valve, clefts may occur in conjunction with atrioventricular septal defects and cause atrioventricular valve regurgitation. Thus, these patients are at risk of infective endocarditis. A raised venous pressure with dominant V wave may reflect either mitral regurgitation or direct left ventricular to right atrial shunting. Pregnancy is usually well tolerated but atrial arrhythmias occasionally develop and require treatment.

Atrioventricular canal defects are sometimes familial.

Pulmonary stenosis

Mild or moderate pulmonary valve stenosis is common and usually causes no trouble during pregnancy. No deaths or serious complications have been reported.[15,16] Even severe pulmonary stenosis can be tolerated; however, congestive features may appear from superimposition of a gestational volume overload on a hypertrophied and stiffened right ventricle. Percutaneous balloon valvuloplasty with maximum uterine shielding may be considered for the rare patient with symptomatic severe pulmonary valve stenosis, with systemic or suprasystemic pressure in the right ventricle, seen first during pregnancy. The procedure carries little risk of serious complication although hypotension, arrhythmias and transient right bundle-branch block have been reported. Balloon valvuloplasty should be delayed until the second trimester, after organogenesis is complete if possible. Pulmonary balloon valvuloplasty is the procedure of choice for the treatment of pulmonary stenosis and is now usually carried out in childhood.

Infundibular pulmonary stenosis with or without a restrictive VSD, or a double-chambered right ventricle, is similarly well tolerated during pregnancy, but much rarer. The treatment of pregnant patients depends on the functional class and severity of stenosis. These types of obstruction are not amenable to percutaneous intervention. If symptomatic deterioration occurs during pregnancy, operative repair is recommended.

Patients with pulmonary valve stenosis or right ventricular outflow tract obstruction should receive antibiotic prophylaxis to cover dental treatment or complicated delivery.

Persistent ductus arteriosus

Narrow arterial ducts with only small shunts and normal pulmonary artery pressure give rise to no hemodynamic difficulties during pregnancy. Women with larger shunts may develop congestive heart failure and these bigger ducts should be closed before pregnancy is contemplated.

Most ducts cause a typical machinery murmur and the continuous flow is readily identified on continuous wave Doppler. Patients with patent ductus arteriosus should receive antibiotic prophylaxis.

Uncorrected widely patent ducts with pulmonary hypertension may be complicated by the development of a pulmonary artery aneurysm (of which persistent ductus is the most common single cause). Dissecting aneurysm of the main pulmonary artery may develop, with spontaneous rupture during pregnancy or post partum.[17,18] Cystic medial necrosis and atheroma are usually found and both are related to severe pulmonary hypertension. Both systemic and pulmonary arterial dissections seem to have an increased incidence in pregnancy perhaps as a result of increased uptake of water by connective tissue mucopolysaccharides.[18] All patients with pulmonary hypertension should be counseled to avoid pregnancy.

Ventricular septal defect

Patients with small VSDs usually tolerate pregnancy without difficulty. The degree of left-to-right shunting is not significantly altered if baseline pulmonary vascular resistance is normal.[3,7] The increase in systemic vascular resistance, which occurs during labour, may increase the degree of left-to-right shunting. Small VSDs are noisy and the loud pansystolic murmur at the lower left sternal edge is usually discovered before pregnancy. Some small VSDs may be identified first in pregnancy. Many of these murmurs may previously have been dismissed as innocent and the VSD missed even on echocardiography until the advent of color flow Doppler.

Patients with unoperated non-restrictive VSDs and 'obligatory' pulmonary hypertension, who are still acyanotic, shunting left to right and have no symptoms, are occasionally encountered during pregnancy. They are usually quite well and may give no history of infantile heart failure or failure to thrive. Such patients may tolerate pregnancy without difficulty. However, if seen before pregnancy, these patients should be counseled to avoid pregnancy because of the recognized high risk of morbidity and mortality. Accelerated progression of pulmonary vascular disease is a hazard although not inevitable. Heart failure is not a risk because the shunt is usually small and the heart not volume loaded before pregnancy. Provided that the patient remains acyanotic fetal growth is normal. Acute blood loss or vasodilatation during delivery can lead to shunt reversal. This is avoided by generous volume replacement and avoidance of systemic vasodilators. Vasoconstricting oxytocic agents are well tolerated.

The risk of pregnancy after closure of a VSD does not differ from that in patients without heart disease unless there is residual pulmonary hypertension. Infants and children who have large non-restrictive VSDs closed may be left with pulmonary hypertension, particularly when the surgical closure occurred when the patient was aged over 2 years. Such patients need to be considered individually. Some patients with stable pulmonary hypertension and no symptoms may go through pregnancy without trouble. Others behave more as patients with primary-type pulmonary hypertension, with progression of right ventricular decompensation and a high risk of morbidity and mortality.[19] The risk of pregnancy should be considered high if the pulmonary artery pressure is over three-quarters systemic. These patients should be counseled to avoid pregnancy as a result of the high risk of mortality, estimated to be 30–50% (Chapter 6).

Occasionally a patient with pulmonary hypertension becomes pregnant and refuses a termination. The cardiovascular management of the patient during pregnancy is critically important. Close cardiovascular follow-up is essential. The functions of the left and right ventricles should receive close attention. Impairment is occasionally seen, particularly in patients who had operative intervention early in the surgical experience. The right ventricle is most vulnerable to failure of myocardial protection, and impaired function combined with residual pulmonary hypertension may seriously compromise cardiovascular reserve. During pregnancy, the patient with pulmonary hypertension should rest as much as possible and be seen frequently for evaluation of right and left ventricular function, both clinically and by echocardiography. Admission to hospital is needed for any patient with significant pulmonary vascular disease with a view to delivery by cesarean section under general anesthetic.[20] The puerperium is the time of greatest risk even in patients who seem to have tolerated pregnancy and delivery well. Consideration should be given to administering nitric oxide or nebulized prostacyclin prenatally, to try to prevent the postnatal rise in pulmonary vascular resistance that sometimes occurs.

The recurrence of VSDs among offspring of mothers with them is reported to be between 4 and 11%.[14,21] Patients with VSDs should be considered for endocarditis prophylaxis at the time of a complicated delivery.

Aortic stenosis (Table 4.2)

Severe aortic valve stenosis is seldom encountered during pregnancy and there are few published reports.[22] Congenital aortic valve disease is about five times as prevalent in male as in female individuals. Patients with a normally functioning or mildly abnormal bicuspid aortic valve have a favorable pregnancy prognosis provided that they receive appropriate care, and have no associated complicating factors such as coarctation or aortopathy.[15]

Table 4.2 Aortic stenosis and pregnancy

Signs of trouble
Onset of:
• Tachycardia
• New dyspnea
• Angina
• ECG deterioration
• Fall in peak aortic velocity
• Deterioration in left ventricular function
• Pulmonary congestion or edema
• Congestive failure

Pregnancy in women with severe left ventricular outflow tract obstruction is not recommended. The increase in blood volume and stroke volume leads to an increase in left ventricular pressure and pressure gradient across the obstruction. The increase in left ventricular work demands augmentation of coronary blood flow. Women who were free of symptoms before pregnancy may develop angina, left ventricular failure or pulmonary edema, or die suddenly. Aortic stenosis can be hazardous in pregnancy, but the risk is dependent on the severity of the obstruction. Patients with an aortic valve area <1 cm^2 should be advised against pregnancy or should have aortic valve intervention before proceeding with pregnancy as a result of the increased maternal and fetal risk.[22]

Patients with mild or moderate aortic stenosis do well and pregnancy need not be discouraged.[23] Such women should plan to complete their families before their valves deteriorate and the stenosis worsens, in order to avoid a complication during pregnancy and to avoid pregnancy in the setting of a valve prosthesis.[5]

Patients with severe aortic valve stenosis may not be seen until they are already pregnant and, if the pregnancy is advanced or a termination refused, they require careful supervision through the pregnancy. Pregnant patients with severe asymptomatic aortic stenosis should be followed closely from the cardiac and obstetric standpoint during pregnancy, and delivered in a tertiary center with possible hemodynamic monitoring during labour and delivery. These patients may demonstrate symptomatic deterioration during pregnancy and often respond well to bedrest and occasionally also beta blockers. Every effort should be made to bring the pregnancy to term. If the mother's condition is still giving cause for alarm, the baby should be delivered by cesarean section under general anesthesia *before* proceeding with aortic valve surgery. This may be followed by improvement in the mother's condition, and may even allow surgery to be delayed. The pregnant patient with severe aortic stenosis is extremely intolerant of changes in left ventricular preload. A fall caused by hemorrhage or regional anesthesia can lead to cardiogenic shock and a rise may precipitate pulmonary edema.

Percutaneous balloon aortic valvuloplasty can be a safe and effective palliative procedure during pregnancy, but should be attempted only at centers that have extensive experience and surgical back-up.[12,24] Special considerations for balloon valvuloplasty in the gravid state include radiation exposure and pregnancy outcome. There has been no increase in the incidence of reported congenital malformations or abortions with fetal radiation exposure of less than 5 rads, which can be achieved by shielding the gravid uterus and keeping fluoroscopy time to a minimum. Transesophageal or intracardiac echocardiographic guidance has also been utilized during the procedure to reduce radiation exposure.

The risk of open-heart surgery to the fetus remains high particularly if the mother's condition is poor.[25] There is a risk of fetal loss during induction of anesthesia if this causes hemodynamic instability, with swings in blood pressure, heart rate and output, or the fetus may die during cardiopulmonary bypass despite modern technological improvements with membrane oxygenators and pulsatile flow, especially if this is prolonged. Cardiopulmonary bypass for valve replacement during pregnancy after the fetus is viable not only jeopardizes the fetus unnecessarily, but also increases the hazard to the mother because of tissue edema, high diaphragms and poor operating conditions for the surgeon. Every measure should be taken to avoid cardiac surgery during pregnancy. However, when cardiac surgery cannot be avoided, management at a tertiary center with multidisciplinary cardiology, cardiac anesthesia and cardiac surgical experience is recommended.

Congenital aortic valve stenosis is usually the result of a variety of bicuspid aortic valve with varying degrees of valve thickening and commissural fusion. There may be some narrowing of the aortic root, asymmetry of the sinuses of Valsalva or aortic root dilatation. Aortic valve regurgitation is usually absent or mild. Other left-sided lesions, such as coarctation of the aorta, supravalvar mitral stenosis or subaortic stenosis (Shone syndrome), may also occur together with a congenitally abnormal aortic valve. Left ventricular systolic function is usually normal but this may be impaired in the setting of critical aortic valve stenosis. Low-output, low-gradient aortic stenosis may present with a low Doppler aortic valve velocity and gradient in the presence of reduced left ventricular systolic function. This may reflect severe valve stenosis that needs urgent relief. Left ventricular dysfunction in the setting of aortic stenosis is sometimes the result of endocardial fibroelastosis, which, if seen in combination with mild or moderate aortic stenosis, is a concern as a result of left ventricular dysfunction rather than outflow tract obstruction. Table 4.2 shows what to look out for in pregnant patients with aortic stenosis.

Mutations in diverse genes with dissimilar inheritance patterns are responsible for the development of bicuspid aortic valve in different families.[27] In a recent series, the prevalence of bicuspid aortic valve in the relatives of patients with bicuspid aortic valve was 24%.[26]

Left ventricular outflow tract obstruction may be valvular or supravalvular, or caused by discrete membranous or tunnel-type subvalvular aortic stenosis. Outflow tract gradients associated with hypertrophic cardiomyopathy are considered in Chapter 13. Rheumatic aortic valve stenosis is rare in pregnancy (see Chapter 7) and invariably associated with mitral stenosis, usually in older women. The management of these lesions is similar to the management of patients with congenital aortic stenosis during pregnancy.

Supravalvar aortic stenosis, either with or without the Williams–Beuren syndrome, is rarely seen in pregnancy. Peripheral pulmonary artery branch stenoses may be associated, as well as peripheral arterial dysplasia.[27] When the gradient across the supravalvar stenosis is small and other serious vascular stenoses are absent, the prognosis is good.

Endocarditis prophylaxis should be considered around the time of delivery in patients with left ventricular outflow tract obstruction (Chapter 9).

Coarctation of the aorta

Most patients with coarctation of the aorta who reach child-bearing age have had previous surgical intervention. Although prior surgical repair of coarctation has a favorable effect on overall prognosis and outcome of pregnancy by correcting hypertension or making it possible to treat the hypertension more effectively, long-term risks remain. The outcome of pregnancy with coarctation of the aorta depends on the severity of coarctation and associated cardiac lesions, such as bicuspid aortic valve and aortopathy. Both maternal and fetal outcomes are usually favorable in aortic coarctation. Cases of severe hypertension, congestive heart failure, aortic dissection, rupture of an intracranial berry aneurysm and infective endocarditis have been reported. These are the complications that caused a 17% mortality rate in the first reports, but less than 3% in recent ones.[28,29]

Late complications after coarctation repair are uncommon but should be considered in any woman with a history of repaired coarctation who wishes to become pregnant.[30] Comprehensive pre-pregnancy evaluation should include evaluation of the integrity of the coarctation repair, looking for residual or recurrent obstruction, or an aneurysm, either at the site of repair or in the ascending aorta. In addition, the aortic valve and left ventricle should be evaluated. If a patient with coarctation or repaired coarctation is referred during pregnancy with a suspected aortic complication, the investigation of choice is magnetic resonance imaging.

Drug treatment of hypertension may be unsatisfactory in patients with uncorrected coarctation. Untreated, the resting blood pressure tends to fall slightly in pregnancy as in normal women, but considerable rises in systolic pressure and pulse pressure occur on exercise with attendant risks. Blood pressure-lowering agents, such as hydralazine, methyldopa, labetalol or metoprolol, may be used to temper this, but over-enthusiastic blood pressure reduction will diminish placental perfusion and be detrimental to fetal growth. Ideally, coarctation intervention should be carried out before pregnancy. However, when a pregnant patient with uncorrected coarctation is encountered, strenuous exercise should be avoided in an effort to minimize stress on the arterial wall, because surges in blood pressure and pulse pressure with exercise are not wholly prevented by blood pressure-lowering drugs.

Patients with coarctation of the aorta have an abnormal aortic wall and are prone to aortic dissection. The risk of aortic dissection increases during pregnancy as a result of the physiological, hemodynamic and hormonal changes that occur. Limiting physical activity and controlling blood pressure with beta-blocker therapy probably reduces the risk of dissection during pregnancy and delivery. Vaginal delivery is feasible in most patients with coarctation of the aorta, but it is important for the second stage to be curtailed to minimize arterial stress. If there is any doubt on obstetric grounds or in patients with unstable aortic lesions, cesarean delivery should be considered. Fetal development is usually normal, indicating adequate maintenance of uteroplacental blood flow through the collateral circulation. Pre-eclamptic toxemia increases in patients with coarctation but malignant hypertension or papilledema is rare.[29]

Surgical repair of coarctation during pregnancy should be limited to cases of aortic dissection or severe uncontrollable hypertension or heart failure.[30] The mechanism of aortic enlargement after percutaneous dilatation for coarctation is stretching and tearing of the aortic wall. Pregnancy is a condition that predisposes to dissection, so percutaneous angioplasty or stenting of coarctation of the aorta should be avoided in the pregnant patient or the patient planning future pregnancy.

Endocarditis prophylaxis should be considered in the peripartum period for patients with coarctation of the aorta. A bicuspid aortic valve increases the risk of endocarditis. When endocarditis occurs it is nearly always on the bicuspid valve rather than on the coarctation.

A recent study reported congenital heart disease in 3% of infants born to patients with corrected coarctation.[30] A higher incidence of congenital heart disease has been reported in the infants of mothers with uncorrected coarctation compared with mothers with corrected coarctation.[21]

Congenitally corrected transposition

Corrected transposition (atrioventricular discordance with ventriculoarterial discordance, congenitally corrected transposition or l-TGA) is usually accompanied by other defects, particularly VSD and subpulmonary and pulmonary valve stenosis or an Ebstein-like malformation of the left-sided tricuspid valve with or without regurgitation. Although l-TGA is an uncommon congenital anomaly, survival into adulthood is frequent either after surgery or with isolated l-TGA. The morphological right ventricle supports the systemic circulation in this condition, so up to half of adult patients have systemic ventricular dysfunction or systemic atrioventricular valve regurgitation, or frequently both. As many women with l-TGA reach child-bearing age, a comprehensive cardiovascular evaluation must be undertaken at the time of pregnancy counseling. Particular attention must be paid to the functional class, systemic ventricular function, degree of atrioventricular valve regurgitation and any associated lesions. Those with an ejection fraction <40% or with significant systemic atrioventricular valve regurgitation should be counseled against pregnancy. Successful pregnancy can, however, be achieved in those with good haemodynamics.[31] Heart block may develop at any time in life and may complicate pregnancy in patients with l-TGA.

Endocarditis prophylaxis should be considered. There appears to be an increased risk of congenital heart disease in the offspring of these patient.

Ebstein's anomaly of the tricuspid valve

Ebstein's anomaly is associated with caudal displacement of the septal and posterior leaflets of the tricuspid valve, together with a sail-like abnormality, elongation and variable tethering of a normally attached anterior tricuspid valve leaflet. An interatrial communication, either patent foramen ovale or septal

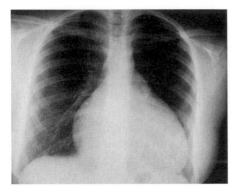

Figure 4.2 Chest X ray picture of a young woman with acyanotic Ebstein's anomaly who presented with an embolic stroke presumed to have been caused by paradoxical embolism. Transthoracic and transesophageal echocardiography showed no evidence of intra-atrial thrombus and there was no history of arrhythmia.

defect, is present in over 50% of affected individuals. Right and, less commonly, left ventricular dysfunction are also often present.

Women with Ebstein's anomaly often reach child-bearing age. They are usually acyanotic and tolerate pregnancy well. Complications may include atrial tachycardia caused by right-sided pre-excitation.[32] Paradoxical embolism can occur even in the asymptomatic patient (Figure 4.2) or late development of cyanosis ('cyanosis tardive') with reduction in the prospect of a successful pregnancy (see Chapter 5). Pregnancy after surgical repair is often also well tolerated. The risk of congenital heart disease in the offspring of women with Ebstein's anomaly is about 6%.[33]

Endocarditis prophylaxis should be considered in the peripartum period for patients with Ebstein's anomaly and associated tricuspid valve regurgitation.

Prosthetic valves

Prosthetic valves which are implanted in adults usually accommodate the increased blood flow during pregnancy without hemodynamic problems. Not many young women are seen through pregnancy after prosthetic heart valve replacement in infancy or childhood and experience is anecdotal. They form a diverse group from valve bearing conduits for complex congenital defects to isolated single valve prostheses. Mechanical valves are more durable and offer a larger effective orifice than bioprostheses in the smaller sizes so have often been chosen for replacement of left heart valves in infancy and childhood and are likely to become outgrown.

History and examination with ECG, (chest X ray) and echocardiography need back-up with establishment of cardiovascular reserve by exercise testing. Transvalvular velocity (for gradient) and (for left-sided prostheses) pulmonary artery pressure should be measured at rest and after exercise. Valve orifice areas which would be adequate with a native valve are likely to prove inadequate with a prosthetic valve. If the pulmonary artery pressure rises on exercise the patient will not sustain pregnancy.

Lack of symptoms and an apparently adequate prosthetic valve orifice are not enough. Analogy with native valve disease is inappropriate. There can be no rescue by balloon. Echo studies should be repeated at each monthly visit between 8 and 20 weeks gestation. Termination is safer than continuation. Bed rest (with prophylactic heparin if not already on anticoagulant) and titrated dosage of a beta blocker may hold a patient with a stenotic aortic or mitral prosthesis. Surgery should, if possible, be deferred until the fetus is viable. It should be delivered by cesarean section *before* the maternal surgery.

Patients who are going to need re-do surgery should defer pregnancy (Chapter 9).

Conclusions

More women with congenital heart disease are now considering pregnancy. Despite potential complications associated with congenital heart disease in pregnancy, careful cardiac and obstetric management in a tertiary referral center results in good maternal and fetal outcomes in most cases.[5] A multidisciplinary approach at a tertiary care center is mandatory for the high-risk pregnant patient with congenital heart disease and, for the woman in whom pregnancy is not advisable, appropriate contraceptive advice must be given.

References

1 Elkayam U, Gleicher N. Cardiac problems in pregnancy. 1. Maternal aspects: the approach to the pregnant patient with heart disease. *JAMA* 1984;**251**:2838–9.
2 McFaul P, Dornan J, Lamki H, Boyle D. Pregnancy complicated by maternal heart disease: a review of 519 women. *Br J Obstet Gynaecol* 1988;**95**:861–7.
3 Pitkin R, Perloff J, Koos B, Beall M. Pregnancy and congenital heart disease. *Ann Intern Med* 1990;**112**:445–54.
4 Oakley C. Cardiovascular disease in pregnancy. *Can J Cardiol* 1990;**6**:33B–44B.
5 Siu S, Sermer M, Colman J et al. Prospective multicenter study of pregnancy outcomes in women with heart disease. *Circulation* 2001;**104**:515–521.
6 Coleman J, Sermer M, Seaward P, Siu S. Congenital heart disease in pregnancy. *Cardiol Rev* 2000;**8**:166–173.
7 Zuber M, Gautschi N, Oechslin E, Widmer V, Kiowski W, Jenni R. Outcome of pregnancy in women with congenital shunt lesions. *Heart* 1999;**81**:271–5.
8 Harvey J, Teague S, Anderson J, Voyles W, Thadani V. Clinically silent atrial septal defects with evidence for cerebral embolisation. *Ann Intern Med* 1986;**105**:695–7.
9 Pinto FJ Minisymposium. When and how to diagnose patent foraman ovale. *Heart* 2005;**91**:438–40.
10 Amarenco P Minisymposium. Patent foramen ovale and the risk of stroke: smoking gun by association? *Heart* 2005;**91**:441–3.
11 Flaschkampf FA, Daniel WG. Minisymposium. Closure of patent foramen ovale: is the case really closed as well? *Heart* **91**:449–51.
12 Presibitero P, Prever S, Brusca A. Interventional cardiology in pregnancy. *Eur Heart J* 1996;**17**:182–8.

13 Markman P, Howitt G, Wade EG. Atrial septal defect in the middle-aged and elderly. *Quart J Med* 1965;**34**:409–26.

14 Nora J, McGill C, McNamara D. Empiric recurrence risks in common and uncommon congenital heart lesions. *Teratology* 1970;**3**:325–9.

15 Perloff J, Koos B, Phil D, Beall M. Pregnancy and congenital heart disease. *Ann Intern Med* 1990;**112**:445–54.

16 Siu S, Sermer M, Harrison D et al. Risk and predictors for pregnancy-related complications in women with heart disease. *Circulation* 1997;**96**:2789–94.

17 Hankins G, Brekken A, Davis L. Maternal death secondary to a dissecting aneurysm of the pulmonary artery. *Obstet Gynecol* 1985;**65**:45–8.

18 Guthrie W, MacLean H. Dissecting aneurysms of arteries other than the aorta. *J Pathol* 1972;**108**:210–35.

19 Jackson G, Dildy G, Varner M, Clark S. Severe pulmonary hypertension in pregnancy following successful repair of ventricular septal defect in childhood. *Obstet Gynecol* 1993;**82**:680–2.

20 Avila W, Grinberg M, Snitcowsky R et al. Maternal and fetal outcome in pregnant women with Eisenmenger's syndrome. *Eur Heart J* 1995;**16**:460–4.

21 Wooley C, Sparks E. Congenital heart disease, inheritable cardiovascular disease and pregnancy. *Prog Cardiovasc Dis* 1992;**35**:41–60.

22 Silversides C, Colman J, Sermer M, Farine D, Siu S. Early and intermediate-term outcomes of pregnancy with congenital aortic stenosis. *Am J Cardiol* 2003;**91**:1386–9.

23 Lao TT, Sermer M, MaGee L et al. Congenital aortic stenosis and pregnancy – a reappraisal. *Am J Obstet Gynecol* 1993;**169**:540–45.

24 Bhargava B, Agarwal R, Yadav R, Bahl V, Manchanda S. Percutaneous balloon aortic valvuloplasty during pregnancy: use of the Inoue balloon and the physiologic antegrade approach. *Cathet Cardiovasc Diagn* 1998;**45**:422–5.

25 Bernal J, Miralles P. Cardiac surgery with cardiopulmonary bypass during pregnancy. *Obstet Gynecol Surv* 1986;**41**:1–6.

26 Cripe L, Andelfinger G, Martin L, Shooner K, Benson D. Bicuspid aortic valve is heritable. *J Am Coll Cardiol* 2004;**44**:138–43.

27 Wessel A, Pankau R, Kececioglu D, Ruschewski W, Bursch J. Three decades of follow-up of aortic and pulmonary vascular lesions in the Williams-Beuren syndrome. *Am J Med Genet* 1994;**52**:297–301.

28 Koller M, Rothlin M, Senning A. Coarctation of the aorta: review of 362 operated patients; long-term follow-up and assessment of prognostic variables. *Eur Heart J* 1987;**8**:670–9.

29 Beauchesne L, Connolly H, Ammash N, Warnes C. Coarctation of the aorta. Outcome of pregnancy. *J Am Coll Cardiol* 2001;**38**:1728–33.

30 Saidi A, Bezold L, Altman C, Ayres N, Bricker J. Outcome of pregnancy following intervention for coarctation of the aorta. *Am J Cardiol* 1998;**82**:786–8.

31 Connolly H, Grogan M, Warnes C. Pregnancy among women with congenitally corrected transposition of the great arteries. *J Am Coll Cardiol* 1999;**33**:1692–5.

32 Waickman L, Storton D, Varmer M, Ehmke D, Goplerud C. Ebstein's anomaly in pregnancy. *Am J Cardiol* 1984;**53**:357–8.

33 Connolly H, Warnes CA. Ebstein's anomaly: outcome of pregnancy. *J Am Coll Cardiol* 1994;**23**:1194–8.

CHAPTER 5

Cyanotic congenital heart disease

Carole A Warnes

When cyanosis accompanies congenital heart disease, the underlying anomaly is commonly complex. Many patients with congenital heart disease undergo successful repair in infancy or childhood, but some lesions associated with increased pulmonary vascular resistance (Eisenmenger syndrome) are not amenable to surgical repair. In addition, a number of patients with compensated anomalies survive to adulthood without surgical intervention. These include patients with Ebstein's anomaly and mild tetralogy of Fallot. Sometimes the lesion was unrecognized in childhood but, as more blood was shunted from the right to the left circulation, the patient became progressively cyanosed. Sometimes surgery was refused by the patient or the patient's family.

Cyanotic congenital heart disease can be divided into those lesions associated with low pulmonary blood flow and those associated with high pulmonary blood flow. In both circumstances, cyanosis poses risks for both the mother and the fetus.

Maternal risks

Patients with right-to-left shunts usually have erythrocytosis and, the more severe the hypoxia, the more elevated the hemoglobin and packed cell volume. During pregnancy, as there is increased platelet adhesiveness and decreased fibrinolysis, there is an increased risk of thrombotic complications for the cyanotic mother. Overzealous treatment with diuretics should therefore be avoided because of the risk of hemoconcentration and abnormal renal function. A study by Presbitero et al. evaluated pregnancy outcomes in 44 cyanotic patients who had 96 pregnancies.[1] In this series, patients with Eisenmenger syndrome were excluded because it was considered that elevated pulmonary vascular resistance is a greater hazard than the presence of cyanosis. Two patients in this series had thrombotic complications (pulmonary and cerebral); their hemoglobin concentrations were 170 and 180 g/L. Cardiovascular complications occurred in fourteen patients (32%); eight patients developed heart failure, three requiring hospital admission at 32–36 weeks of gestation; and peripartum bacterial endocarditis occurred in two patients (4–5%), both with palliated tetralogy of Fallot.

If cyanotic patients develop thrombophlebitis or deep venous thrombosis, they are at risk not only of pulmonary, but also of paradoxical embolism. There must therefore be meticulous attention to leg care during pregnancy, and this is particularly important during labour and the puerperium. These risks can be minimized by arranging coordinated care with cardiologists, obstetricians and anesthetists throughout pregnancy and during labour and delivery. Patients should be adequately hydrated during labour. Elastic support stockings or compression pumps should be used, and patients mobilized early. Anticoagulation should not be used routinely in cyanotic patients because they are also at risk of bleeding. This is because they are usually deficient in the clotting factors produced in the liver, and the platelet count may be low and platelet function abnormal. It is possible, however, that the use of low-dose aspirin after the first trimester is safe without increasing the risk of bleeding, and perhaps may help to reduce thrombotic complications. It does not have an adverse effect on the fetus. Prophylactic doses of heparin may be used during the period of greatest risk while the patient is in hospital and are safe.

Fetal risk

Cyanosis also poses a substantial risk to the fetus, and results in increased fetal loss, prematurity and small birthweight. Neill and Swanson reported that, with increasing cyanosis, as reflected in the maternal hemoglobin, the incidence of spontaneous abortion increased and the handicap to fetal growth was more pronounced.[2] In their series, no infant survived if the maternal hemoglobin was greater than 180g/L, and most babies were lost in the first trimester. Whittemore estimated maternal hypoxia using the packed cell volume (PCV), and showed that infants born to mothers with a PCV > 0.44 were all below the 50th percentile of birthweight for gestational age.[3] The study by Presbitero et al. also demonstrated that, with increasing maternal hypoxia, as reflected by the mother's hemoglobin, the percentage of live-born infants fell and, when the mother's hemoglobin exceeded 200g/L, only 8% of children were live born (Table 5.1).[1] Similarly, when the maternal oxygen saturation was ≤85%, only 2 of 17 pregnancies (12%) resulted in live-born infants. In total, 41 of the 96 pregnancies (43%) produced a live birth: 26 of these babies reached term and 15 were premature. There were 49 spontaneous abortions and 6 stillbirths, again reflecting the high risk that cyanotic congenital heart disease poses for the fetus. Congenital heart disease was found in 2 of 41 live infants (4.9%).

Tetralogy of Fallot

Tetralogy of Fallot consists of a ventricular septal defect immediately beneath the aortic valve and an overriding aorta that lies over the ventricular septal defect. Pulmonary outflow tract obstruction usually occurs at infundibular level and often with associated pulmonary valve stenosis, and this causes secondary right ventricular hypertrophy. As a result of the right ventricular outflow tract ob-

Table 5.1 Fetal outcome in cyanotic congenital heart disease and its relationship to maternal cyanosis

	No. of pregnancies	No. of live births	Percentage born alive
Hemoglobin (g/L)[a]			
≤ 160	28	20	71
170–190	40	18	45
≥ 200	26	2	8
Arterial oxygen saturation (%)[b]			
≤ 85	17	2	12
85–89	22	10	45
≥ 90	13	12	92

Reproduced from Presbitero et al. with permission.[1]

[a]Hemoglobin concentration unknown in two pregnancies.

[b]Arterial oxygen saturation unknown in 44 pregnancies.

struction, there is a right-to-left shunt through the ventricular septal defect and blue blood enters the aorta. Patients with mild tetralogy of Fallot may survive into adulthood without substantial symptoms but usually the pulmonary stenosis progresses, increasing the right-to-left shunt and the severity of cyanosis.

As a result of the fall in peripheral vascular resistance that occurs during a normal pregnancy, there may be an increase in the right-to-left shunt, with subsequent increase in the cyanosis. Thus, even mothers with mild cyanosis may notice a deterioration during pregnancy. Labour and delivery are a particularly hazardous time, because the blood loss associated with delivery may induce hypotension and again exaggerate the right-to-left shunt.

Right and left heart failure may occur during pregnancy, particularly when there is associated aortic regurgitation.[4] Aortic regurgitation tends to be progressive in patients with tetralogy of Fallot who have not undergone surgery because the aortic valve leaflets have no support and prolapse into the defect. In addition, the aorta itself is usually larger than normal because it is carrying increased blood flow. Further problems may occur during pregnancy with the onset of atrial arrhythmias, which are more common in the third and fourth decade.[5] Rarely, pulmonary stenosis has been surgically palliated during pregnancy.[6] Presbitero et al. reported the outcome of 21 patients with 46 pregnancies who had either tetralogy of Fallot or pulmonary atresia with aortopulmonary collaterals.[1] There were 15 live births (33%) and 9 babies were premature. There were 26 abortions and 5 stillbirths. In addition 8 of the mothers experienced cardiovascular complications, including 2 with peripartum bacterial endocarditis.

The risk of a congenital heart defect in the offspring of a parent with tetralogy has been reported to be 2.5–8.3%.[7–10] In the largest series reported so far, of 127 parents (62 women, 65 men), congenital heart defects occurred in 3 (1.2%) of the 253 children.[11] One of these children had tetralogy of Fallot, one a ventricular septal defect and the other truncus arteriosus. The reasons for these discrepancies in risks depend on many factors, including ascertainment bias, environmental factors and how vigorously congenital heart disease in the offspring is sought (e.g. physical examination compared with echocardiography).

After successful surgical repair of tetralogy of Fallot, the outcome is considerably improved.[12] Singh et al. reported 40 pregnancies in 27 patients with surgically repaired tetralogy of Fallot.[8] There were no serious complications in any of the pregnancies, and the incidence of miscarriage was no higher than that in the general population. Of 31 pregnancies about which detailed information was available, 30 resulted in normal infants, the one abnormal infant having pulmonary atresia.

The Mayo Clinic group reported the outcomes of 43 women with tetralogy of Fallot who had 112 pregnancies.[13] Six patients had pulmonary hypertension, three moderate or severe right ventricular dysfunction and thirteen severe right ventricular dilatation secondary to severe pulmonary regurgitation. Six patients had cardiovascular complications during pregnancy. All six had one of the following: severe right ventricular (RV) dilatation, RV dysfunction (or both), RV hypertension from outflow obstruction or pulmonary hypertension. Complications included supraventricular tachycardia in two, heart failure in two, pulmonary embolism in a patient with pulmonary hypertension and progressive right ventricular dilatation in a patient with pulmonary regurgitation. Some 16 patients had 30 miscarriages (27%) and one term stillbirth. Mean overall birthweight was satisfactory at 3.2 kg. Eight women had unrepaired tetralogy at the time of their 20 pregnancies: 5 of them were cyanotic during 12 pregnancies. Unrepaired tetralogy was predictive of low infant birthweight, as was a morphological pulmonary artery abnormality. Five of the offspring (6%) in this series had congenital anomalies. These data emphasize that, although many women with repaired tetralogy can have a successful outcome during pregnancy, those with significant structural or hemodynamic problems are more likely to experience adverse cardiovascular complications. This was also confirmed in a series from the Netherlands: 50 successful pregnancies occurred in 26 patients with repaired tetralogy. Complications occurred in 5 patients (19%) and were either symptomatic right heart failure or arrhythmias or both.[14] Both patients who developed symptomatic right heart failure had severe pulmonary regurgitation, which is the most common residual hemodynamic sequela currently seen in adults after tetralogy repair. It is a lesion easily missed on clinical examination because the murmur is soft and short, and can be missed on echocardiographic examination because the pulmonary regurgitant flow is laminar rather than turbulent.

Each patient should be assessed before conception with careful history taking to determine functional status, exercise capacity, and the presence or absence of other lesions.[15] The presence of a 22q11.2 microdeletion should also be considered because this may occur in 6–22% of patients with tetralogy and other conotruncal anomalies. A recent report suggests that the typical clinical features may be difficult to detect in the adult population, and so there should be some consideration and discussion with the potential parent about the pros and cons of screening, the implications if positive and appropriate genetic counseling if necessary.[16] Echocardiography should be done to delineate the hemodynamics and find out whether or not there is any RV outflow tract obstruction, pulmonary regurgitation or RV dysfunction. Any residual defects, such as ventricular septal defect or aortic regurgitation, should also be discovered, in addition to assessment of left ventricular function. If necessary, exercise testing should be done to assess functional capacity. Provided that there are no major residual defects, it is likely that pregnancy and delivery will be uncomplicated.[14]

Pulmonary atresia

Pulmonary atresia represents an extreme form of Fallot's tetralogy in which there is congenital absence of the pulmonary valve and main pulmonary artery, and the lungs receive their blood supply from collateral arteries arising from the descending aorta. Patients rarely survive to adulthood without surgical intervention, or more commonly after a palliative shunt. Little information is available about the outcome of pregnancy in women with pulmonary atresia. Connolly et al. reported 14 patients with complex pulmonary atresia who had 24 pregnancies resulting in 10 live births (including a twin pregnancy).[17] There was one neonatal death from abruptio placentae at 27 weeks. Six pregnancies were terminated in women with unoperated pulmonary atresia.

Six patients had successful pregnancies: two unoperated patients had three deliveries (including twins—four births), two palliated patients had three deliveries, and two patients had two successful and two unsuccessful pregnancies after complete repair. One pregnancy was complicated by high RV pressure from conduit obstruction and one unoperated patient had congestive heart failure requiring admission to hospital in the last month of pregnancy. No pregnancy-related maternal deaths occurred. The mean maternal hemoglobin in patients with successful pregnancies was 149 g/L (SD 13 g/L) compared with 183 (21) g/L in patients who terminated pregnancy ($p = 0.01$) and 164 (22) g/L in patients with unsuccessful pregnancies. None of the offspring had congenital heart disease. Thus, pregnancy in patients with complex pulmonary atresia can be accomplished successfully, but there is an increased risk of fetal loss even without maternal hypoxia (miscarriage rate 50%).

Assessment of pulmonary pressures and degree of cyanosis is necessary before pregnancy is contemplated; for those patients, after radical repair, ventricular and conduit function must also be evaluated.

Ebstein's anomaly

This malformation consists of an inferior displacement of the tricuspid valve with resulting tricuspid regurgitation and enlargement of the right heart chambers. At least 50% of patients with Ebstein's anomaly have either an atrial septal defect or a patent foramen ovale, and may therefore be cyanosed. Although Ebstein's anomaly is an uncommon congenital malformation, many patients survive to adulthood without surgical intervention; their functional status varies widely, however, depending on the degree of tricuspid regurgitation and RV dysfunction. Several small series have reported the outcome of pregnancy in women with Ebstein's anomaly.[18,19] The largest series was reported by Connolly and Warnes who reported the outcome of 44 women with Ebstein's anomaly who had pregnancies (Figure 5.1):[20] 44 women had 111 pregnancies, resulting in 85 live births (76%). The pregnancy outcomes are shown in Figure 5.2. Eighteen women were cyanotic at the time of pregnancy (16 had documented interatrial communication; 2 did not have an atrial septal defect or patent foramen ovale). The 18 cyanotic women had 52 pregnancies resulting in 39 live births (75%). Among the 39 live births were 12 pre-term infants born to 6 cyanotic women (31%). The outcome of pregnancy of the cyanotic patients compared with the acyanotic women is shown in Table 5.2.

The mean birthweight of infants born to cyanotic women was significantly lower than that of infants born to acyanotic women (2530–3140 g, $p < 0.001$). This difference persisted when pre-term infants were excluded from the analysis. In this study, the miscarriage and fetal loss rates were only slightly increased at 18% (19/104), compared with the expected rate of 10–15%.[21] Although arrhythmias are a common complication in patients with Ebstein's anomaly, particularly as accessory conduction pathways are often associated, none of the patients in this series had significant arrhythmias during pregnancy. Of the 83 offspring, 5 had congenital heart disease, an incidence of 6%. Two had aortic

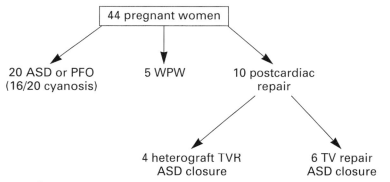

Figure 5.1 Characteristics of 44 women with Ebstein's anomaly who had pregnancies: 20 had an interatrial communication (either atrial septal defect [ASD] or patent foramen ovale [PFO]) at the time of pregnancy; 16 were cyanotic. Five women had one or more accessory pathways (Wolff–Parkinson–White syndrome [WPW]). Ten women had pregnancies after successful cardiac repair, all had ASD closure and reduction atrioplasty; six had tricuspid valve (TV) repair, and the remaining four had tricuspid valve replacement (TVR) with a heterograft prosthesis. (Reproduced from Connolly and Warnes[20] with permission.)

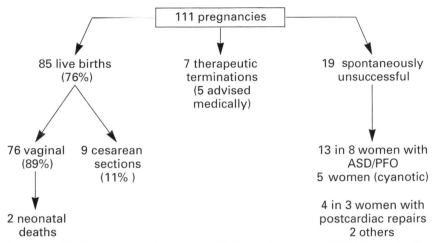

Figure 5.2 Of 111 pregnancies in women with Ebstein's anomaly, 85 (76%) resulted in live births. Of these, 76 children (89%) were born by vaginal delivery and 9 (11%) by cesarean section (C-section). Of the 19 spontaneously unsuccessful pregnancies, 13 occurred in women with atrial septal defect (ASD) or patent foramen ovale (PFO); 5 of the 8 women with ASD or PFO were cyanotic. Four unsuccessful pregnancies occurred in three women after successful cardiac repair and two occurred in women who had no ASD or PFO and had not had cardiac repair. (Reproduced from Connolly and Warnes[20] with permission.)

Table 5.2 Outcome of pregnancy in Ebstein's anomaly: cyanotic compared with acyanotic women

	Cyanotic (n = 18)	Acyanotic (n = 26)	P
Pre-term delivery	3 (17)	8 (31)	0.627
Miscarriage	4 (22)	4 (15)	0.928
Pre-term + miscarriage	3 (17)	2 (8)	0.733
Total	10 (56)	14 (54)	0.844

Reproduced from Connolly and Warnes with permission.[20]

Figures are numbers with percentages in parentheses.

valve abnormalities, one had pulmonary atresia with intact ventricular septum, and two had ventricular septal defects that closed spontaneously.

As Ebstein's anomaly may encompass a wide spectrum of anatomical and functional severity, it is recommended that all patients have a thorough evaluation before they become pregnant, with particular reference to ventricular size and function. Many cyanotic patients with Ebstein's anomaly may be amenable to surgical repair with a good functional result.[22] As the Connolly study showed, pregnancy is well tolerated after tricuspid valve repair or replacement, and the risk of paradoxical embolism is obviated after closure of the atrial septal defect. Therefore, although there is an increased risk of fetal loss, prematurity and a low-birthweight infant, in most cases one can be optimistic about the outcome of pregnancy.

Single ventricle/tricuspid atresia

Patients with a morphological single ventricle (univentricular atrioventricular connection) may have atresia of one or other atrioventricular valve (commonly tricuspid atresia). There may be two atrioventricular valves entering the main ventricular chamber (double-inlet left ventricle), or one large atrioventricular valve entering the main ventricular chamber (commonly a morphological right ventricle). Few patients survive to reproductive age without surgery, although some cases have been reported.[23] Most commonly, patients survive because of previous palliative surgery in the form of a shunt or after definitive repair. The presence of pulmonary hypertension is a major determinant of maternal risk. Some of these patients survive to adulthood with pulmonary vascular disease, but most have pulmonary stenosis. If there is modest pulmonary stenosis and good ventricular function associated with a moderate degree of cyanosis, pregnancy may be possible, but it is associated with an increased risk, for both the mother and the fetus. There are only a few isolated reports in the literature regarding pregnancy and a single ventricle.

Stiller et al. reported a patient with double-inlet left ventricle and significant pulmonary stenosis with a systolic gradient of 89 mmHg.[24] She delivered a healthy infant at 30 weeks' gestation weighing 2353 g. Leibbrandt et al. reported a 29-year-old woman with a single ventricle and transposed great arteries who had only mild stenosis, but who tolerated two pregnancies.[25] Collins et al. reported a 23-year-old woman with tricuspid atresia and a previous Blalock–Taussig shunt who delivered a low-birthweight infant but survived the pregnancy.[26] Two years later, however, she became pregnant again, had a stroke and subsequently aborted a 2-month fetus. Finally, in another pregnancy, she had two pulmonary emboli, refused termination and at 24 weeks delivered a pre-term infant, who did not survive. After delivery she had another pulmonary embolus but survived.

The important determinants of maternal and fetal survival are therefore ventricular function and degree of cyanosis. The pulmonary artery pressure must be assessed before pregnancy. For those with moderate pulmonary stenosis, pregnancy may be tolerated with an increased risk and particular caution to avoid hypotension during pregnancy and labour.

The definitive repair for both tricuspid atresia and single ventricle is the Fontan operation or one of its modifications.[27,28] This operation is designed to separate the systemic and pulmonary venous returns and to reduce the volume load on the left ventricle. This is accomplished by a right atrial to pulmonary artery anastomosis or a modification to divert caval blood to the pulmonary circuit. For those women who have had a successful Fontan operation, pregnancy may be successfully accomplished provided that there are no significant residual lesions.[29] There is, however, an increased risk of fetal loss.

One multicentre study reported 28 pregnancies in 11 mothers after the Fontan operation.[29] Of these eleven women, seven had the Fontan operation for tricuspid atresia and two for a single ventricle, and two had complex anomalies. There were 12 (43%) live births. One had two term pregnancies. There were nine (32%) first trimester miscarriages, five elective abortions and two women are currently pregnant. The gestational age of the infants averaged 36.2 weeks and their mean weight was 2331 g (range 1050–3575 g). One infant had an atrial septal defect. None of the mothers experienced any cardiac complications.

Each case must be assessed before pregnancy, including evaluation of functional capacity and echocardiography to assess residual lesions and ventricular function. For those patients with considerable right atrial enlargement, there is an increased risk of atrial arrhythmias, thrombus formation within the right atrium and thromboembolism. This may be particularly true if spontaneous echo contrast is noted. Early delivery is frequently necessary to prevent decompensation of the single ventricle.

Transposition of the great vessels

In this anomaly, the aorta arises from the morphological right ventricle and the pulmonary artery from the morphological left ventricle, with a communication between the two circulations in the form of an atrial septal defect, a ventricular septal defect or a patent ductus arteriosus. These patients do not survive to adulthood without surgical intervention, but, with the development of reparative surgery, most female infants now survive to reach child-bearing age. The most common type of repair seen in women of child-bearing age is the Mustard operation, which was introduced in the 1960s.[30] The Mustard atrial baffle repair directs pulmonary venous return to the right ventricle and the transposed aorta, and the systemic venous blood is directed to the mitral valve and left ventricle, and hence out to the pulmonary artery. This allows the blood to go in the appropriate direction but through the incorrect ventricle, so the right ventricle is left to support the systemic circulation.

There have been several reports of successful pregnancy after a Mustard procedure.[31,32] Lynch-Salamon et al. reported three women who had Mustard operations in childhood and each had a successful pregnancy.[31] Two of the pregnancies were complicated by failure of the systemic ventricle and one by preterm labour.

Clarkson et al. reviewed nine women with 15 pregnancies after Mustard procedures.[33] They were symptom free before pregnancy and remained so during each pregnancy. There were twelve live births, two spontaneous abortions and one intrauterine death. None of the live born infants had evidence of congenital heart disease. As anticipated, RV volumes increased during pregnancy, as is the case in normal individuals, but none had overt failure. The authors concluded that, in this group with good functional capacity, pregnancy was well tolerated. Although many patients do well for two or three decades after the Mustard procedure, the degree of RV dysfunction is variable, and this needs to be carefully assessed at the time of pregnancy counseling. Echocardiography should be done to assess the degree of RV dilatation, dysfunction and tricuspid regurgitation. Associated residual lesions should also be looked for and, if necessary, exercise testing done to assess the functional capacity. The good outcome of pregnancy in the cohorts reported should not always be extrapolated to women who show evidence of RV impairment before pregnancy; RV function may deteriorate, sometimes irreversibly, and tricuspid regurgitation may also progress with no recovery in some.[34]

The Rastelli procedure is a type of surgical repair for patients with transposition and pulmonary stenosis, and many patients who have had this operation also survive to child-bearing age.[35] The procedure involves placing a conduit between the right ventricle and the pulmonary artery to relieve the pulmonary stenosis, and closing the ventricular septal defect in such a way as to divert the blood from the left ventricle into the aorta. Provided that ventricular function is adequate and there are no residual lesions (such as subaortic stenosis or conduit obstruction), a pregnancy may be tolerated after this procedure.

Congenitally corrected transposition with ventricular septal defect and pulmonary stenosis

Congenitally corrected transposition (atrioventricular discordance with ventriculoarterial discordance) is commonly associated with ventricular septal defect, pulmonary stenosis and left atrioventricular valve regurgitation. A common additional problem is congenital complete heart block. When a ventricular septal defect exists with pulmonary stenosis, right-to-left shunting can occur, causing cyanosis. Few data are available about pregnancy in this condition. Presbitero et al. reported five patients with ten pregnancies, producing six live births (60%).[1] There were four spontaneous abortions and two babies were pre-term. Comparing the outcome of these pregnancies, however, with those with single ventricle or tricuspid atresia or both, and with those with tetralogy of Fallot or pulmonary atresia, the outcome was considerably better (60% versus 31% and 33%, respectively). As the morphological right ventricle is supporting the systemic circulation in this condition, the volume load of pregnancy may induce ventricular failure. Therefore functional capacity as well as ventricular function and degree of cyanosis must be evaluated at pre-pregnancy counseling.

Eisenmenger syndrome

Eisenmenger syndrome is associated with high pulmonary vascular resistance and a reversed or bidirectional shunt, at a ventricular, aortopulmonary or atrial level.[36] The degree of pulmonary vascular obstructive disease, therefore, determines the degree of cyanosis. Many women with Eisenmenger syndrome survive to reproductive age but often get increasing symptoms in the third decade. Pulmonary vascular disease in pregnancy poses significant risks because it limits the RV output through the lungs, and the systemic vasodilatation that occurs favors right-to-left shunting and therefore exaggerates the degree of cyanosis. Thus, even a minor fall in blood pressure, such as vasovagal faint or minor blood loss, can precipitate sudden death.[37] Clinical experience with Eisenmenger syndrome in a single institution is limited, and a number of published cases are unsatisfactorily or incompletely documented. Gleicher et al. reviewed 44 well-documented published cases of Eisenmenger syndrome and these women had 70 pregnancies.[38] Of these women 52% died in connection with one of their pregnancies. There was no difference in maternal mortality among the first, second and third pregnancies, suggesting that, if a woman has one success-ful pregnancy, this should not be taken as a positive predictor for further preg-nancies. A particularly high incidence of maternal death was associated with hypovolemia, thromboembolic phenomena and pre-eclampsia. Thirty-four per cent of all vaginal deliveries, three of four cesarean sections and only one of fourteen pregnancy interruptions (the only one by hysterotomy) resulted in maternal death. The number having cesarean section was small and it may be that they were a high-risk group already in hemodynamically compromised states. Only 25.6% of all pregnancies reached term and 54.9% of all deliveries occurred pre-term. The perinatal mortality rate was 28.3% and was strongly as-sociated with prematurity. The conclusion from this study was that the progno-sis for any woman with Eisenmenger syndrome and pregnancy was extremely grave and that elective abortion was considerably safer than any kind of deliv-ery. Labour and delivery may be a particularly precarious time. Even if the mother has a successful delivery, death often occurs in the next few days from either deteriorating hemodynamics or pulmonary infarction.[39–41]

A summary of published reports of pregnant patients with pulmonary vascu-lar disease from various countries, from 1978 to 1996, also noted a high mater-nal mortality rate of 36% in those with Eisenmenger syndrome ($n = 73$) and a similar mortality in patients with primary pulmonary hypertension ($n = 27$).[42] Of 26 fatalities, 23 died within 30 days of delivery, and late diagnosis and late hospital admission were predictive risk factors for mortality. The cause of death was reportedly pulmonary hypertensive crisis with refractory heart failure ($n = 13$), sudden death ($n = 7$), pulmonary thromboembolism confirmed by post-mortem examination ($n = 1$), cerebral thromboembolism ($n = 1$), and dissection and rupture of the pulmonary artery ($n = 1$). The authors suggested that mater-nal risks of pregnancy in this setting have changed little over the past two decades.

One single-center experience from Brazil reported slightly better out-comes:[43] 12 women with 13 pregnancies were associated with 2 maternal deaths before 28 weeks' gestation, and only 7 pregnancies reached the end of the second trimester. Patients were admitted to hospital for bed rest and careful monitoring and all received prophylactic heparin. cesarean section was per-formed in all using general anesthesia. One patient died 30 days post partum. Thus women with Eisenmenger syndrome should be advised strongly against pregnancy.

If a patient becomes pregnant against medical advice, she should be advised to have the pregnancy terminated. A first trimester dilatation and curettage appears to be the procedure of choice for interruption of pregnancy.[38] A cardiac anesthetist should be consulted to participate in the anesthetic management. If the patient insists on continuing the pregnancy, the following management strategy may be considered:

1 Careful and coordinated follow-up between the cardiologist and obstetrician with frequent observation to detect early hemodynamic deterioration. A coordinated approach is also essential with the anesthetist at the time of labour and delivery.

2 Bedrest is encouraged to reduce the cardiac demands. Rest should be undertaken in the lateral position to avoid fetal compression of the inferior vena cava and so maintain venous return. Complete bedrest should be considered with admission to hospital in the third trimester.

3 Oxygen delivered by facemask may be administered during episodes of dyspnea,[44] although there is little evidence that it improves either the maternal or the fetal outcome.[45,46]

4 Fetal well-being must be carefully monitored with estriol estimations and fetal ultrasonography to evaluate growth.

5 Congestive heart failure, if it occurs, can be treated with digoxin and diuretics, but diuretics must be used with caution to avoid hemoconcentration.

6 There is controversy over the use of heparin during pregnancy, and no consensus has been established.[38,47] Although there is certainly a hypercoagulable state during pregnancy, these patients are also paradoxically at increased risk of bleeding because of the inherent hemostatic diathesis secondary to their cyanotic heart disease. Prophylactic doses of heparin should be used during the period of bedrest in hospital when the risk is highest, but no case comparison exists and the literature is anecdotal. The largest single-center series reported a strategy of heparin anticoagulation before delivery by cesarean section under general anesthesia with warfarin anticoagulation started post partum.[43]

7 In early series, vaginal delivery appears to have been chosen more often than elective cesarean section.[38] Blood loss with cesarean section is greater than with vaginal delivery. Although a normal patient may tolerate blood loss of 500–1000 mL without difficulty, a patient with Eisenmenger syndrome may not be able to adjust her pulmonary circulation to a sudden fall in peripheral resistance[38] so that blood lost should be replaced immediately volume for volume. In recent years, however, scheduled cesarean section is more commonly the preferred method of delivery, with either general anesthesia[48] or combined spinal–epidural anesthesia. There is little evidence, however, of any benefit from this approach, and both the mode of delivery and the anesthetic management remain debated.[49] The author's personal preference is cesarean section delivery with general anesthesia administered by an experienced cardiac anesthetist.

8 Labour and delivery should take place in an operating room close to an intensive care unit. Cardiac monitoring should be continuous, with intravenous lines and intra-arterial lines and frequent measurements of arterial blood gases. A central venous pressure catheter may be helpful, and allow rapid detection of changes in shunt flow and facilitate hemodynamic assessment; changes in shunt flow can be monitored by pulse oximetry.[41,45] A Swan–Ganz catheter may also be used, but there may be complications in implanting this device.[50]

9 Epidural anesthesia appears to be safe, provided that there is no hypotension. Any fall in blood pressure should immediately be counteracted by the administration of norepinephrine (noradrenaline), and loss of blood by transfusion.[46] Spinal anesthesia should be used only in low dose and with extreme caution because of the risk of hypotension, and single-shot spinal anesthesia is contraindicated.[51]

10 If vaginal delivery is elected, low-dose epidural analgesia is considered of paramount importance because it reduces the adverse hemodynamic consequences of labor.[49,52] The second stage of delivery should be kept short, assisted by elective forceps or a vacuum extractor.

11 The patient should be kept in bed and monitored continuously for at least the first day after delivery and then gradually activated. Thromboguard compression pumps may be helpful in preventing venous stasis and thrombosis in the legs.

12 The patient should stay in hospital for at least 14 days after delivery because of the continued risk of sudden death.

Role of pulmonary vasodilators

Isolated case reports have suggested a more favorable maternal outcome with the use of pulmonary vasodilators such as intravenous epoprostenol and inhaled nitric oxide.[53–55] Nitric oxide can be administered via a nasal cannula, but is more commonly given via a facemask or endotracheal tube. Reduction in pulmonary pressure has been accomplished in some patients with successful deliveries by both vaginal and cesarean section approaches. If nitric oxide is used, maternal methemoglobin must be monitored during its administration.

References

1 Presbitero P, Somerville J, Stone S et al. Pregnancy in cyanotic congenital heart disease. Outcome of mother and fetus. *Circulation* 1994;**89**:2673–6.

2 Neill CA, Swanson S. Outcome of pregnancy in congenital heart disease. *Circulation* 1961;**24**:1003.

3 Whittemore R. Congenital heart disease: its impact on pregnancy. *Hosp Pract* 1983;**18**:65–74.

4 Higgins CB, Mulder DG. Tetralogy of Fallot in the adult. *Am J Cardiol* 1972;**29**:837–46.

5 Meyer EC, Tulsky AS, Sigmann P et al. Pregnancy in the presence of tetralogy of Fallot. Observations on two patients. *Am J Cardiol* 1964;**14**:874–9.

6 Baker JL, Russell CS, Grainger RG et al. Closed pulmonary valvotomy in the management of Fallot's tetralogy complicated by pregnancy. *J Obstet Gynecol* 1963;**70**:154–7.

7 Dennis NR, Warren, J. Risks to the offspring of patients with some common congenital heart defects. *J Med Genet* 1981;**18**:8–16.

8 Singh H, Bolton PJ, Oakley CM. Pregnancy after surgical correction of tetralogy of Fallot. *BMJ* 1982;**285**:168–70.

9 Ando M, Takao A, Mori K. Genetic and environmental factors in congenital heart disease. In: Inouye E, Nishimura H (eds), *Gene–Environment Interaction in Common Diseases*. Baltimore, MD: University Park Press, 1977: pp 71–88.

10 Nora JJ, Nora AH. Recurrence risks in children having one parent with a congenital heart disease. *Circulation* 1976;**53**:701–2.

11 Zellers TM, Driscoll DJ, Michels VV. Prevalence of significant congenital heart defects in children of parents with Fallot's tetralogy. *Am J Cardiol* 1990;**65**:523–6.

12 Gersony WM, Batthany S, Bowman FO Jr et al. Late follow-up of patients evaluated hemodynamically after total correction of tetralogy of Fallot. *J Thorac Cardiovasc Surg* 1973;**66**:209–13.

13 Veldtman GR, Connolly HM, Grogan M et al. Outcomes of pregnancy in women with tetralogy of Fallot. *J Am Coll Cardiol* 2004;**44**:174–80.

14 Meijer JM, Pieper PG, Drenthen W et al. Pregnancy, fertility, and recurrence risk in corrected tetralogy of Fallot. *Heart* 2005;**91**:801–5.

15 Stout K. Pregnancy in women with congenital heart disease: the importance of evaluation and counselling. *Heart* 2005;**91**:713–14.

16 Beauchesne LM, Warnes CA, Connolly HM et al. Prevalence and clinical manifestations of 22q11.2 microdeletion in adults with selected conotruncal anomalies. *J Am Coll Cardiol* 2005;**45**:595–8.

17 Connolly HM, Warnes CA. Outcome of pregnancy in women with complex pulmonary atresia. *Am J Cardiol* 1997;**79**:519–21.

18 Waickman LA, Skorton DJ, Varner MW et al. Ebstein's anomaly and pregnancy. *Am J Cardiol* 1984;**53**:357–8.

19 Donnelly JE, Brown JM, Radford DJ. Pregnancy outcome and Ebstein's anomaly. *Br Heart J* 1991;**66**:368–71.

20 Connolly HM, Warnes CA. Ebstein's anomaly: outcome of pregnancy. *J Am Coll Cardiol* 1994;**23**:1194–8.

21 Beischer NA, MacKay EV. *Obstetrics and the Newborn*. Sydney: WB Saunders, 1986: pp 406–20.

22 Danielson GK, Driscoll DJ, Mair DD et al. Operative treatment of Ebstein's anomaly. *J Thorac Cardiovasc Surg* 1992;**104**:1195–202.

23 Ammash NA, Warnes CA. Survival into adulthood of patients with unoperated single ventricle. *Am J Cardiol* 1996;**77**:542–4.

24 Stiller RJ, Vintzileos AM, Nochimson DJ et al. Single ventricle in pregnancy: case report and review of the literature. *Obstet Gynecol* 1984;**64**(3 suppl):18S–20S.

25 Leibbrandt G, Munch U, Gander M. Two successful pregnancies in a patient with single ventricle and transposition of the great arteries. *Int J Cardiol* 1982;**1**:257–62.

26 Collins ML, Leal J, Thompson NJ. Tricuspid atresia and pregnancy. *Obstet Gynecol* 1977;**50**(1 suppl):72s–3s.

27 Fontan F, Baudet E. Surgical repair of tricuspid atresia. *Thorax* 1971;**26**:240–8.

28 Kreutzer G, Galindez E, Bono H et al. An operation for the correction of tricuspid atresia. *J Thorac Cardiovasc Surg* 1973;**66**:613–21.

29 Canobbio M, Mair D. Pregnancy outcome following Fontan operation. *Circulation* 1993;**88**:1–290.

30 Mustard WT. Successful two-stage correction of transposition of the great vessels. *Surgery* 1964;**55**:469–72.

31 Lynch-Salamon DI, Maze SS, Combs CA. Pregnancy after Mustard repair for transposition of the great arteries. *Obstet Gynecol* 1993;**82**(4 Pt 2 suppl):676–9.

32 Warnes CA, Somerville J. Transposition of the great arteries: late results in adolescents and adults after the Mustard procedure. *Br Heart J* 1987;**58**:148–55.

33 Clarkson PM, Wilson NJ, Neutze JM et al. Outcome of pregnancy after the Mustard operation for transposition of the great arteries with intact ventricular septum. *J Am Coll Cardiol* 1994;**24**:190–3.

34 Guedes A, Mercier LA, Leduc L et al. Impact of pregnancy on the systemic right ventricle after a Mustard operation for transposition of the great arteries. *J Am Coll Cardiol* 2004;**44**:433–7.

35 Rastelli GC, McGoon DC, Wallace RB. Anatomic correction of transposition of the great arteries with ventricular septal defect and subpulmonary stenosis. *J Thorac Cardiovasc Surg* 1969;**58**:545–52.

36 Wood P. The Eisenmenger syndrome or pulmonary hypertension with reversed central shunt. I. *BMJ* 1958;**46**:701–9.

37 Warnes CA. Pregnancy and pulmonary hypertension. *Int J Cardiol* 2004;**97**(suppl 1):11–13.

38 Gleicher N, Midwall J, Hochberger D et al. Eisenmenger's syndrome and pregnancy. *Obstet Gynecol Surv* 1979;**34**:721–41.

39 Lieber S, Dewilde P, Huyghens L et al. Eisenmenger's syndrome and pregnancy. *Acta Cardiol* 1985;**40**:421–4.

40 Heytens L, Alexander JP. Maternal and neonatal death associated with Eisenmenger's syndrome. *Acta Anaesthesiol Belg* 1986;**37**:45–51.

41 Arias F. Maternal death in a patient with Eisenmenger's syndrome. *Obstet Gynecol* 1977;**50**(1 suppl):76s–80s.

42 Weiss BM, Zemp L, Seifert B et al. Outcome of pulmonary vascular disease in pregnancy: a systematic overview from 1978 through 1996. *J Am Coll Cardiol* 1998;**31**:1650–7.

43 Avila WS, Grinberg M, Snitcowsky R et al. Maternal and fetal outcome in pregnant women with Eisenmenger's syndrome. *Eur Heart J* 1995;**16**:460–4.

44 Neilson G, Galea EG, Blunt A. Eisenmenger's syndrome and pregnancy. *Med J Aust* 1971;**1**:431–4.

45 Midwall J, Jaffin H, Herman MV et al. Shunt flow and pulmonary hemodynamics during labour and delivery in the Eisenmenger syndrome. *Am J Cardiol* 1978;**42**:299–303.

46 Bitsch M, Johansen C, Wennevold A et al. Eisenmenger's syndrome and pregnancy. *Eur J Obstet Gynecol Reprod Biol* 1988;**28**:69–74.

47 Pitts JA, Crosby WM, Basta LL. Eisenmenger's syndrome in pregnancy: does heparin prophylaxis improve the maternal mortality rate? *Am Heart J* 1977;**93**:321–6.

48 O'Hare R, McLoughlin C, Milligan K et al. Anaesthesia for caesarean section in the presence of severe primary pulmonary hypertension. *Br J Anaesth* 1998;**81**:790–2.

49 Bonnin M, Mercier FJ, Sitbon O et al. Severe pulmonary hypertension during pregnancy: mode of delivery and anesthetic management of 15 consecutive cases. *Anesthesiology* 2005;**102**:1133–7.

50 Devitt JH, Noble WH, Byrick RJ. A Swan–Ganz catheter related complication in a patient with Eisenmenger's syndrome. *Anesthesiology* 1982;**57**:335–7.

51 Blaise G, Langleben D, Hubert B. Pulmonary arterial hypertension: pathophysiology and anesthetic approach. *Anesthesiology* 2003;**99**:1415–32.

52 Easterling TR, Ralph DD, Schmucker BC. Pulmonary hypertension in pregnancy: treatment with pulmonary vasodilators. *Obstet Gynecol* 1999;**93**:494–8.

53 Stewart R, Tuazon D, Olson G et al. Pregnancy and primary pulmonary hypertension: successful outcome with epoprostenol therapy. *Chest* 2001;**119**:973–5.

54 Lust KM, Boots RJ, Dooris M et al. Management of labour in Eisenmenger syndrome with inhaled nitric oxide. *Am J Obstet Gynecol* 1999;**181**:419–23.

55 Goodwin TM. Favorable response of Eisenmenger syndrome to inhaled nitric oxide during pregnancy.[See comment.] *Am J Obstet Gynecol* 1999;**180**(1 Pt 3):S208–13.

CHAPTER 6

Pregnancy and pulmonary hypertension

Joseph G Parambil, Michael D McGoon

Pulmonary hypertension (PH) may present initially during pregnancy or may be identified in women contemplating becoming pregnant. Women with idiopathic pulmonary arterial hypertension outnumber men by a ratio of 1.7 : 1, and the median age range of affected individuals encompasses fertile women.[1] Accordingly, the clinical impact of pulmonary hypertension on pregnant women warrants careful consideration and appropriate medical responses.

The interaction between the hemodynamic consequences of PH, whatever its cause, and the normal hemodynamic profile of pregnancy produce an excessive mortality risk to both the mother and the fetus. An increased blood volume and demand for a higher cardiac output associated with pregnancy, combined with elevated pulmonary vascular resistance, leads to a constellation of increased right ventricular work as a result of pressure and volume overload, inadequate left ventricular filling and systemic hypotension. These hemodynamic perturbations lead to further deleterious sequelae: elevated myocardial oxygen demand, right ventricular ischemia resulting from diminished right coronary artery flow, further reduction in left ventricular function because of interventricular dependence, decreased cardiac output and ultimately the development of cardiogenic shock.

This chapter discusses the causes of PH, its recognition and treatment, and the implications that it presents for counseling and managing women (and their partners) who are considering or have become pregnant.

Definition and classification of pulmonary hypertension

Pulmonary hypertension is a progressive hemodynamic condition characterized by elevation in the blood pressure of the arteries of the lungs. The median value of mean pulmonary arterial pressure (mPAP) in a general population is 12–16 mmHg, but it is unlikely that a minimal elevation of mPAP is clinically significant. Consequently, an mPAP >25 mmHg at rest is generally accepted as indicative of PH.[2,3] Systolic pulmonary artery pressure >35 mmHg is also suggestive of PH. The term 'pulmonary arterial hypertension' (PAH) implies that the PH is entirely or predominantly the result of pre-capillary resistance, whereas post-capillary PH is a factor when the pulmonary venous pressure (as measured by the pulmonary capillary wedge pressure [PCWP]) exceeds 15 mmHg. Pre-capillary PH therefore exhibits an elevated transpulmonary gradient that is reflected in a pulmonary arterial resistance (PAR) of >3 Wood units, where:

PAR = (mPAP – PCWP)/Pulmonary blood flow.

This distinction between pre-capillary and post-capillary PH is important in identifying underlying causes and initiating appropriate treatment.

Pulmonary hypertension refers only to a hemodynamic observation that implies the presence of an underlying pathologic etiology. Currently, pulmonary hypertensive disorders are classified based on a combination of pathologic features, clinical findings, hemodynamics, and response to pharmacologic intervention.[4] This system abandons the term 'primary pulmonary hypertension' in light of growing recognition of subgroups with similar histopathology but distinct clinical, hemodynamic and genetic associations. 'Idiopathic pulmonary arterial hypertension' now refers to PAH of unknown cause, whereas other forms of PAH are characterized by specific additional attributes (Table 6.1). The classification also eliminates the general concept of 'secondary pulmonary hypertension' in favor of more specifically descriptive terminology with regard to the mechanistic substrate (Table 6.1).

All forms of PAH share histopathologic features of endothelial cell proliferation in small and medium-sized pulmonary arteries, causing intimal thickening and fibrosis, vascular smooth muscle cell proliferation and extension, causing medial hypertrophy, and the frequent presence of disordered endothelial growth in the form of plexiform lesions (Figure 6.1).[5]

Diagnosis of PAH

As the issue of pregnancy in the pulmonary hypertensive state is most likely to arise in patients with PAH (category 1 in Table 6.1), this chapter focuses on the recognition and treatment of these conditions, and on its implications with respect to the pregnant woman. PAH is diagnosed based on suspicions deduced from the clinical examination and by echocardiography, and confirmed by right heart catheterization (RHC).

Symptoms

Patients with PAH may be discovered before the development of symptoms, but generally present with a spectrum of complaints attributable to impaired oxygen transport, reduced cardiac output and right ventricular pressure overload. Exertional dyspnea is the most frequent presenting symptom. This symptom can be easily overlooked in pregnancy because exertional intolerance may be common as a result of normal anatomic and functional alterations in the cardiovascular and respiratory systems. In the pregnant patient with PAH, decreased exercise capacity, fatigue and generalized weakness may be subtle initially, but become more pronounced and tend to progress as the pregnancy

Table 6.1 Classification of pulmonary arterial hypertension (PAH)

---

1 Pulmonary arterial hypertension
   1.1 Idiopathic (IPAH)
   1.2 Familial (FPAH)
   1.3 Associated with (APAH):
      1.3.1 Collagen vascular disease
      1.3.2 Congenital systemic-to-pulmonary shunts
      1.3.3 Portal hypertension
      1.3.4 HIV infection
      1.3.5 Drugs and toxins
      1.3.6 Other (thyroid disorders, glycogen storage disease, Gaucher's disease, hereditary hemorrhagic telangiectasia, hemoglobinopathies, chronic myeloproliferative disorders, splenectomy)
   1.4 Associated with significant venous or capillary involvement
      1.4.1 Pulmonary veno-occlusive disease (PVOD)
      1.4.2 Pulmonary capillary hemangiomatosis (PCH)
   1.5 Persistent pulmonary hypertension of the newborn

2 Pulmonary hypertension with left heart disease
   2.1 Left-sided atrial or ventricular heart disease
   2.2 Left-sided valvular heart disease

3 Pulmonary hypertension associated with lung diseases and/or hypoxemia
   3.1 Chronic obstructive pulmonary disease
   3.2 Interstitial lung disease
   3.3 Sleep-disordered breathing
   3.4 Alveolar hypoventilation disorders
   3.5 Chronic exposure to high altitude
   3.6 Developmental abnormalities

4 Pulmonary hypertension caused by chronic thrombotic and/or embolic disease (CTEPH)
   4.1 Thromboembolic obstruction of proximal pulmonary arteries
   4.2 Thromboembolic obstruction of distal pulmonary arteries
   4.3 Non-thrombotic pulmonary embolism (tumor, parasites, foreign material)

5 Miscellaneous
Sarcoidosis, histiocytosis X, lymphangiomatosis, compression of pulmonary vessels (adenopathy, tumor, fibrosing mediastinitis)

---

advances. As a result of the combined influence of right ventricular pressure overload caused by high pulmonary resistance and volume overload resulting from increased cardiac output, leg swelling, abdominal bloating and distension, anorexia, plethora and more profound fatigue develop as right ventricular dysfunction and tricuspid valve regurgitation (TR) evolve. Dyspnea may be present even at rest.

Anginal chest pain occurs in about a third of patients because of increased right ventricular myocardial oxygen demand resulting from elevated wall stress, and because of reduced coronary blood flow caused by reduced aortic to

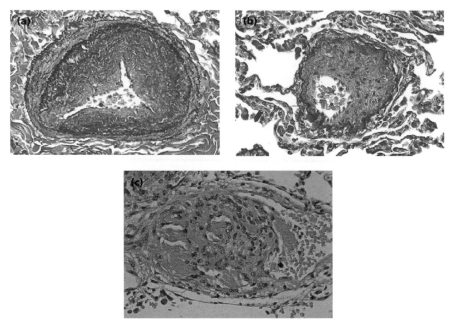

Figure 6.1 Histological sections from a patient with advanced idiopathic pulmonary arterial hypertension, showing (a) endothelial proliferation causing intimal hypertrophy and fibrosis, (b) pulmonary vascular smooth muscle proliferation causing medial hypertrophy and (c) a plexiform lesion.

right ventricular endomyocardial pressure gradient.[6] Some patients have compression of the left main coronary artery by the dilated central pulmonary artery.[7–10] Syncope also may occur in a third of patients resulting either from arrhythmias or from systemic vasodilatation. Syncope may be more likely in pregnant patients because of the potential for impeded venous return to the heart, decreasing right ventricular diastolic filling.

As PH may be associated with a variety of co-morbid conditions, symptomatic evidence of a related illness should be considered. Orthopnea and paroxysmal nocturnal dyspnea suggest elevated pulmonary venous pressures and pulmonary congestion resulting from left-sided cardiac disease. Raynaud's phenomenon, arthralgias, swollen hands or other symptoms raise the possibility of PAH associated with connective tissue diseases. A history of snoring or apneic spells provided by the patient's partner warrants evaluation for sleep-disordered breathing as a potential causative or contributory factor.[11] Because of the recognized genetic component of PAH,[12,13] inquiry into whether other family members have had symptoms or an established diagnosis of PAH may lead to recognition of clinical disease. Potential toxic exposures should be explored, especially a history of use of appetite suppressants.[14] Known or suspected exposure to HIV infection should be explored.[15] Although a history of pulmonary embolism or deep vein thrombosis in a patient with diagnosed or suspected PH requires a meticulous search for unresolved chronic thromboembolic disease, chronic thromboembolic pulmonary hypertension (classification 4 in Table 6.1) may occur even in the absence of a recognized history of venous thromboembolism or acute pulmonary embolism.

Physical examination

Signs of PH on physical examination can also be subtle, especially in the pregnant patient, and are often overlooked. An accentuated pulmonary component of the second heart sound (which becomes audible at the apex) is noted in 90% of patients with PAH, reflecting an increased force of pulmonary valve closure resulting from elevated pulmonary artery pressures. Physical signs of more advanced disease include the diastolic murmur of pulmonary regurgitation and the holosystolic murmur of tricuspid regurgitation. Tricuspid regurgitation can also be detected by an elevated jugular venous pressure with accentuated 'v' waves and by a pulsatile liver. The presence of a right ventricular S3 gallop, marked distension of the jugular veins, pulsatile hepatomegaly, peripheral edema and ascites is indicative of right ventricular failure, although in the pregnant patient, peripheral edema is usually present as a result of inferior vena cava compression. Abdominal distension caused by the gravid uterus may obscure the detection of ascites.

The physical examination also may provide insights into the etiology. Cyanosis suggests right-to-left shunting, severely reduced cardiac output or a marked impairment in intrapulmonary gas transfer. The presence of digital clubbing should raise the possibility of congenital heart disease, pulmonary veno-occlusive disease or fibrosing lung diseases. Inspiratory crackles or decreased breath sounds point to pulmonary fibrosis or pleural effusion, respectively, and expiratory wheezes or prolonged exhalation implies airway-centered disorders. Obesity and enlarged tonsils suggest sleep-disordered breathing as a potential causative or contributory factor. Scleroderma skin changes or other rashes, nailfold capillary abnormalities, arthritis and other stigmata are suggestive of an underlying connective tissue disease. Peripheral venous insufficiency or obstruction warrants investigation for venous thrombosis and pulmonary thromboembolic disease.

Chest radiograph and electrocardiogram

Chest radiography and electrocardiography may provide support for the presence of pulmonary hypertension, but are not sufficient confidently to establish or exclude the diagnosis. However, the presence of prominent hilar pulmonary arteries, relatively clear peripheral lung fields and right ventricular enlargement on chest radiograph are compelling evidence for pulmonary hypertension (Figure 6.2). Similarly, right ventricular hypertrophy and strain, right axis deviation and right atrial enlargement on the EKG warrant further exploration (Figure 6.3).

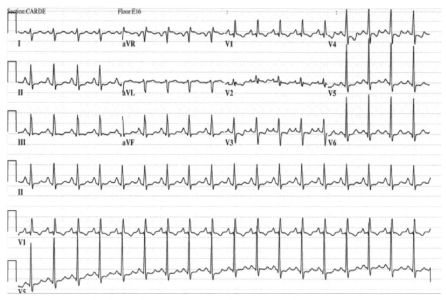

Figure 6.2 A 12-lead ECG from a 31-year-old woman with pulmonary arterial hypertension caused by hemoglobin SC disease, demonstrating right atrial enlargement, right ventricular hypertrophy and right axis deviation.

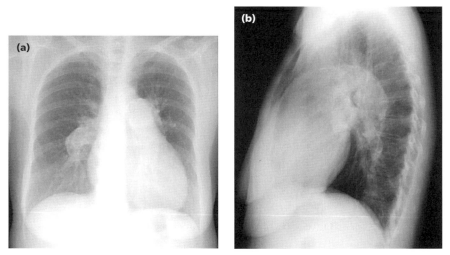

Figure 6.3 (a) Posteroanterior and (b) lateral chest radiographs from a 45-year-old woman with pulmonary arterial hypertension resulting from an atrial septal defect with physiology of Eisenmenger syndrome, demonstrating bilateral, dilated, calcified, pulmonary arteries with right ventricular enlargement.

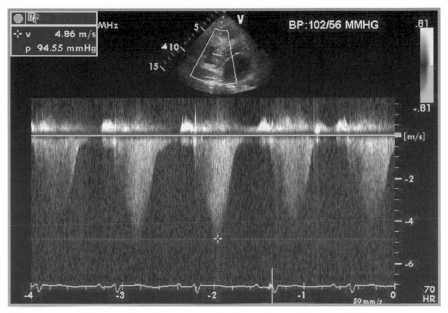

Figure 6.4 Cardiac Doppler ultrasonography in a patient with severe pulmonary arterial hypertension. Tricuspid regurgitant velocity of 4.9 m/s is measured. By application of the modified Bernoulli equation, and assuming a right atrial pressure of 10 mmHg, right ventricular systolic pressure is estimated at $4(4.9)^2 + 10 = 106$ mmHg.

Echocardiogram

Echocardiography is the pivotal screening procedure in the evaluation of possible PAH. Transthoracic Doppler echocardiography (TTE) estimates pulmonary artery systolic pressure (PASP)[16] and can provide additional information about the cause and consequences of PH. The PASP is equivalent to the right ventricular systolic pressure (RVSP) in the absence of pulmonary outflow obstruction. The RVSP is approximated by adding the measured systolic regurgitant tricuspid flow velocity 'v' to an estimate of the right atrial pressure (RAP) applied in the modified Bernoulli equation (Figure 6.4):

$$RVSP = 4v^2 + RAP.$$

RAP is either a standardized, or an estimated, value from characteristics of the inferior vena cava or internal jugular venous distension.[17] Pulmonary hemodynamics can also be estimated from the pulmonary regurgitant Doppler signal, right ventricular outflow patterns and time intervals, including pre-ejection period, acceleration and deceleration times, and relaxation and contraction times.

Right heart catheterization

Right heart catheterization is required to confirm the diagnosis of PAH and this can be safely performed in the pregnant patient. Cardiac output, determined by thermodilution or Fick (with measured oxygen consumption) techniques during RHC, is also needed to calculate pulmonary vascular resistance. The RHC characterizes intracardiac shunting and measures pulmonary venous pressure. An elevated PCWP supports the presence of left heart disease or pulmonary vein obstruction, although a normal pulmonary capillary wedge pressure does not rule out pulmonary veno-occlusive disease.

Functional assessment

Objective definition of exercise tolerance is an important part of the evaluation of patients with PAH. Functional assessment is most commonly by 6-minute walk testing, in which the distance a patient can walk at a free pace for 6 minutes is measured. This test may reveal limitations that the patient may have minimized or been unaware of. The results provide prognostic information: studies have shown that a distance of less than 330 meters is associated with a significantly worse survival over 3–5 years.[18] During therapy, comparison of 6-minute walk distances with baseline reflect treatment efficacy, and therefore this parameter has been the primary endpoint for most clinical drug trials.

Formal cardiopulmonary treadmill exercise testing may provide additional information about exercise characteristics and limitations, but many patients with severe PAH are unable to negotiate the demands of a conventional treadmill test and results vary significantly between institutions.

Classification of functional status according to criteria outlined by the World Health Organization (WHO) conference is shown in Table 6.2.

Other tests

Further tests are usually required to determine the underlying cause of PAH. These include HIV blood tests, antinuclear antibody serology to rule out connec-

Table 6.2 World Health Organization classification of functional status of patients with pulmonary hypertension

---

Class I
Patients with pulmonary hypertension (PH) in whom there is no limitation of usual physical activity; ordinary physical activity does not cause increased dyspnea, fatigue, chest pain, or presyncope

Class II
Patients with PH who have mild limitation of physical activity. There is no discomfort at rest, but normal physical activity causes increased dyspnea, fatigue, chest pain, or presyncope

Class III
Patients with PH who have a marked limitation of physical activity. There is no discomfort at rest, but less than ordinary activity causes increased dyspnea, fatigue, chest pain, or presyncope

Class IV
Patients with PH who are unable to perform any physical activity at rest and who may have signs of right ventricular failure. Dyspnea and/or fatigue may be present at rest, and symptoms are increased by almost any physical activity

---

tive tissue diseases, transthoracic or transesophageal Doppler echocardiograms with contrast (agitated saline) injection to look for right-to-left shunt and liver function assessment to screen for possible portopulmonary hypertension. Non-PAH causes of pulmonary hypertension must also be evaluated with echocardiography to determine whether left heart or valvular disease may be causative, pulmonary function tests and arterial blood gases to evaluate possible obstructive or interstitial lung diseases, overnight oximetry and possible polysomnography to work up sleep apnea, and ventilation–perfusion scintigraphy or contrast-enhanced computer tomography of the chest to screen for chronic thromboembolic disease, followed by pulmonary angiography if necessary.

Treatment of PAH

The spectrum of medical treatment for PAH has expanded significantly in the last decade and can now provide improved life expectancy with more stable and tolerable symptoms.[19] While providing benefits, including increased longevity for many patients, the available therapies remain essentially palliative. As a result of their complex nature, the use of these agents has been largely focused in multidisciplinary referral centers with dedicated PH clinics and specialized personnel who provide follow-up, including careful reassessment and modification of treatment. Specific treatment is dictated by multiple factors: severity of disease and symptoms; specific type of PH; access to and ability to use expensive, complex medications; and acute vasodilator responsiveness.

Vasodilator assessment

Right heart catheterization, including assessment of response to pulmonary vasodilators, is a pivotal component of the evaluation of PH. After careful assessment of baseline hemodynamics and confirmation of pre-capillary pulmonary hypertension, a pulmonary vasodilator (inhaled nitric oxide or infused epoprostenol) is administered and the peak effect is noted. About 50% of patients with PAH who acutely respond to vasodilators (by demonstration of a decrease in mPAP $\geq 10\,\mathrm{mmHg}$ to a value $<40\,\mathrm{mmHg}$) have improved symptoms and survival when treated with calcium channel blockers (CCBs). However, only 10–12% have an acute vasodilator response.[20] Virtually no patients with PAH associated with connective tissue disease or congenital heart disease respond acutely to a vasodilator trial. Patients who are unstable, or have WHO class IV symptoms or severe right heart failure never do well with CCBs and need not undergo vasodilator assessment. These patients and vasodilator nonresponders require treatment with an alternate agent.

Since 1996, five drugs have been approved by the US Food and Drug Administration (FDA) for use in patients with PAH.

Epoprostenol

Prostacyclin, a potent endogenous vasodilator and platelet function inhibitor produced from arachidonic acid in endothelial cells by prostacyclin synthase, is deficient in patients with PAH. Epoprostenol sodium, a synthetic prostacyclin analog, improves exercise capacity, quality of life and hemodynamics in IPAH and PAH associated with scleroderma, and improves survival in patients with IPAH. The survival rates of IPAH patients treated with epoprostenol therapy are 85–88%, 70–76% and 63% at 1, 2 and 3 years, respectively (compared with expected survival rates of 59, 46 and 35%).[21–23]

Epoprostenol (Flolan) treatment is complicated and expensive. As a result of a half-life of several seconds, the drug must be given by continuous intravenous infusion through an indwelling central line. It is unstable at room temperature, so the supply must be changed frequently (at least three times a day) or kept cool, necessitating ice packs surrounding an administration pump. Patients are exposed to significant side effects and risks. Common side effects of epoprostenol include headache, flushing, jaw pain, diarrhea, nausea, dermatitis and painful leg discomfort. Infection of the central venous catheter may occur. Sudden interruption of the infusion may cause severe rebound PH and death. Despite the improvements in symptoms, longevity and exercise capacity (as measured by the distance that an individual can walk on a level surface in 6 minutes) seen in many patients, hemodynamic improvements tend to be relatively modest. Benefit in some, if not most, patients may be the result of stabilization and prevention of progression of the disease with its attendant right heart failure. Many investigators feel that much of the benefit over time may result from its anti-proliferative properties, which lead to beneficial vascular reverse remodeling. A salutary inotropic effect of the drug has also been postulated.

Treprostinil

Treprostinil (Remodulin) is a prostacyclin analog with a half-life of over 3 hours; it is stable at room temperature, so it can be administered by a tiny subcutaneous catheter using a small pump that does not require an ice pack. The medication is provided in usable form, rather than requiring daily mixing of active compound with a diluent (as epoprostenol does). Compared with placebo, treprostinil tends to improve exercise capacity on 6-minute walk testing, quality of life and hemodynamics, but the benefits are quite limited.[24,25] At higher doses and among more symptomatic patients, the beneficial effects are more pronounced. Treprostinil exhibits a similar side-effect profile to epoprostenol; an additional concern is the frequent occurrence of pain at the infusion site, which may limit the ability to raise doses to a level that is most likely to produce optimal benefit. As a result of this the drug has also been approved for intravenous use. The expense of treprostinil is also similar to epoprostenol.

Iloprost

A third prostacyclin analog is iloprost (Ventavis), which is administered as an inhaled aerosol. Inhaled therapy delivers the drug to ventilated alveolar units, where local pulmonary arterioles vasodilate, enhancing ventilation–perfusion matching. Iloprost improves functional class, exercise capacity and pulmonary hemodynamics,[26] with side effects of flushing, headache and cough in some patients. The relatively short duration of action of inhaled iloprost requires between six and nine 5- to 15-minute inhalations daily to obtain a sustained clinical benefit. Co-administration of iloprost with other pulmonary vasoactive agents such as sildenafil augments and prolongs the duration of action.[27,28]

Bosentan

Bosentan (Tracleer) is a non-selective endothelin receptor antagonist, blocking the action of endothelin-1 (ET-1), a potent vasoconstrictor and smooth muscle mitogen, at endothelin receptor subtypes A and B (ET_A and ET_B). Its therapeutic effect is the result of reduction of vasoconstriction and pulmonary vascular hypertrophy caused by increased plasma levels of ET-1 in patients with PAH, probably mediated predominantly via ET_A receptors on vascular smooth muscle cells. As with the prostanoids, the demonstrable clinical vasodilatory effect of the drug is quite modest in patients with established PAH, but clinical studies of bosentan have demonstrated an augmented 6-minute walk distance compared with placebo and improved functional classification.[29–31] Some of its benefit may be related to anti-proliferative and anti-fibrotic effects that stabilize the disease process and promote remodeling. Side effects associated with bosentan include syncope, flushing and a dose-dependent elevation of transaminases, reflecting hepatic toxicity. Drug interactions with glyburide (glibenclamide) and ciclosporin are recognized; bosentan may also interfere with the action of hormonal contraceptives. Concomitant administration of sildenafil increases the plasma concentration of bosentan and decreases sildenafil concentration.[32] The medication is administered orally in pill form twice daily and liver function tests are monitored monthly. It, too, is very expensive.

Sildenafil

Sildenafil (Viagra) is a phosphodiesterase-5 inhibitor that augments the vasodilatory effect of the nitric oxide (NO) pathway. NO is an endogenous vasodilator produced from L-arginine by nitric oxide synthase (NOS) in endothelial cells. It has a central function in regulating basal vascular resistance. In vascular smooth muscle cells, it promotes conversion of GTP to cyclic GMP (cGMP), which is a second messenger that leads to a cascade of cell membrane and intracellular events, reducing entry of calcium ions into smooth muscle cells and thereby producing vasodilatation. Intracellular cGMP levels are regulated by phosphodiesterases that catalyze its degradation to 5'-GMP. Agents that inhibit the predominant phosphodiesterase-5 (PDE5) in the pulmonary vasculature consequently have a net effect of boosting the pulmonary vascular response to endogenous NO. Sildenafil is a potent and highly specific PDE5 inhibitor used for treatment of erectile dysfunction because PDE5 is present in the corpus cavernosum. Sildenafil improves 6-minute walk distance and symptoms in PAH.[33] After approval of the drug for use in PAH it was reformulated in a different dose size (20 mg) and renamed for this purpose as Revatio. It is administered three times daily.

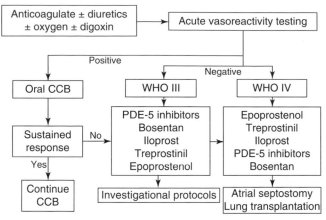

Figure 6.5 Treatment guideline for management of pulmonary arterial hypertension, modified from American College of Chest Physicians' (ACCP) guidelines.[19]

Adjunctive therapy

In general, patients with PAH are treated with warfarin in conservative doses aiming for an international normalized ratio (INR) of 2.0–2.5. The use of chronic anticoagulation is predicated on the results of two retrospective studies that demonstrate an apparent survival benefit, possibly as a result of minimization of *in situ* small vessel thrombosis.[34,35] Inotropic support with digoxin may be appropriate when right ventricular failure is present, and diuretics are frequently required to manage resulting intravascular volume overload, peripheral edema, ascites and hepatic congestion. Hypoxemia caused by reduced diffusing capacity, low cardiac output and low mixed venous oxygen saturation, suboptimal ventilation–perfusion matching and right-to-left shunting of blood through a patent foramen ovale may necessitate the use of supplemental oxygen.

Treatment strategy

Recommended guidelines for treatment of PAH have been published by the American College of Chest Physicians (Figure 6.5).[19]

Combined hemodynamic effects of pulmonary hypertension and pregnancy

The normal hemodynamic adjustments of pregnancy both affect and are affected by the coexistence of elevated pulmonary resistance and result in a hemodynamically unstable milieu with increased clinical risk.

Hemodynamic perturbations in pregnancy

Pregnancy normally induces profound changes in the maternal hemodynamics. Cardiovascular changes begin in the first trimester of a normal pregnancy and continue into the postpartum period. Maternal blood volume increases progressively to a maximum of about 40% over the pre-gravid level by the third trimester, mediated primarily by an increase in plasma volume by 45–50% and red cell mass by 20–30%. The increased blood volume is associated with a 30–50% augmentation of cardiac output by 25 weeks.[36] Systemic vascular resistance decreases by 20–30% as a result of the combined effects of gestational hormones, circulating prostaglandins and the low resistance vascular bed in the placenta; these lead to a further increase in cardiac output as a result of left ventricular afterload reduction. Both heart rate and, to a lesser extent, stroke volume increase and reach maximal values of 10–30% above baseline values by 32 weeks, and remain constant until term. During labour and delivery, pain and uterine contractions result in additional elevation of cardiac output and increased blood pressure. Immediately after delivery, relief of inferior vena caval compression and autotransfusion from the emptied and contracted uterus produce further increase in cardiac output. Most of these hemodynamic changes of pregnancy resolve by 2 weeks post partum.

Structural changes in the heart occur during pregnancy as well. Left atrial size increases, correlating with the change in blood volume. Left ventricular end-diastolic dimension increases, whereas the left ventricular end-systolic dimension decreases mildly as a result of changes in cardiac contractility and reduced afterload. Left ventricular wall thickness increases by 28% and left ventricular mass by 52%, which reduces left ventricular distensibility.[37]

Effects of normal gestational hemodynamics on abnormal pulmonary hemodynamics

Several of the hemodynamic changes that occur during normal pregnancy contribute to the high maternal mortality in patients with pulmonary vascular disease. The progressive increase in plasma volume superimposes an excess volume burden on a compromised, pressure-overloaded, right ventricle and may precipitate right heart failure. Increased left ventricular mass and leftward shift of the interventricular septum as a result of right ventricular enlargement from chronic pressure overload combine to exacerbate left ventricular diastolic impairment.

Effects of abnormal pulmonary hemodynamics on gestational systemic hemodynamics

Pulmonary vasculopathy restricts the ability of blood flow to increase in response to gestation, increases right ventricular work and decreases cardiac output, thereby predisposing to systemic hypotension and inadequate perfusion pressure to vital organs and the fetus. When an intracardiac left-to-right shunt is present, as occurs in patients with congenital heart disease and Eisenmenger syndrome physiology, decreased systemic vascular resistance of pregnancy augments right-to-left shunting (decreases Qp/Qs ratio) and leads to worsening hypoxemia, which in turn causes more pulmonary vasoconstriction.

Unlike the left ventricle, the right ventricular myocardium normally receives most of its coronary blood flow during systole because of the pressure gradient between the endocardium and aorta during systole. With PAH, the gradient is reduced and coronary blood flow is compromised. Resulting right ventricular ischemia leads to systolic dysfunction and further diminished blood flow to the fetus and vital organs.

During labour and delivery, tachycardia or hypotension resulting from hypovolemia caused by blood loss or from a vasovagal response to pain may worsen systemic hypotension and pre-existing right ventricular ischemia. These abrupt changes predispose the patient to sudden cardiac death from ventricular arrhythmias or right ventricular infarction. Metabolic acidosis that occurs during the second stage of labour may further increase pulmonary vascular resistance. In addition, the hypercoagulable state induced by pregnancy may predispose to pulmonary thromboembolism or *in situ* thrombosis and further pulmonary pressure elevation or even pulmonary infarction.

The mutually aggravating effect of PAH and the otherwise normal hemodynamic adjustments of pregnancy place the patient at serious risk of a spiraling course of deterioration, which may be abrupt and difficult or impossible to reverse.

Clinical implications of PAH and pregnancy

The presence of PAH poses a substantial risk to the pregnant female and the fetus. Before the current era of pharmacological therapy, the reported maternal mortality rate among patients affected by severe pulmonary hypertension was 36% for Eisenmenger syndrome, 30% for idiopathic PAH and 56% for pulmonary hypertension related to a variety of underlying causes. The patients included in this literature review had markedly abnormal hemodynamics, with reported pulmonary artery systolic pressures of 108 ± 26 mmHg among 73 Eisenmenger syndrome patients, 85 ± 20 mmHg in 27 patients with idiopathic PAH and 83 ± 18 mmHg in 25 secondary pulmonary hypertension patients. These figures, reported in 1998,[38] do not reflect any significant improvement in risk compared with the 52% mortality rate among 70 patients reported in 1979.[39] Successful pregnancy earlier in life does not assure that subsequent pregnancies will be uncomplicated.[39]

Among published experience, most maternal deaths occurred within 30 days of delivery, rather than during pregnancy, labour or delivery.[38] The high incidence of maternal death was frequently attributed to resistant right heart failure and cardiogenic shock precipitated by pulmonary hypertension. Other identifiable causes included sudden cardiac death due to malignant arrhythmias, pulmonary thromboembolism, cerebral thromboembolism, and dissection and rupture of the pulmonary artery. In an earlier series of patients with Eisenmenger syndrome mortality was associated most often with thromboembolic events or hypovolemia.[39] Patients with Eisenmenger syndrome or idiopathic PAH both exhibited high mortality rates with either vaginal (29% and 20%, respectively) or operative delivery (38% and 42%, respectively).[40] Subsequent reports and observational series have suggested greater control over hemodynamics and better outcomes with elective cesarean sections under general anesthesia than with vaginal deliveries.[41–43] Despite these publications, expert opinions still suggest that termination of pregnancy is a safer option, although pregnancy interruptions in patients with PAH are also associated with an elevated risk of maternal death. If termination of pregnancy is desired, dilatation and curettage in the first trimester is probably the procedure of choice, preferably with general anesthesia.

Limited data on fetal outcomes among patients with Eisenmenger syndrome from small series suggest that more than half of all deliveries occur prematurely with almost a third of all infants showing intrauterine growth retardation.[44] However, neonatal survival surpasses maternal survival under these circumstances (about 90% versus 50–70%, respectively).[38,40]

No systematic studies are available on outcome of pregnancy in patients with PAH treated with vasodilators. Case reports have noted variable outcomes using pulmonary vasodilators, including successful management of labour and delivery, but frequently with subsequent maternal death within days to weeks.[45–53] No suggestion of drug-related fetal or neonatal complications has been reported.

Pregnancy and PAH management issues

Pregnancy prevention

In view of high maternal and fetal risk of pregnancy in the setting of PAH, the prevention of pregnancy is paramount in risk management. The degree of PAH that significantly augments risk of pregnancy is uncertain, although it is likely that risk increases with severity of PAH, evidence of right ventricular dysfunction or presence of symptoms. Among these patients, effective contraception is mandatory. As PAH is seldom sufficiently reversed by optimal therapy to a point where the risk of pregnancy is acceptable, permanent sterilization of the woman (or long-term partner) should be considered. Otherwise, double barrier contraception is advisable in order to minimize the chances of pregnancy. Oral contraceptives cannot be considered to be contraindicated (especially compared with pregnancy) but carry a potential risk of venous thromboembolic events. Bosentan interacts with oral contraception, reducing reliability when used concomitantly. The risks imposed by pregnancy are high enough that elective termination counseling should be provided for patients in whom pregnancy occurs despite precautions or who are found to have PAH after pregnancy. Risks of elective interruption of pregnancy, however, may be 4–6%.[40]

Prenatal management

As a result of the high mortality from PAH in pregnancy and the progression of pre-existing PAH during pregnancy, pulmonary vasodilation should be attempted in symptomatic patients despite the lack of well-designed safety trials for the various therapeutic agents available for the treatment of this disorder. Drug initiation and careful monitoring in centers with expertise in PAH, adult

congenital disease and high-risk obstetrics is warranted. Cautious anticoagulant treatment is recommended in pregnant patients with PAH because of the
potential for *in situ* pulmonary thrombosis from the hypercoagulable state induced by pregnancy. Anticoagulation can be obtained with warfarin despite a
small risk to the fetus with the goal of international normalized ratio (INR)
being no higher than 2.0. Pulse oximetry should be used to detect any fall in systemic oxygen saturation and supplemental oxygen via nasal cannulae should
be used to promote oxygen transport and pulmonary vasodilation.

Mainstays of management throughout pregnancy include:
- Early recognition of PAH and early admission (second trimester) to a quali-
fied center.
- Multidisciplinary approach involving high-risk obstetric team, cardiologist,
pediatrician and anesthesiologist.
- Liberal oxygen supplementation throughout with careful monitoring of systemic oxygen saturation.
- Antithrombotic management including compression stockings or pumps,
and strong consideration of low-molecular-weight heparin to counteract the
effects of hypercoagulability and inactivity.

Management of delivery

Slowing of fetal growth or maternal deterioration may bring a need for early delivery. Elective cesarean section is preferable to vaginal delivery because it is
quicker and avoids pain and physical exertion, thereby protecting the fetus
from hypoxemia and the maternal pulmonary circulation from the untoward
effects of acidosis, which develops during the second stage of labour. Although
epidural analgesia has been employed for delivery of patients with heart
disease, general anesthesia may be preferable for anyone with a fixed low cardiac
output in whom vasodilatation may precipitate a drop in blood pressure or increase right-to-left shunting and hypoxemia. Moreover, many PAH patients
may be anticoagulated and epidural anesthesia can be associated with an increased risk of spinal hematomas. During epidural anesthesia the patient is
awake and worried and the opiate infusion usually given is a venodilator, which
further reduces an already compromised venous return. Most epidural agents
are also systemic vasodilators. This combination tends to redistribute blood out
of the thorax and into the periphery, which, combined with any uncorrected
blood loss, may cause a precipitous decline in blood pressure and cardiac arrest
may follow.

General anesthesia, on the other hand, provides rest with reduced metabolic
demand, maximum oxygenation and minimal interference with the forces
conserving a fragile circulatory reserve. A number of anesthetic protocols have
been described.[54] Vasodilatation and shifts in the distribution of the blood volume can also be minimized. During induction, agents with a negative inotropic
effect should be avoided and intravascular volume repletion should be generous. Blood loss should be immediately corrected because maintenance of cardiac output is dependent on a high right ventricular filling pressure.

After delivery patients should be returned to the ICU with continued monitoring of venous and arterial blood pressure and arterial saturation, followed by slow mobilization and resumption of anticoagulant treatment. Swan–Ganz catheterization and an intra-arterial line are not usually necessary because the systemic blood pressure and the central venous pressure are the best guidelines. Right ventricular failure may resolve dramatically after delivery.

Conclusions

- Normal physiologic changes associated with pregnancy conspire with the circulatory abnormalities of significant PAH to produce an unstable and fragile hemodynamic state, which markedly increases risk of maternal mortality and adverse fetal and neonatal outcome.
- Early recognition of PAH is essential in avoiding or minimizing risk of pregnancy. Late diagnosis and late admission to hospital for management are predictive of an adverse outcome.
- Pharmacologic management of PAH includes prostacyclin analogues, endothelin antagonists and phosphodiesterase inhibitors. Adjunctive therapy may include oxygen, anticoagulation, diuretics, nitric oxide and inotropic agents.
- Maternal risk caused by pregnancy of patients with PAH remains high (up to 50%).
- Among pregnancies that proceed to delivery, maternal mortality exceeds neonatal mortality.
- The majority of maternal deaths occur within the first 30 days after delivery.
- A high-risk multidisciplinary approach is mandatory for managing pregnant patients with PAH.

References

1 Rich S, Dantzker DR, Ayres SM, et al. Primary pulmonary hypertension: a national prospective study. *Ann Intern Med* 1987;**107**:216–23.
2 McGoon MD, Gutterman D, Steen V, et al. Screening, early detection, and diagnosis of pulmonary arterial hypertension: ACCP evidence-based clinical practice guidelines. *Chest* 2004;**126**(suppl 1):14S–34S.
3 Barst RJ, McGoon MD, Torbicki A, et al. Diagnosis and differential assessment of pulmonary arterial hypertension. *J Am Coll Cardiol* 2004;**43**(suppl 12):S40–7.
4 Simonneau G, Galiè N, Rubin L, et al. Clinical classification of pulmonary hypertension. *J Am Coll Cardiol* 2004;**43**(suppl 12):S5–12.
5 Voelkel NF, Cool C. Pathology of pulmonary hypertension. *Cardiol Clin* 2004;**22**: 343–51.
6 Gomez A, Bialostozky D, Zajarias A, et al. Right ventricular ischemia in patients with primary pulmonary hypertension. *J Am Coll Cardiol* 2001;**38**:1137–42.
7 Kawut S, F. S, Ferrari V, et al. Extrinsic compression of the left main coronary artery by the pulmonary artery in patients with long-standing pulmonary hypertension. *Am J Cardiol* 1999;**83**:984–6.

8 Mesquita S, Castro C, Ikari N, Oliveira S, Lopes A. Likelihood of left main coronary artery compression based on pulmonary trunk diameter in patients with pulmonary hypertension. *Am J Med* 2004;**116**:369–74.

9 Rich S, McLaughlin VV, O'Neill W. Stenting to reverse left ventricular ischemia due to left main coronary artery compression in primary pulmonary hypertension. *Chest* 2001;**120**:1412–15.

10 Bonderman D, Fleischmann D, Prokop M, Klepetko W, Lang IM. Left main coronary artery compression by the pulmonary trunk in pulmonary hypertension. *Circulation* 2002;**105**:265.

11 Parish JM, Somers VK. Obstructive sleep apnea and cardiovascular disease. *Mayo Clinic Proc* 2004;**79**:1036–46.

12 Loyd JE. Genetics and gene expression in pulmonary hypertension. *Chest* 2002;**121**:46S–50S.

13 Deng Z, Morse JH, Slager SL, et al. Familial primary pulmonary hypertension (gene PPH1) is caused by mutations in the bone morphogenetic protein receptor-II gene. *Am J Human Genet* 2000;**67**(electronically published).

14 Abenhaim L, Moride Y, Brenot F, et al. Appetite-suppressant drugs and the risk of primary pulmonary hypertension. *N Engl J Med* 1996;**335**:609–16.

15 Mesa R, Edell E, Dunn WF, W. E. Human immunodeficiency virus infection and pulmonary hypertension: two new cases and a review of 86 reported cases. *Mayo Clinic Proc* 1998;**73**:37–45.

16 Currie PJ, Seward JB, Chan KL. Continuous wave Doppler determination of right ventricular pressure: a simultaneous Doppler-catheterization study in 127 patients. *J Am Coll Cardiol* 1985;**6**:750–6.

17 Ommen SR, Nishimura RA, Hurrell DG, Klarich KW. Assessment of right atrial pressure with 2-dimensional and Doppler echocardiography: a simultaneous catheterization and echocardiographic study. *Mayo Clinic Proc* 2000;**75**:24–9.

18 Miyamoto S, Nagaya N, Satoh T, et al. Clinical correlates and prognostic significance of six-minute walk test in patients with primary pulmonary hypertension: comparison with cardiopulmonary exercise testing. *Am J Respir Crit Care Med* 2000;**161**:487–92.

19 Badesch DB, Abman SH, Ahearn GS, et al. Medical therapy for pulmonary arterial hypertension: ACCP evidence-based clinical practice guidelines. *Chest* 2004; **126**(suppl 1):35S–62S.

20 Sitbon O, Humbert M, Jais X, et al. Long-term response to calcium channel blockers in idiopathic pulmonary arterial hypertension. *Circulation* 2005;**111**:3105–11.

21 Sitbon O, Humbert M, Nunes H, et al. Long-term intravenous epoprostenol infusion in primary pulmonary hypertension: prognostic factors and survival. *J Am Coll Cardiol* 2002;**40**:780–8.

22 McLaughlin VV, Shillington A, Rich S. Survival in primary pulmonary hypertension: the impact of epoprostenol therapy. *Circulation* 2002;**106**:1477–82.

23 Barst RJ, Rubin LJ, McGoon MD, Caldwell EJ, Long WA, Levy PS. Survival in primary pulmonary hypertension with long-term continuous intravenous prostacyclin. *Ann Intern Med* 1994;**121**:409–15.

24 McLaughlin VV, Gaine SP, Barst RJ, et al. Efficacy and safety of treprostinil: an epoprostenol analogue for primary pulmonary hypertension. *J Cardiovasc Pharmacol* 2003;**41**:293–9.

25 Oudiz R, Schilz RJ, Barst RJ, et al. Treprostinil, a prostacyclin analogue, in pulmonary arterial hypertension associated with connective tissue disease. *Chest* 2004;**126**: 420–7.

26 Olschewski H, Simonneau G, Galie N, et al. Inhaled iloprost for severe pulmonary hypertension. *N Engl J Med* 2002;**347**:322–9.

27 Ghofrani HA, Rose F, Schermuly RT, et al. Oral sildenafil as long-term adjunct therapy to inhaled iloprost in severe pulmonary arterial hypertension. *J Am Coll Cardiol* 2003;**42**:158–64.

28 Wilkens H, Guth A, Konig J, et al. Effect of inhaled iloprost plus oral sildenafil in patients with primary pulmonary hypertension. *Circulation* 2001;**104**:1218–22.

29 Channick RN, Simonneau G, Sitbon O, et al. Effects of the dual endothelin-receptor antagonist bosentan in patients with pulmonary hypertension: a randomised placebo-controlled study. *Lancet* 2001;**358**:1119–23.

30 Rubin LJ, Badesch DB, Barst RJ, et al. Bosentan therapy for pulmonary arterial hypertension. *N Engl J Med* 2002;**346**:896–903.

31 Sitbon O, Badesch DB, Channick RN, et al. Effects of the dual endothelin receptor antagonist bosentan in patients with pulmonary arterial hypertension: a 1-year follow-up study. *Chest* 2003;**124**:247–54.

32 Paul GA, Gibbs JS, Boobis AR, Abbas AE, Wilkins MR. Bosentan decreases the plasma concentration of sildenafil when coprescribed in pulmonary hypertension. *Br J Clin Pharmacol* 2005;**60**:107–12.

33 Galie N, Ghofrani A, Torbicki A, et al. Sildenafil citrate therapy for pulmonary arterial hypertension. *N Engl J Med* 2005;**353**(20):2148–57.

34 Fuster V, Frye RL, Gersh BJ, McGoon MD, Steele PM. Primary pulmonary hypertension: natural history and the importance of thrombosis. *Circulation* 1984;**70**:580–7.

35 Rich S, Kaufmann E, Levy PS. The effect of high doses of calcium-channel blockers on survival in primary pulmonary hypertension. *N Engl J Med* 1992;**327**:76–81.

36 Crapo RO. Normal cardiopulmonary physiology during pregnancy. *Clin Obstet Gynecol* 1996;**39**:3–16.

37 Oakley CM. Cardiovascular disease in pregnancy. *Can J Cardiol* 1990;**6**:3–9.

38 Weiss BM, Zemp L, Seifert B, Hess OM. Outcome of pulmonary vascular disease in pregnancy: a systematic overview from 1978 through 1996. *J Am Coll Cardiol* 1998;**31**:1650–7.

39 Gleicher G, Midwall J, Hochberger D, Jaffin H. Eisenmenger's syndrome and pregnancy. *Obstet Gynecol* 1979;**34**:721–41.

40 Weiss B, Hess OM. Pulmonary vascular disease and pregnancy: current controversies, management strategies, and perspectives. *Eur Heart J* 2000;**21**:104–15.

41 Rout CC. Anesthesia and analgesia for the critically ill parturient. *Best Pract Res Clin Obstet Gynecol* 2001;**15**:507–22.

42 Duggan AB, Katz SG. Combined spinal and epidural anesthesia for cesarean section in a parturient with severe primary pulmonary hypertension. *Anesth Intens Care* 2003;**31**:565–9.

43 Bonnin M, Mercier FJ, Sitbon O, et al. Severe pulmonary hypertension during pregnancy. *Anesthesiology* 2005;**102**:1133–7.

44 Avila WS, Grinberg M, Snitcowsky R, Faccioli R, Da Luz PL, Pileggi F. Maternal and fetal outcome in pregnant women with Eisenmenger's syndrome. *Eur Heart J* 1995;**16**(4):460–4.

45 Lacassie HJ, Germain AM, Valdes G, Fernandez MS, Allamand F, Lopez H. Management of Eisenmenger syndrome in pregnancy with sildenafil and L-arginine. *Obstet Gynecol* 2004;**103**(5 Pt 2):1118–20.

46 Goodwin TM, Gherman RB, Hameed A, Elkayam U. Favorable response of Eisenmenger syndrome to inhaled nitric oxide during pregnancy.[See comment.] *Am J Obstet Gynecol* 1999;**180**(1 Pt 1):64–7.

47 Lust KM, Boots RJ, Dooris M, Wilson J. Management of labour in Eisenmenger syndrome with inhaled nitric oxide. *Am J Obstet Gynecol* 1999;**181**:419–23.

48 Decoene C, Boursoufi K, Moreau D, Narducci F, Crepin F, Krivosic-Horber R. Use of inhaled nitric oxide for emergency cesarean section in a woman with unexpected primary pulmonary hypertension. *Canadian J of Anesthesia* 2001;**48**(6):584–7.

49 Avdalovic M, Sandrock C, Hoso A, Allen R, Albertson TE. Epoprostenol in pregnant patients with secondary pulmonary hypertension: two case reports and a review of the literature. *Treatment Respir Med* 2004;**3**(1):29–34.

50 Badalian SS, Silverman RK, Aubry RH, Longo J. Twin pregnancy in a woman on long-term epoprostenol therapy for primary pulmonary hypertension. A case report. *J Reprod Med* 2000;**45**(2):149–52.

51 Stewart R, Tuazon D, Olson G, Duarte AG. Pregnancy and primary pulmonary hypertension: successful outcome with epoprostenol therapy. *Chest* 2001;**119**:973–5.

52 Nootens M, Rich S. Successful management of labour and delivery in primary pulmonary hypertension. *Am J Cardiol* 1993;**71**:1124–5.

53 Torres PJ, Gratacos E, Magrina J, Martinez-Crespo JM. Primary pulmonary hypertension and pre-eclampsia: a successful pregnancy. *Br J Obstet Gynaecol* 1994;**101**: 163–5.

54 Blaise G, Langleben D, Hubert B. Pulmonary arterial hypertension: pathophysiology and anesthetic approach. *Anesthesiology* 2003;**99**:1415–32.

CHAPTER 7
Rheumatic heart disease

Bernard Iung

Rheumatic heart disease is the most frequent acquired heart disease encountered in pregnant women. The tolerance of pregnancy-induced hemodynamic changes differs dramatically according to the type of valvular heart disease and this is a heterogeneous group. The management of such patients requires a careful analysis of the severity of the valve disease itself, as well as its tolerance according to the term of pregnancy. The risks of medical therapy and, even more, of interventional procedures, should be weighed against the risk of maternal and fetal complications.

Epidemiology

There has been a major decrease in the incidence of rheumatic fever during the last decades in western countries, leading to a decrease in the prevalence of chronic rheumatic heart valve disease. However, rheumatic fever remains endemic in a number of developing countries. In school surveys performed in India and Nepal, the prevalence of rheumatic heart disease was estimated as between 1 and 5.4 per 1000 between 1984 and 1995, whereas the corresponding figure was below 0.5 per 1000 in western countries.[1,2] In rural Pakistan, a recent survey, including a systematic clinical screening and confirmation by Doppler echocardiography, led to a consistent prevalence of 5.7 per 1000, with higher figures, between 8 and 12 per 1000, in women of child-bearing age.[3] More than 80% of the patients who had rheumatic heart disease were not aware of the diagnosis, 78% had few or no symptoms (New York Heart Association or NYHA class I or II), and only 8% received rheumatic prophylaxis.[3] The lack of adherence to prophylaxis has been observed in other countries and is a probable explanation for why the prevalence of rheumatic heart disease has not decreased in developing countries.

Valvular heart disease is the second most frequent heart disease after congenital heart disease, during pregnancy, in western countries and the most frequent in developing countries.[4,5] Rheumatic heart disease is the main cause of valvular disease in young women and mitral stenosis is the most frequently encountered, which is particularly important because it is the most poorly tolerated valvular disease during pregnancy.[5,6]

Although far less prevalent than degenerative etiologies, rheumatic heart disease still represents 27% of native valve diseases in Europe.[7] As the prevalence of degenerative diseases is low in young women, rheumatic heart disease accounts for the majority of acquired heart valve diseases which are poorly tolerated during pregnancy.[4] This is particularly the case in immigrants who have not had optimal access to health care facilities and in whom valve disease has frequently not been diagnosed. Nevertheless, the absolute number of cases is far lower than in developing countries and this may account for the trend towards a decreased awareness of valve disease in pregnant women.

Stenotic left-sided heart valve diseases

Pathophysiology

Pregnancy-induced hemodynamic changes are detailed in Chapter 2. The main consequence of the increase in cardiac output across a stenotic valve is a sharp increase in the gradient, and therefore a pressure overload in the cardiac chamber located above the valve. This explains why stenotic heart valve diseases are poorly tolerated during pregnancy, in particular because of the physiological increase in cardiac output, which reaches 30–50% at the beginning of the second trimester.[8] In a series of 221 women with heart disease who had 276 pregnancies, the presence of left heart obstruction was a significant predictor of the occurrence of cardiac events during pregnancy.[9]

Hemodynamic deterioration is directly related to the increase in cardiac output and, therefore, most frequently develops during the second trimester. The postpartum period remains a period at risk of hemodynamic complications because cardiac output and loading conditions only normalize after 3–5 days. In addition, the relief of the inferior vena cava compression and secondary blood shift to the placenta and uterine contraction results in an increase in preload.[10]

Pregnancy-induced hemodynamic modifications are poorly tolerated in mitral stenosis because, in addition to the increase in cardiac output, tachycardia reduces the length of diastole, thereby contributing to the increase in mean mitral gradient.

Mitral stenosis

Clinical presentation

Pregnancy in a patient with severe mitral stenosis is nearly always associated with a marked deterioration of clinical status.[6,11] The diagnosis of mitral stenosis may be made for the first time with the onset of cardiac symptoms during pregnancy in a previously asymptomatic patient (Figure 7.1).[12] If mitral stenosis has not been relieved before pregnancy, close follow-up is necessary at 3 months and every month thereafter, including clinical and systematic echocardiographic evaluations. Given the risk of worsening clinical status during pregnancy, prophylactic treatment of severe mitral stenosis, in particular using percutaneous mitral commissurotomy, is frequently considered in women of child-bearing age.

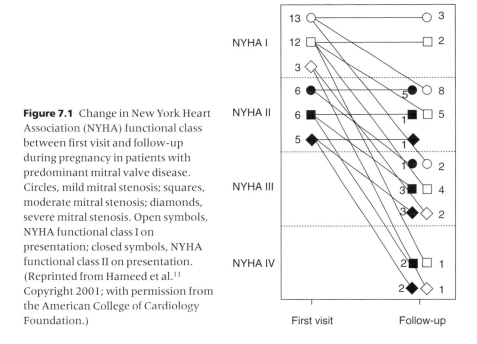

Figure 7.1 Change in New York Heart Association (NYHA) functional class between first visit and follow-up during pregnancy in patients with predominant mitral valve disease. Circles, mild mitral stenosis; squares, moderate mitral stenosis; diamonds, severe mitral stenosis. Open symbols, NYHA functional class I on presentation; closed symbols, NYHA functional class II on presentation. (Reprinted from Hameed et al.[11] Copyright 2001; with permission from the American College of Cardiology Foundation.)

Hemodynamic tolerance is generally good during the first trimester because tachycardia and increase in cardiac output are still moderate. Symptoms generally begin during the second trimester. Pulmonary edema may be the first symptom, in particular if mitral stenosis is complicated by atrial fibrillation; however, progressively increasing shortness of breath is the most common.

Theoretically, clinical diagnosis should be easier during pregnancy because the intensity of the murmur tends to increase with cardiac output. However, the perception of the murmur may be difficult because of tachycardia. Moreover, the decrease in the prevalence of mitral stenosis in western countries has rendered practitioners less aware of this disease and its auscultatory characteristics.

Echocardiographic examination

The reference measurement of the severity of mitral stenosis is measurement of the mitral valve area as assessed by planimetry using two-dimensional echocardiography.[13] Doppler estimation of the valve area using the pressure half-time method is widely used because it is easier to perform than planimetry. The pressure half-time method is influenced by loading conditions, and this can be of importance given the hemodynamic changes occurring during pregnancy. However, recent reports suggest that the half-time method is applicable in pregnant women.[14] Mitral valve area is a strong determinant of the risk of pulmonary edema during pregnancy. The commonly utilized threshold for severe mitral stenosis is $1.5\,cm^2$, or $1\,cm^2/m^2$ of body surface area, although there is no consensus for the latter value.[15-17] The mitral gradient increases after the increase in cardiac output and, thus, it is a marker of the tolerance of mitral stenosis but not of its severity.[18] However, the measurement of mean mitral gradient is useful for patient follow-up and evaluation of the effect of medical therapy. The estimation of systolic pulmonary artery pressure using Doppler examination of the tricuspid regurgitant flow is the other important echocardiographic marker of tolerance to mitral stenosis.

Echocardiographic evaluation of the anatomy of the mitral valve has important implications because it is one of the determinants of whether percutaneous mitral commissurotomy can be performed and is likely to succeed. Leaflet thickening or calcification and the degree of involvement of the subvalvular apparatus are usually combined in different scoring systems that have been shown to be predictors of the immediate and late results of balloon commissurotomy.[19] When patients present with mitral re-stenosis after earlier surgical or percutaneous commissurotomy, anatomical analysis should assess the degree of commissural re-fusion. A repeat commissurotomy can be effective only if re-stenosis is caused by a recurrence of commissural fusion. If re-stenosis is related to valvular and/or subvalvular rigidity with both commissures still open, balloon commissurotomy would bring little or no benefit and is not indicated.[13]

Echocardiographic examination should pay particular attention to other valvular lesions. Functional tricuspid regurgitation is characterized by the absence of structural change in the leaflets. It is frequent and does not modify patient management during pregnancy. It should be differentiated from rheumatic tricuspid disease, which may have its own implications in the therapeutic strategy, particularly in the case of tricuspid stenosis. Rheumatic aortic regurgitation is frequently associated but does not have implications for patient management. Conversely, rheumatic aortic stenosis contributes to worsen hemodynamic tolerance. Its severity may be underestimated because the association with mitral stenosis may decrease aortic gradient. This underlines the need for a careful estimation of aortic valve area using the continuity equation.

Transesophageal echocardiography should be avoided as a first-line examination in pregnant women. Its main application is to rule out left atrial thrombosis before percutaneous mitral commissurotomy. In such cases, it is best to perform transesophageal echocardiography under anesthesia, possibly during the interventional procedure itself.[13]

Principles of treatment
Medical therapy
Treatment with beta blockers is advised in women with severe mitral stenosis who become symptomatic or whose estimated systolic pulmonary artery pressure, according to Doppler examination, exceeds 50 mmHg.[20] Propranolol is the

reference treatment but selective drugs such as atenolol or metoprolol may be preferred to reduce the risk of interaction with uterine contractions. The dose should be adjusted according to heart rate, functional tolerance, and the evolution of mean mitral gradient and systolic pulmonary artery pressure on serial Doppler–echocardiographic examinations. Given the increase in catecholaminergic activity during pregnancy, high doses of beta blockers may be required, in particular during the last trimester. The fetal tolerance of the use of beta blockers is generally good. However, the obstetric and pediatric teams should be aware of the treatment at delivery because of the risk of fetal bradycardia.

Beta blockers may also reduce the risk of atrial arrhythmia. The tolerance of atrial fibrillation is particularly poor in pregnant patients with severe mitral stenosis and, given the concerns related to the use of anti-arrhythmic drugs during pregnancy, electric cardioversion is the treatment of choice and is safe for the fetus.[17]

In patients with paroxysmal or permanent atrial fibrillation, anticoagulant therapy is mandatory whatever the severity of mitral stenosis. This is true for any patient with mitral stenosis, but even more during pregnancy because it is associated with a hypercoagulable state. Vitamin K antagonists can be used safely during the second and third trimester, provided that heparin is substituted at week 36 or a cesarean section is planned.[17] During the first trimester, the risk of embryopathy and fetal hemorrhage with vitamin K antagonists (especially for women who need high dosage) should be balanced against the less satisfactory protection from thromboembolic complications when using long-term heparin treatment.[21] The management of anticoagulant therapy during pregnancy is detailed in Chapter 9.

When dyspnea and/or congestive heart failure persists despite the use of beta blockers, loop diuretics may be added. Dose adjustment should be gradual to avoid an excessive decrease in blood volume.

Vaginal delivery can generally be performed safely in women with well-tolerated mitral stenosis, in NYHA class I or II, and when systolic pulmonary artery pressure remains below 50 mmHg. Epidural anesthesia is frequently advised to reduce the hemodynamic stress inherent to delivery. Beta-blocker therapy should be adapted to heart rate during delivery and the early postpartum period. The use of short half-life beta blockers, such as esmolol, can be useful in this setting. Vaginal delivery can be performed even in patients in NYHA class III or IV using hemodynamic monitoring with a pulmonary artery catheter.[10] However, the current preference is to perform percutaneous mitral commissurotomy during pregnancy in women with severe symptomatic mitral stenosis. Cardiologists, obstetricians and anesthetists should collaborate closely to plan the mode of delivery. This is detailed in Chapters 19 and 20.

Patients with moderate mitral stenosis (valve area >1.5 cm^2) have a good prognosis, but may experience dyspnea caused by an increase in mitral gradient and pulmonary arterial pressure.[6,11] Beta blockers may be needed in certain cases.

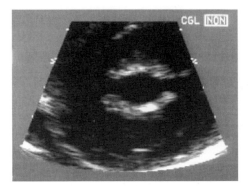

Figure 7.2 Mitral stenosis: opening of both commissures after percutaneous mitral commissurotomy. Transthoracic echocardiography, short-axis view.

Valvular interventions

The persistence of severe dyspnea and, even more serious, signs of congestive heart failure despite medical therapy are associated with a high risk of pulmonary edema at delivery or during the early postpartum period, thereby threatening the life of both the mother and the fetus.[5,10] This leads to consideration of valvular intervention during pregnancy to relieve mitral stenosis before delivery. Closed mitral valvotomy has been for a long time the procedure of choice because of the fetal hazard of valvular surgery under cardiopulmonary bypass. The fetal mortality rate is estimated to be between 20 and 30%, and signs of distress have been shown using fetal monitoring during cardiopulmonary bypass.[22,23] Problems related to cardiac surgery during pregnancy are detailed in Chapter 21. In a recent series, the maternal mortality after closed-heart commissurotomy during pregnancy was almost 0 but the fetal mortality rate ranged from 2% to 10%.[24]

During the 1990s, percutaneous mitral commissurotomy emerged as a feasible and efficient treatment of severe symptomatic mitral stenosis during pregnancy (Figure 7.2).[25–29] Percutaneous mitral commissurotomy was already accepted as an alternative to surgical commissurotomy. However, its performance during pregnancy initially raised concerns about the fetal tolerance of the procedure and the potential risk related to radiation, because the procedure is monitored using fluoroscopy. In our experience, the use of cardiac fetal monitoring during the procedure showed that percutaneous mitral commissurotomy during pregnancy was not associated with signs of fetal distress.[26] Semi-quantitative radiation dose assessment showed that the radiation dose remains below very low levels and this is unlikely to have any consequence on the short- as well as the long-term outcome of the fetus.[26] The alternative of performing the procedure uniquely under transesophageal echocardiography has

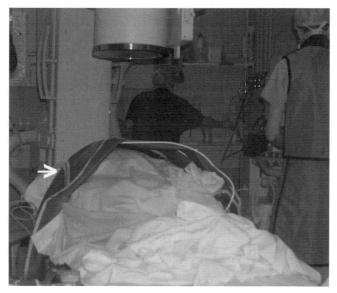

Figure 7.3 Preparation of a procedure of percutaneous mitral commissurotomy in a pregnant women. The patient's abdomen is protected by a lead apron (arrow).

been proposed in a short series. However, this was associated with a high complication rate, including tamponade. This approach is, therefore, not recommended.

Particularly during pregnancy, percutaneous mitral commissurotomy should be performed by experienced operators to keep the risk of complications as low as possible and to shorten the duration of the procedure and fluoroscopy time. The use of the Inoue balloon facilitates this. The abdomen of the patient should be wrapped in a lead apron during the procedure (Figure 7.3). The monitoring of valve opening relies on echocardiographic examination, thereby avoiding the use of cardiac catheterization and angiography.[13]

There have now been more than 300 published reports of percutaneous mitral commissurotomy during pregnancy. This procedure enables valve function and, therefore, clinical status, to be dramatically improved. The course of the remaining pregnancy and peripartum period is uneventful in most patients and vaginal delivery can be performed safely after successful percutaneous mitral commissurotomy. In rare cases, balloon commissurotomy can be performed as an emergency procedure in critically ill pregnant patients.

It should not be forgotten that percutaneous mitral commissurotomy is an interventional procedure and carries inherent risks. Thromboembolic complications are rare but may be favored by the hypercoagulability present during pregnancy. Traumatic mitral regurgitation related to leaflet tearing is the most frequent severe complication and occurs in approximately 5% of the procedures.[19] Its consequences can be particularly harmful in pregnant patients because severe, acute, mitral regurgitation is poorly tolerated, given the increase in blood volume and cardiac output. Urgent valvular surgery is frequently needed in such cases, with the inherent risk for the fetus. As a result of the poor prognosis of patients who remain symptomatic despite medical therapy, the benefit from percutaneous mitral commissurotomy during pregnancy outweighs its risks. However, pregnancy outcome and fetal prognosis are good in patients who are in NYHA class I or II,[4,5,12] so there is no reason to advise systematic balloon commissurotomy during pregnancy in women who have severe mitral stenosis without either severe symptoms or pulmonary hypertension.

Despite the efficacy of percutaneous mitral commissurotomy, closed mitral commissurotomy remains widely used during pregnancy because of economic constraints in certain developing countries where mitral stenosis remains frequent in young women.[30]

Aortic stenosis

Clinical presentation

Severe aortic stenosis of rheumatic origin is uncommon in young patients. Severe symptoms seldom occur in patients who were asymptomatic before pregnancy (Figure 7.4). Conversely, patients with severe, symptomatic aortic stenosis face a high maternal and fetal risk.[11]

There is frequently little or no valve calcification, which may explain why the second aortic sound can be present, even in patients with severe stenosis.

Echocardiographic evaluation

The severity of aortic stenosis is quantified by the measurement of aortic valve area using the continuity equation. Aortic stenosis is severe if valve area is <1.0 cm^2 or, better, 0.6 cm^2/m^2 body surface area.[15,16] Mean aortic gradient is a less reliable marker of the severity of aortic stenosis because it is dependent on cardiac output. In the particular case of pregnancy, the mean aortic gradient tended to overestimate the degree of aortic stenosis. However, the estimation of the mean gradient is important because of its prognostic value.

The analysis of valve anatomy has no direct implications for patient management, but it is of importance for differential diagnosis. It is important to rule out bicuspid aortic valve, which is the main other cause of aortic stenosis in young women, and may have specific implications for patient management when enlargement of the ascending aorta is associated.

Echocardiographic examination should search for other valve disease, in particular mitral stenosis, which is usually present in cases of aortic stenosis of rheumatic origin.

Principles of treatment

Asymptomatic patients with a mean aortic gradient that remains <50 mmHg during pregnancy have a good prognosis and require only close follow-up.[11]

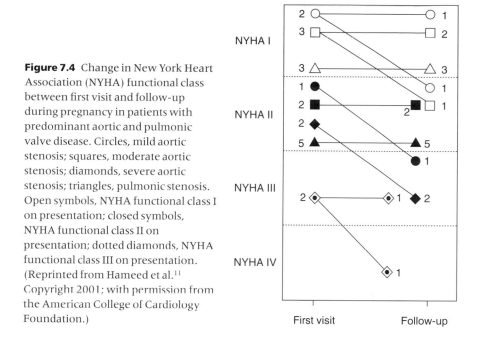

Figure 7.4 Change in New York Heart Association (NYHA) functional class between first visit and follow-up during pregnancy in patients with predominant aortic and pulmonic valve disease. Circles, mild aortic stenosis; squares, moderate aortic stenosis; diamonds, severe aortic stenosis; triangles, pulmonic stenosis. Open symbols, NYHA functional class I on presentation; closed symbols, NYHA functional class II on presentation; dotted diamonds, NYHA functional class III on presentation. (Reprinted from Hameed et al.[11] Copyright 2001; with permission from the American College of Cardiology Foundation.)

Whatever the etiology of aortic stenosis, vaginal delivery under close monitoring can generally be performed in those patients. The administration of epidural anesthesia must be cautious and slow because the decrease in peripheral vascular resistance may be harmful and spinal block should be avoided. The stability of hemodynamic conditions is paramount during delivery when aortic stenosis is present. In particular, hypovolemia should be avoided during delivery and the postpartum period. Therefore, some authors advise cesarean section in cases of severe aortic stenosis to avoid abrupt increases in arterial pressure and cardiac output, and to shorten the duration of delivery.[6]

Patients who experience severe dyspnea are treated with diuretics. In such cases, the main problem is the risk of worsening of cardiac status during delivery. Patients who have severe aortic stenosis and severe symptoms despite medical therapy (NYHA class III or IV) or signs of congestive heart failure raise the question of an intervention during pregnancy to relieve aortic stenosis. Aortic valve replacement under cardiopulmonary bypass should be avoided if possible because of the fetal risk.[31] However, if required, it is advised to perform aortic valve replacement when the fetus is viable. The fetus should be delivered by cesarean section just before cardiac surgery under cardiopulmonary bypass. Although it has been almost abandoned for the treatment of aortic stenosis in adults, percutaneous balloon aortic valvotomy can be considered in certain cases.[31-34] Its main advantage is to avoid cardiopulmonary bypass. As rheumatic aortic stenosis in young women is generally associated with commissural fusion and only a moderate amount of valve calcification, a transient improvement of aortic valve function is likely to be obtained in order to manage the peripartum period safely and to postpone aortic valve replacement until after delivery. When attempted during pregnancy, percutaneous balloon aortic valvuloplasty should be carried out with the same measures to reduce radiation dose as in percutaneous mitral commissurotomy, and its performance should be restricted to centers with a great deal of experience.

Regurgitant left-sided heart valve diseases

Pathophysiology

The progressive increase in blood volume and cardiac output, which occurs during pregnancy, tends to increase the regurgitant volume in patients who have aortic or mitral regurgitation. However, other physiological changes, such as tachycardia and the decrease in systemic arterial resistances, tend to increase forward stroke volume and to compensate in part for the consequences of valvular regurgitation.[8]

Most often, even severe valvular regurgitation is well tolerated during pregnancy, provided that it is chronic, associated with dilatation of the left ventricle and preserved left ventricular function. Acute regurgitation is poorly tolerated because of the sharp increase in filling pressures, but is very seldom encountered in patients with rheumatic valve disease (except in the context of infective endocarditis).

Rare cases of long-standing aortic or mitral regurgitation complicated by severe left ventricular dysfunction may decompensate during pregnancy. The prognosis and management of such patients during pregnancy is similar to those with cardiomyopathy.[17] When present, left ventricular dysfunction seems to be more the consequence of chronic volume overload than the late evolution of rheumatic lesions in the myocardium itself. The possibility of rheumatic myocarditis has been mentioned in patients presenting with ventricular dysfunction during acute rheumatic fever. However, this seems to be more probably the consequence of concomitant severe valvular regurgitations than of direct rheumatic myocardial lesions.[35]

Clinical presentation

Severe symptoms or signs of congestive heart failure are seldom encountered. The most frequent situation is the systematic follow-up of a pregnant patient who has a previously known regurgitant murmur. In patients with mitral regurgitation, the frequency of atrial premature beats may increase during pregnancy. In patients with aortic regurgitation, clinical interpretation of the severity of the regurgitation may be difficult because the increase in stroke volume during pregnancy may produce bounding pulses in the absence of heart disease.

Echocardiographic evaluation

The principles do not differ from the usual echocardiographic examination of regurgitant heart valve diseases.[36] Given the particular hemodynamic conditions during pregnancy, the use of qualitative Doppler echocardiography to assess regurgitant volume and effective regurgitant orifice area should be preferred over qualitative methods.

The interpretation of left ventricular dimensions should take into account the possibility of a normal mild left ventricular enlargement because of the increase in blood volume during pregnancy.

Echocardiographic analysis of valve anatomy will generally not influence management during pregnancy. However, it contributes to determining the feasibility of mitral valve repair in patients with rheumatic mitral regurgitation who will need surgical treatment after pregnancy. In patients with aortic regurgitation, a careful analysis of the aortic valve and the ascending aorta is needed to confirm the diagnosis of rheumatic aortic regurgitation. It is necessary to eliminate alternative diagnoses, in particular Marfan syndrome or bicuspid aortic valve associated with enlargement of the ascending aorta, given their different prognostic implications during pregnancy.

Principles of treatment

Most patients with severe mitral or aortic regurgitation do not need any medical therapy. When severe symptoms or signs of congestive heart failure occur, in particular during the third trimester, clinical tolerance improves with medical therapy using diuretics and vasodilators. Angiotensin-converting enzyme (ACE) inhibitors and angiotensin receptor antagonists are contraindicated throughout pregnancy. As hydralazine is not commercially available in certain countries, the most frequently used vasodilators during pregnancy are nitrates and dihydropyridine calcium-channel blockers.[37]

Even in patients who develop dyspnea or signs of heart failure, treatment is medical and surgery should be avoided during pregnancy.[17] Cardiac surgery using cardiopulmonary bypass carries a particularly high risk for the fetus and this is not justified given the good prognosis of regurgitant heart valve disease during pregnancy, including the peripartum period. Cardiac surgery should be considered only in the very rare cases of severe valvular regurgitation complicated by refractory heart failure.

Vaginal delivery may be carried out in most patients, even in patients who have experienced symptoms. The same treatment is used during the peripartum period. The indication for surgery after pregnancy is discussed according to guidelines following a complete re-evaluation of the severity and tolerance of the valve disease.

When valve replacement is needed after delivery, the choice of valve substitute should include weighing the durability of a mechanical prosthesis against the risk of a subsequent pregnancy under anticoagulant therapy.

In the rare cases of valvular regurgitation complicated by severe and poorly tolerated left ventricular dysfunction (ejection fraction <40%), early termination of pregnancy may be considered given the risk of worsening heart failure during pregnancy, as in patients with cardiomyopathy.[17]

Tricuspid valve diseases

Pathophysiology

Rheumatic tricuspid valve disease is never isolated and it is generally associated with mitral stenosis. Tricuspid regurgitation determines an increase in right atrial and venous pressure according to the severity of the regurgitation itself and the level of pulmonary arterial pressure. Predominant tricuspid stenosis is less frequently encountered than tricuspid regurgitation. Tricuspid stenosis determines a tricuspid gradient, an increase in right atrial pressure and a decrease in cardiac output.

Clinical presentation

A systolic murmur of tricuspid regurgitation is frequent in patients with mitral stenosis, but in most cases it is related to functional regurgitation. The auscultatory diagnosis of tricuspid stenosis is frequently difficult. Tricuspid valve disease may be suspected in patients who have predominant signs of right heart failure, whereas signs of left heart failure are classically attenuated.

Echocardiographic examination

Two-dimensional echocardiography shows leaflet thickening, which is frequently associated with reduced motion and chordal thickening. This differentiates rheumatic tricuspid disease from functional tricuspid regurgitation, which is more frequent and in which the anatomy of leaflets and chordae is normal. Commissural fusion is frequently associated with cases of tricuspid stenosis.

Quantification of regurgitation or stenosis depends on loading conditions. Tricuspid stenosis is considered significant if the mean gradient exceeds 5 mmHg. As a result of the increased blood volume and cardiac output, the severity of tricuspid regurgitation may be overestimated. The difficulty in the accurate quantification of right-sided valve disease during pregnancy explains that their hemodynamic relevance is frequently assessed from the presence of clinical signs of right heart failure.

Principles of treatment

Diuretics can be used in the case of clinical signs of congestive heart failure. Beta blockers are efficient in tricuspid stenosis, as in mitral stenosis. However, the persistence or signs of heart failure under medical therapy should lead to consideration of intervention on the valves, as is the case for isolated mitral stenosis.

In non-pregnant patients, severe rheumatic tricuspid valve disease is generally considered a contraindication to percutaneous mitral commissurotomy and combined tricuspid and mitral surgery is indicated. However, in the particular case of pregnancy, given the fetal hazard of surgery under cardiopulmonary bypass, percutaneous mitral commissurotomy may be considered, either isolated or associated with tricuspid balloon valvotomy when there is an association with severe tricuspid stenosis.[38]

Fetal outcome

The analysis of fetal outcome should take into account valvular heart disease, as well as co-morbidity or obstetric risk factors for neonatal complications, which are more frequent in pregnant patients with heart disease than in the general population.[4]

Relatively high rates of fetal complications, in particular fetal growth retardation, pre-term delivery and low birthweight, have been reported in a number of series of pregnant patients with rheumatic heart disease (Table 7.1).[5,11,12,14,39]

In a series of 312 pregnancies in patients with rheumatic heart disease compared with 321 controls, there were significantly higher frequencies of intrauterine growth retardation, pre-term delivery, low birthweight and Apgar score <8, but no significant differences in congenital abnormalities and stillbirth.[39]

Functional class is a strong determinant of the risk of fetal complications, which occur mainly in patients who are in NYHA class III or IV during pregnancy.[4,5,12]

Conclusion

The wide range of situations that may occur during pregnancy in women with rheumatic heart disease emphasizes the need for close cooperation between obstetricians and cardiologists at every stage:

- Before pregnancy, when preventive treatment of the valve disease is indicated, in particular in women with severe mitral stenosis.
- During pregnancy, particularly after the beginning of the second trimester, reacting promptly to any change in symptomatic status.
- At delivery, when the modality should be debated and planned, in concert with the anesthetists, and during the first days of the postpartum period.

Key points

- Echocardiographic evaluation is mandatory in any young woman who has a cardiac murmur, even if she is asymptomatic.
- Preventive treatment of severe mitral stenosis ($<1.5 \, cm^2$) should be considered in women who wish to be pregnant, even in the absence of symptoms, in particular when the conditions are favorable to percutaneous mitral commissurotomy.
- In the case of severe aortic stenosis ($<1.0 \, cm^2$) before pregnancy, surgery is mandatory in symptomatic patients and should be considered in

Table 7.1 Maternal and fetal outcome in recent series of pregnant patients with valvular heart disease

Series	Country	No. of pregnancies	Mitral stenosis (%)	Initial NYHA class (%)	Maternal outcome			IUGR (%)	Fetal outcome		
					Heart failure (%)	Arrhythmias (%)	Mortality rate (%)		Pre-term (%)	Low birthweight (%)	Stillbirth (%)
Hameed et al.[11]	USA	66	70	I: 55 II: 42 III: 3	38	15	2	21	23	–	3
Silversides et al.[14]	Canada	80	100	I–II: 89 III–IV: 11	31	11	0	8	21	–	3
Bhatla et al.[12]	India	207	57[a]	I: 53 II: 28 III: 14 IV: 5	5	5	0	18	25	39	1
Sawhney et al.[5]	India	480	89	I–II: 77 III–IV: 23	–	–	2	18	12	29	2
Malhotra et al.[39]	India	312	76	I: 56 II: 31 III: 8 IV: 5	5	7	3	6	48	44	3

[a]Eleven per cent of patients had congenital heart disease.

IUGR, intrauterine growth retardation; NYHA, New York Heart Association.

asymptomatic patients, weighing the risks of complications during pregnancy against the drawbacks of a valve prosthesis.

- In women with uncorrected heart valve disease who become pregnant, close follow-up is mandatory from the beginning of the second trimester.
- Regurgitant valvular lesions are generally well tolerated during pregnancy. These patients should be managed medically, even if they become symptomatic.
- Stenotic valve disease carries a high risk of maternal and fetal complications during pregnancy when patients become symptomatic.
- Mitral stenosis is the most frequent rheumatic heart disease encountered in young women as well as the most prone to becoming decompensated during pregnancy, even in previously asymptomatic patients.
- The first-line treatment of severe symptomatic mitral stenosis during pregnancy is medical, mainly with beta blockers.
- Percutaneous mitral commissurotomy should be considered in women with severe mitral stenosis who have severe symptoms (NYHA class III or IV) or pulmonary artery pressure >50 mmHg despite medical therapy during pregnancy.
- Heart valve surgery under cardiopulmonary bypass should be considered only when the mother's life is threatened. Prior delivery is indicated if the fetus is viable to avoid the high risk of fetal death during induction of anesthesia.
- Delivery should be planned after close collaboration of the obstetrician, anesthetist and cardiologist on the basis of recent evaluation of tolerance of the heart valve disease.

References

1 Padmavati S. Present status of rheumatic fever and rheumatic heart disease in India. *Indian Heart J* 1995;**47**:395–8.
2 Bahadur KC, Sharma D, Shresta MP et al. Prevalence of rheumatic and congenital heart disease in schoolchildren of Kathmandu valley in Nepal. *Indian Heart J* 2003;**55**:615–18.
3 Rizvi SFH, Khan MA, Kundi A, Marsh DR, Samad A, Pasha O. Current status of rheumatic heart diseases in rural Pakistan. *Heart* 2004;**90**:394–9.
4 Siu SC, Coleman JM, Sorensen S et al. Adverse neonatal and cardiac outcomes are more common in pregnant women with cardiac disease. *Circulation* 2002;**105**: 2179–84.
5 Sawhney H, Aggarwal N, Suri V, Vasishta K, Sharma Y, Grover A. Maternal and perinatal outcome in rheumatic heart disease. *Int J Gynecol Obstet* 2003;**80**:9–14.
6 Lesniak-Sobelga A, Tracz W, Kostiewicz M, Podolec P, Pasowicz M. Clinical and echocardiographic assessment of pregnant women with valvular heart diseases. Maternal and fetal outcome. *Int J Cardiol* 2004;**94**:15–23.
7 Iung B, Baron G, Butchart EG et al. A prospective survey of patients with valvular heart disease in Europe: the Euro Heart Survey on valvular heart disease. *Eur Heart J* 2003;**24**:1231–43.
8 Hunter S, Robson SC. Adaptation of the maternal heart in pregnancy. *BMJ* 1992;**68**:540–3.

9 Siu SC, Sermer M, Harrison DA et al. Risk and predictors for pregnancy-related complications in women with heart disease. *Circulation* 1997;**96**:2789–94.

10 Clark S, Phelan JP, Greenpoon J, Aldahl D, Horenstein J. Labour and delivery in the presence of mitral stenosis: central hemodynamic observation. *Am J Obstet Gynecol* 1985;**152**:984–8.

11 Hameed A, Karaalp IS, Tummala PP et al. The effect of valvular heart disease on maternal and fetal outcome during pregnancy. *J Am Coll Cardiol* 2001;**37**:893–9.

12 Bhatla N, Lal S, Behera G et al. Cardiac disease in pregnancy. *Int J Gynecol Obstet* 2003;**82**:153–9.

13 Vahanian A, Iung B, Cormier B. Mitral valvuloplasty. In: Topol EJ (ed.), *Textbook of Interventional Cardiology*, 4th edn. Philadelphia: WB Saunders, 2002: pp 921–40.

14 Silversides CK, Colman JM, Sermer M, Siu SC. Cardiac risk in pregnant women with rheumatic mitral stenosis. *Am J Cardiol* 2003;**91**:1382–5.

15 Bonow RO, Carabello B, DeLeon AC et al. ACC/AHA guidelines for the management of patients with valvular heart disease. *J Am Coll Cardiol* 1998;**32**:1486–588.

16 Iung B, Gohlke-Bärwolf C, Tornos P et al. Recommendations on the management of the asymptomatic patient with valvular heart disease. Working Group Report on behalf of the Working Group on Valvular Heart Disease. *Eur Heart J* 2002;**23**:1253–66.

17 Oakley C, Child A, Iung B et al. Expert consensus document on management of cardiovascular diseases during pregnancy. *Eur Heart J* 2003;**24**:761–81.

18 Bryg RJ, Gordon PR, Kudesia VS et al. Effect of pregnancy on pressure gradient in mitral stenosis . *Am J Cardiol* 1989;**63**:384–6.

19 Vahanian A, Palacios IF. Percutaneous approaches to valvular disease. *Circulation* 2004;**109**:1572–9.

20 Al Kasab SM, Sabag T, Al Zaibag M et al. Beta-adrenergic receptor blockade in the management of pregnant women with mitral stenosis. *Am J Obstet Gynecol* 1990;**163**: 37–40.

21 Bates SM, Greer IA, Hirsh J, Ginsberg JS. Use of antithrombotic agents during pregnancy: the Seventh ACCP Conference on Antithrombotic and Thrombolytic Therapy. *Chest* 2004;**126**(3 suppl):627S–44S.

22 Arnoni RT, Arnoni AS, Bonini RC et al. Risk factors associated with cardiac surgery during pregnancy. *Ann Thorac Surg* 2003;**76**:1605–8.

23 Lamb MP, Ross K, Johnstone AM, Manners JM. Fetal heart monitoring during open heart surgery. Two case reports. *Br J Obstet Gynecol* 1981;**88**:669–74.

24 Pavankumar P, Venugopal P, Kaul U et al. Closed mitral valvotomy during pregnancy. A 20-year experience. *Scand J Thor Cardiovasc Surg* 1988;**22**:11–15.

25 Esteves CA, Ramos AIO, Braga SLN, Harrison JK, Sousa JE. Effectiveness of percutaneous balloon mitral valvotomy during pregnancy. *Am J Cardiol* 1991;**68**:930–4.

26 Iung B, Cormier B, Elias J et al. Usefulness of percutaneous balloon commissurotomy for mitral stenosis during pregnancy. *Am J Cardiol* 1994;**73**:398–400.

27 Ben Farhat M, Gamra H, Betbout F et al. Percutaneous balloon mitral commissurotomy during pregnancy. *Heart* 1997;**77**:564–7.

28 Fawzy ME, Kinsara AJ, Stefadouros M et al. Long-term outcome of mitral balloon valvotomy in pregnant women. *J Heart Valve Dis* 2001;**10**:153–7.

29 Routray SN, Mishra TK, Swain S, Patnaik UK, Behera M. Balloon mitral valvuloplasty during pregnancy. *Int J Gynecol Obstet* 2004;**85**:18–23.

30 Aggarwal N, Suri V, Goyal A, Malhotra S, Manoj R, Dhaliwal RS. Closed mitral valvotomy in pregnancy and labour. *Int J Gynecol Obstet* 2005;**88**:118–21.

31 Ben-Ami M, Battino S, Rosenfeld T, Marin G, Shalev E. Aortic valve replacement during pregnancy. A case report and review of the literature. *Acta Obstet Gynaecol Scand* 1990;**69**:651–3.

32 Banning AP, Pearson JF, Hall RJ. Role of balloon dilatation of the aortic valve in pregnant patients with severe aortic stenosis. *Br Heart J* 1993;**70**:544–5.

33 Bhargava B, Agarwal R, Yadav R, Bahl VK, Manchanda SC. Percutaneous balloon aortic valvuloplasty during pregnancy: use of the Inoue balloon and the physiologic antegrade approach. *Cathet Cardiovasc Diagn* 1998;**45**:422–5.

34 Myerson SG, Mitchell AR, Ormerod OJ, Banning AP. What is the role of balloon dilatation for severe aortic stenosis during pregnancy? *J Heart Valve Dis* 2005;**14**: 147–50.

35 Kamblock J, Payot L, Iung B et al. Does rheumatic myocarditis really exist? Systematic study with echocardiography and cardiac troponin I blood levels. *Eur Heart J* 2003;**24**:853–60.

36 Zoghbi WA, Enriquez-Sarano M, Foster E et al. Recommendations for evaluation of the severity of native valvular regurgitation with two-dimensional and Doppler echocardiography. *J Am Soc Echo* 2003;**16**:777–802.

37 Sheikh F, Rangwala S, DeSimone C, Smith HS, O'Leary AM. Management of the parturient with severe aortic incompetence. *J Cardiothorac Vasc Anesth* 1995;**9**:575–7.

38 Ribeiro PA, Zaibag M, Idris M. Percutaneous double balloon tricuspid valvotomy: three year follow-up study. *Eur Heart J* 1990;**11**:1109–12.

39 Malhotra M, Sharma JB, Tripathii R, Arora P, Arora R. Maternal and fetal outcome in valvular heart disease. *Int J Gynecol Obstet* 2004;**84**:11–16.

CHAPTER 8
Mitral valve prolapse

Bernard Iung

Mitral valve prolapse has been the subject of particular interest in the field of heart disease during pregnancy because certain studies suggested a high prevalence in young women and a potentially poor prognosis. Echocardiographic analyses using strict criteria and community-based studies now enable the burden and prognosis of this disease to be better assessed.

Epidemiology

Mitral valve prolapse is the main mechanism of degenerative mitral regurgitation. With the decline in the incidence of rheumatic fever, degenerative diseases are now the most frequent etiology of acquired heart valve disease in western countries.

Mitral regurgitation is the second most frequent heart valve disease after aortic stenosis. In the Euro Heart Survey on valvular heart disease, which was conducted in 2001 in 25 European countries, mitral regurgitation accounted for 32% of all single native left-sided heart valve disease.[1] Degenerative etiology was the cause of 61% of more than trivial (grade ≥ 2/4) mitral regurgitation and the corresponding figure was 75% when considering western Europe.[1]

The prevalence of mitral valve prolapse has been debated. Series from the 1970s and 1980s reported high prevalence rates, between 5 and 15%, in particular in young women. However, these estimations have been challenged because of concerns about diagnostic criteria and selection bias. More recently, a large community-based study reported a prevalence of 2.4%, and age and sex distribution did not differ from those in the general population.[2]

Pathological features

Mitral valve prolapse is an abnormality of the systolic motion of the mitral valve characterized by leaflet billowing across the plane of the mitral annulus, and can occur with or without mitral regurgitation. Mild billowing, or bowing, of structurally normal-looking mitral valves is considered as normal. The term 'floppy valve' designates marked billowing associated with excess tissue and elongated chordae, whereas the term 'flail leaflet' is restricted to cases with ruptured chordae.[3] The term 'prolapse' now tends to be used to cover all presentations of such degenerative abnormalities of the mitral valve.

The abnormal motion of valve prolapse is usually the consequence of structural abnormalities of the leaflets and subvalvular apparatus. The most typical abnormality is myxomatous degeneration, sometimes called 'Barlow's disease', which is associated with increased leaflet thickness, excess tissue with redundancy of the mitral leaflets, and elongation or rupture of chordae tendinae. The other cause of prolapse is fibroelastic degeneration, in which leaflets are thin, without excess tissue.[4]

Histologically, myxomatous valves are characterized by an expansion of the extracellular matrix in the spongiosa, which is the central layer of the leaflet. Abnormalities of the other two layers are a decrease in collagen content in the fibrosa and a fragmentation of elastic fibers in the atrialis.[5] Extracellular matrix remodeling is mediated by metalloproteases synthesized by interstitial valvular cells, which have common features with myofibroblasts.[5] Annular dilatation contributes to mitral regurgitation. Calcification of the mitral annulus is rare. The mechanical consequences are a decreased strength of chordae in myxoid valves, whereas leaflets are more extensible and less stiff than normal leaflets.[6,7]

The most frequent form is primary valve prolapse, i.e. without associated systemic or cardiac disease. No risk factors have been identified so far, unlike in degenerative aortic stenosis. Thus, the term 'degenerative' is not appropriate because it is used for heterogeneous valve diseases and suggests that valvular abnormalities are passive consequences of aging, even though they involve active valvular remodeling. Familial clustering is seldom observed, but it enables inheritable forms with autosomal transmission to be studied. Different genes have been identified, suggesting that even familial forms of valve prolapse are heterogeneous.[8]

Secondary valve prolapse is less frequent. It is associated with connective tissue disorders or other cardiac diseases. Hereditary connective tissue disorders are Marfan syndrome, Ehlers–Danlos syndrome type IV, osteogenesis imperfecta and pseudoxanthoma elasticum. Cardiac diseases are atrial septal defect, hypertrophic cardiomyopathy, rheumatic carditis and endocarditis.[3]

Clinical presentation

The diagnosis of mitral valve prolapse is often based on auscultatory abnormalities in asymptomatic patients. Dyspnea occurs late in patients who have severe mitral regurgitation. Certain non-specific symptoms have been attributed to mitral valve prolapse, such as chest pain, palpitations or dizziness, even in the absence of any hemodynamic impairment, although recent data do not support a particular association.[2]

Typical auscultation of mitral valve prolapse reveals a mid or late systolic click, followed by a late systolic murmur. These abnormalities vary with loading conditions and tend to increase with tachycardia or upright posture. They tend to decrease during pregnancy.[9] The murmur becomes holosystolic in severe regurgitation, frequently without a click. In patients with posterior leaflet prolapse, the murmur radiates toward the left sternal border and aortic area. In anterior leaflet prolapse, the murmur radiates toward the left scapula.

Atrial fibrillation is uncommon in young patients. Atrial and ventricular premature beats can be present, even in the absence of severe mitral regurgitation.

Examination should look for minor physical abnormalities, in particular straight back, pectus excavatum and joint hypermobility. When physical abnormalities are pronounced, it is necessary to search for diagnostic criteria of Marfan syndrome.[10]

Echocardiographic examination

Echocardiography plays a major role in the diagnosis and risk stratification of mitral valve prolapse. Diagnosis criteria should be strict because valve prolapse tends to be overdiagnosed, in particular from the apical four-chamber view, in which leaflet displacement toward the left atrium can be observed in normal hearts because of non-planarity of the mitral annulus. The echocardiographic diagnosis of mitral valve prolapse requires the consistent observation of exaggerated motion of mitral leaflets toward the left atrium in several views, in particular the parasternal long-axis view. A leaflet displacement >2 mm beyond the mitral annulus is required in long-axis view.[2,11,12] Echocardiographic examination also shows valve thickening and tissue excess with redundancy, particularly in the parasternal short-axis view (Figure 8.1). Valvular thickening is considered significant if >5 mm.[2,11,12]

The diagnosis of the site of valve prolapse provides useful information for assessing its severity and the possibilities of valve repair. It uses a standardized classification dividing each leaflet into three scallops: A1–A3 for the anterior

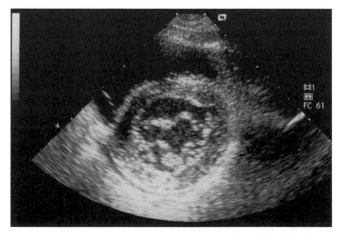

Figure 8.1 Mitral valve prolapse involving anterior and posterior leaflets on a myxomatous valve. Transthoracic echocardiography (parasternal short-axis view): tissue excess with redundant leaflets deforming the shape of the mitral orifice.

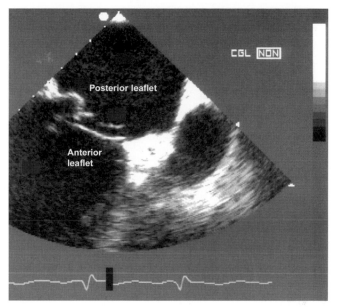

Figure 8.2 Prolapse of the posterior leaflet caused by rupture of chordae. Transesophageal echocardiography.

leaflet and P1–P3 for the posterior leaflet, A2 and P2 corresponding to middle scallops.[13]

The analysis of subvalvular apparatus evaluates chordae elongation and rupture. Chordal rupture is best visualized using transesophageal echocardiography (Figure 8.2).

Color Doppler enables mitral regurgitation to be detected and quantified. The regurgitant jet is generally eccentric and its direction can help to localize the site of prolapse. The regurgitant jet travels along the interatrial septum in posterior leaflet prolapse and along the posterior left atrial wall in anterior leaflet prolapse. Jet eccentricity can make the assessment of severity of mitral regurgitation more difficult, including with quantitative Doppler echocardiography.[14]

Two-dimensional echocardiography facilitates measurement of the left ventricle and left atrium, and of left ventricular function. Careful examination of the ascending aorta is required in patients with Marfan syndrome.

Prognosis

In the general population

The assessment of the prognosis of mitral valve prolapse has been the subject of discrepant estimations, because of inappropriate diagnostic criteria or selection bias. Data from community-based studies now suggest that the outcome is mainly related to the severity and consequences of mitral regurgitation, rather than to the structural valve disease itself. In a series from the Framingham Heart Study,

Table 8.1 Late prognosis of mitral valve prolapse according to risk factors

Risk factors	n	Total mortality rate (%)	Cardiovascular morbidity rate (%)	Valve prolapse-related events (%)[c]
Secondary risk factors[a]				
0 or 1	430	5±2	2±1	2±1
≥2	250	30±5	27±3	15±3
Primary risk factors[b]	153	45±9	61±5	78±6

[a]Secondary risk factors are slight mitral regurgitation, flail leaflet, left atrial diameter > 40 mm, atrial fibrillation, or age ≥ 50 years.

[b]Primary risk factors are left ventricular ejection fraction ≤ 50% or mitral regurgitation ≥ moderate.

[c]Valve prolapse-related events are heart failure resulting from mitral regurgitation, mitral surgery, endocarditis, and death related to valve prolapse.

From Avierinos et al.[12] Ten-year rates of events are given ± standard deviation.

patients who had valve prolapse, most often with mild or no regurgitation, had previously experienced few cardiac events.[2] In a study including 833 patients with initially asymptomatic mitral valve prolapse, 10-year mortality was strongly related to the severity of mitral regurgitation and left ventricular ejection fraction at baseline.[12] Overall mortality, cardiac mortality and cardiovascular morbidity were significantly higher in patients who had a baseline ejection fraction ≤50% or at least a moderate degree of mitral regurgitation (Table 8.1).[12]

During pregnancy

Mitral valve prolapse is well tolerated during pregnancy, even when there is mitral regurgitation.[15] The main physiological hemodynamic changes during pregnancy are increased volume load, increased cardiac output, tachycardia and decreased systemic vascular resistance (see Chapter 2). The increase in cardiac volume due to hypervolemia tends to reduce valvular regurgitation in the particular case of valve prolapse. The decrease in systemic vascular resistance tends to a decrease in the regurgitant volume. Finally, tachycardia increases forward stroke volume, thereby partially compensating for the effect of regurgitation.

Patients with valve prolapse and mild or moderate mitral regurgitation remain asymptomatic during pregnancy and do not experience cardiac complications, including during delivery. Pregnancy tends to increase the frequency of atrial and ventricular premature beats.

Patients with severe mitral regurgitation may experience dyspnea, in particular after the second trimester, which corresponds with the increase in cardiac output. Congestive heart failure is rare. Unlike stenotic heart valve disease, even the occurrence of dyspnea or congestive heart failure in patients with mitral regurgitation does not carry a poor prognosis during pregnancy.[15] Vaginal delivery can be performed in most women, provided that they are in stable hemodynamic condition.

Severe mitral regurgitation can be poorly tolerated during pregnancy only in three rare instances: when acute mitral regurgitation resulting from rupture of major chordae causes a rapid increase in filling pressure;[16] if atrial fibrillation occurs with a very rapid ventricular rate; and when long-standing severe mitral regurgitation is complicated by severe left ventricular dysfunction, the prognosis being comparable to the prognosis of cardiomyopathy.[15]

Principles of treatment

In the general population

There is no need for treatment in asymptomatic patients who have mitral valve prolapse and no severe regurgitation. Beta blockers may be used in the case of severe or highly symptomatic arrhythmias.[15]

When mitral regurgitation is severe, surgical correction is indicated in symptomatic patients.[17] In asymptomatic patients, surgery is indicated in patients when left ventricular ejection fraction is <60% or end-systolic diameter >45 mm.[17,18] There is a current trend to consider surgery at an earlier stage in asymptomatic patients with severe mitral regurgitation, in particular when valve repair is feasible.[18,19]

Mitral valve repair is the preferred treatment for valve prolapse because operative mortality is lower and late results are better than after prosthetic valve replacement.[20,21] However, the feasibility of mitral valve repair depends on valve anatomy. When valve prolapse involves the mid-scallop of the posterior leaflet (P2), valve repair is feasible in most cases and offers good long-term results.[22] Results may be less satisfactory in the case of extensive bivalvular prolapse, in particular when involving commissural areas. Calcification of the mitral annulus can also compromise the feasibility of valve repair. Thus, it is mandatory to take into account the likelihood of valve repair according to echocardiographic analysis and the experience of the surgeon, when considering early surgery in patients with severe mitral regurgitation.[23]

In young women, the desire for pregnancy is a strong incentive to perform mitral valve repair in order to avoid anticoagulation-related complications with a mechanical prosthesis or the deterioration of a bioprosthesis. Given the good tolerance of regurgitant valve diseases during pregnancy, the desire for pregnancy should not lead to advice to undergo surgery at an earlier stage in asymptomatic women with severe mitral regurgitation.

Vasodilator therapy decreases the degree of mitral regurgitation but its clinical efficacy in delaying surgery has not been proven.[24] Endocarditis prophylaxis is indicated in patients with valve prolapse who have mitral regurgitation and/or valve thickening.[25]

During pregnancy

Patients with mild or moderate mitral regurgitation require medical therapy only in rare instances in the case of frequent or poorly tolerated arrhythmias. Beta blockers are well tolerated and effective in this setting.

Patients with severe mitral regurgitation and dyspnea or congestive heart failure should be treated medically using diuretics and vasodilators, taking into account the contraindication to the use of angiotensin enzyme-converting (ACE) inihibitors and angiotensin receptor blockers throughout pregnancy. Even in the case of heart failure, valvular surgery should be avoided during pregnancy. The risk for the fetus, with a 20–30% mortality rate, is not justified by the impairment of maternal prognosis.[15,26] In such cases, mitral valve surgery should be postponed until after delivery.

Antibiotic prophylaxis is discretionary for an uncomplicated delivery, but is administered in most centers.

Key points

- Valve prolapse is the main mechanism of degenerative mitral regurgitation.
- The use of strict echocardiographic criteria avoids over-diagnosis.
- Echocardiographic examination plays a key role in quantifying mitral regurgitation and left ventricular function, which are the main prognostic factors.
- Early surgery should be considered in patients with severe regurgitation, provided that there is a high likelihood of valve repair.
- Mitral regurgitation is well tolerated during pregnancy and should be treated medically.

References

1 Iung B, Baron G, Butchart EG et al. A prospective survey of patients with valvular heart disease in Europe: the Euro Heart Survey on valvular heart disease. *Eur Heart J* 2003;**24**:1231–43.
2 Freed LA, Levy D, Levine RA et al. Prevalence and clinical outcome of mitral valve prolapse. *N Engl J Med* 1999;**341**:1–7.
3 Oakley CM. Mitral valve prolapse. In: Acar J, Bodnar E (eds), *Textbook of Acquired Heart Valve Disease*, Vol 1. London: ICR Publishers, 1995: pp 433–53.
4 Carpentier A. Cardiac valve surgery—the 'French correction'. *J Thorac Cardiovasc Surg* 1983;**86**:323–37.
5 Rabkin E, Aikawa M, Stone JR, Fukumoto Y, Libby P, Schoen FJ. Activated interstitial myofibroblasts express catabolic enzymes and mediate matrix remodeling in myxomatous heart valves. *Circulation* 2001;**104**:2525–32.
6 Barber JE, Ratliff NB, Cosgrove DM 3rd, Griffin BP, Vesely I. Myxomatous mitral valve chordae. I: Mechanical properties. *J Heart Valve Dis* 2001;**10**:320–4.
7 Barber JE, Kasper FK, Ratliff NB, Cosgrove DM 3rd, Griffin BP, Vesely I. Mechanical properties of myxomatous mitral valves. *J Thorac Cardiovasc Surg* 2001;**122**:955–62.
8 Nesta F, Leyne M, Yosefy C et al. New locus for autosomal dominant mitral valve prolapse on chromosome 13. Clinical insights from genetic studies. *Circulation* 2005;**112**:2022–30.
9 Haas JH. The effect of pregnancy on the mid-systolic click and murmur of the prolapsing posterior leaflet of the mitral valve. *Am Heart J* 1976;**92**:407–8.
10 De Paepe A, Devereux RB, Dietz HC, Hennekam RC, Pyeritz RE. Revised diagnostic criteria for the Marfan syndrome. *Am J Med Genet* 1996;**62**:417–26.

11 Levine RA, Stathogiannis E, Newell JB, Harrigan P, Weyman AE. Reconsideration of echocardiographic standards for mitral valve prolapse: lack of association between leaflet displacement isolated to the apical four chamber view and independent echocardiographic evidence of abnormality. *J Am Coll Cardiol* 1988;**11**:1010–19.

12 Avierinos JF, Gersh BJ, Melton III LJ et al. Natural history of mitral valve prolapse in the community. *Circulation* 2002;**106**:1355–61.

13 Pellerin D, Brecker S, Veyrat C. Degenerative mitral valve disease with emphasis on mitral valve prolapse. *Heart* 2002;**88**(suppl IV):IV-20–8.

14 Zoghbi WA, Enriquez-Sarano M, Foster E et al. Recommendations for evaluation of the severity of native valvular regurgitation with two-dimensional and Doppler echocardiography. *J Am Soc Echo* 2003;**16**:777–802.

15 Oakley C, Child A, Iung B et al. Expert consensus document on management of cardiovascular diseases during pregnancy. *Eur Heart J* 2003;**24**:761–81.

16 Hagay ZJ, Weissman A, Geva D, Snir E, Caspi A. Labour and delivery complicated by acute mitral regurgitation due to ruptured chordae tendineae. *Am J Perinatol* 1995;**12**:111–12.

17 Bonow RO, Carabello B, DeLeon AC et al. ACC/AHA guidelines for the management of patients with valvular heart disease. *J Am Coll Cardiol* 1998;**32**:1486–588.

18 Iung B, Gohlke-Bärwolf C, Tornos P et al. Recommendations on the management of the asymptomatic patient with valvular heart disease. Working Group Report on behalf of the Working Group on Valvular Heart Disease. *Eur Heart J* 2002;**23**:1253–66.

19 Enriquez-Sarano M, Avierinos JF, Messika-Zeitoun D et al. Quantitative determinants of the outcome of asymptomatic mitral regurgitation. *N Engl J Med* 2005;**352**:875–83.

20 Mohty D, Orszulak TA, Schaff HV et al. Very long-term survival and durability of mitral valve repair for mitral valve prolapse. *Circulation* 2001;**104**(suppl 1):I1–7.

21 Braunberger E, Deloche A, Berrebi A et al. Very long-term results [more than 20 years] of valve repair with Carpentier's techniques in nonrheumatic mitral valve insufficiency. *Circulation* 2001;**104**(suppl 1):I8–11

22 Monin JL, Dehant P, Roiron C et al. Functional assessment of mitral regurgitation by transthoracic echocardiography using standardized imaging planes: diagnostic accuracy and outcome implications. *J Am Coll Cardiol* 2005;**46**:302–9.

23 Otto CM. Timing of surgery in mitral regurgitation. *Heart* 2003;**89**:100–5.

24 Boon NA, Bloomfield P. The medical management of valvar heart disease. *Heart* 2002;**87**:395–400.

25 Horstkotte D, Follath F, Gutschik E et al. Guidelines on prevention, diagnosis and treatment of infective endocarditis executive summary: The Task Force on Infective Endocarditis of the European Society of Cardiology. *Eur Heart J* 2004;**25**:267–76

26 Arnoni RT, Arnoni AS, Bonini RC et al. Risk factors associated with cardiac surgery during pregnancy. *Ann Thorac Surg* 2003;**76**:1605–8.

CHAPTER 9

Artificial heart valves

James R Trimm, Lynne Hung, Shahbudin H Rahimtoola

The first successful pregnancy and delivery in a patient with a prosthetic heart valve was reported in 1966 in a patient with a Starr–Edwards mitral prosthesis;[1] warfarin embryopathy was reported in 1965.[2] Over the last 40 years, mechanical valves have been documented to be durable and reliable, and the 'best' method of administering warfarin anticoagulant therapy in women with mechanical prostheses during pregnancy has been resolved.[3] Biological valves have been shown to have the advantage of not requiring anticoagulants if sinus rhythm is maintained; however, unlike mechanical prostheses, biological valves lack durability, particularly in young people, and may deteriorate before or during pregnancy.

As there are no perfect choices, women who are likely to need prosthetic heart valves (PHVs) should be encouraged to have their children early before the valve disease deteriorates further to a state where valve replacement becomes necessary.

Mechanical valves

Warfarin

Early reports of oral anticoagulants during pregnancy for a variety of disorders were anecdotal and have been collected together into a much quoted review in the USA, in which experience with warfarin and heparin was compared in patients with various conditions.[4] The use of each was associated with similar fetal loss, prematurity and stillbirth rates, although about two-thirds of the pregnancies were successful.[4,5]

Warfarin embryopathy was first described by Hall in 1965;[2] this syndrome is characterized by nasal hypoplasia and/or stippled epiphyses. Less common features, including central nervous system and eye abnormalities, may be due to warfarin exposure during the second and third trimesters.[4] The fetus is unavoidably overdosed compared with its mother because the fetal liver produces small amounts of vitamin K dependent clotting factors and the molecules of maternal procoagulants are too large to cross the placental barrier. The risk to the fetus is dose dependent and the maternal dose requirement varies widely, but has not been taken into consideration when computing fetal risk.[4]

A higher prevalence of major bleeding complications has been reported in non-pregnant patients with prosthetic valves in the USA compared with in

Europe because the USA was slow to adopt the international normalized ratio (INR). Thromboplastins used in the USA had lower responsiveness than European thromboplastins and resulted in less prolongation of the prothrombin time for the same warfarin dose, resulting in use of higher doses of warfarin. With international sensitivity indices (ISIs) ranging from 1.7 to 2.8, in the USA prothrombin time ratios of between 2.7 and 5.2 may be equivalent to INRs between 5.0 and 10.0. By the 1970s, it was recognized that prothrombin time ratios >2.0 resulted in higher bleeding rates with no further reduction in thromboembolism, but unfortunately this was not generally accepted. As a result, overdosing of American women with warfarin during pregnancy in those with prosthetic valves may have resulted in unduly high rates of fetal complications, and the risk of fetal damage has been greater in reports from the USA because of the use of higher dosages of warfarin in the USA than in Europe.[3] Moreover, it has been shown that INRs controlled to between 2.0 and 3.0 for aortic valves and 2.5 and 3.5 for mitral valves reduces the risk of bleeding complications without increasing the thromboembolic risk in non-pregnant patients.

A wide range of the incidences of warfarin embryopathy has been reported.[6-19] A review published in 2003,[3] which included data from 19 studies comprising almost 1400 pregnancies, showed that the incidence of newborn warfarin embryopathy was 3.9% with a large percentage of the patients having received warfarin in the 6–9 and 12 weeks of pregnancy (Table 9.1). In 779 live births, the incidence of warfarin embryopathy was 7.4%. These comparatively high incidences must be kept in clinical perspective with respect to anticoagulation practices at the time of the studies. Most of the increased incidences seen in these studies were from studies published in the 1960s and 1970s, a time when levels of anticoagulation were much higher than those used later. In 10 of these studies published later, of 427 pregnancies reported, the incidence was actually zero. Four recent studies between 1994 and 1999 reported an incidence of 3 in 189 (1.6%) live births.[3] From the patient's point of view, the incidence per live birth may be more relevant and important. Confirming an earlier report[16] one group has shown that the risk of warfarin embryopathy was extremely low in the 33 women who needed 5 mg or less of warfarin to maintain an adequate INR.[20]

In a recent report 267 women, aged about 31 ± 7 years had mitral mechanical PHV, 30-day mortality was 1.1%. At 25 years, survival was $70 \pm 0.4\%$,

Table 9.1 Incidence of warfarin embryopathy

	No. of pregnancies	No. of live babies	Warfarin embryopathy No. (%) of pregnancies
Total (19 studies)[a]	1399	—	44 (3.9)
	—	779	59 (7.4)
Ten studies	427		0 (0)
Four studies		189	3 (1.6)

[a]From Hung and Rahimtoola.[3]

thromboembolism rate was $25 \pm 0.06\%$ and re-operation rate was $14 \pm 0.04\%$. While receiving warfarin therapy, 35 patients undertook 46 pregnancies and none (zero) experienced adverse cardiac or valve related events. There were 27 healthy babies, 16 spontaneous abortions, 2 stillbirths and 1 baby had ventricular septal defect. Fetal events were less frequent with a daily warfarin doses <5 mg ($p < 0.0001$).[21]

The incidence of warfarin embryopathy is lower with the use of intravenous unfractionated heparin between weeks 6 and 12 of pregnancy; one review concluded that this strategy 'eliminated the risk'.[22] Intravenous unfractionated heparin use in the last 2 weeks of pregnancy is associated with a reduced risk of hemorrhage in the mother during the delivery and the neonatal period, as well as in the baby, because warfarin crosses the placenta and, therefore, the fetus/baby is anticoagulated. To reduce the latter complication, some have suggested elective cesarean section in week 36 of pregnancy.[16,20] An earlier study reported that the incidence of abortion and stillbirths in these patients was higher than in the general population.[9,15]

Intravenous unfractionated heparin

Heparin does not cross the placenta and was thought to be ideal because of its inability to reach the fetus, but its safety and efficacy, when given for a very long time for the prevention of arterial thromboembolism, has not been shown. Its powerful effects, short duration of action, narrow therapeutic index and somewhat unpredictable pharmacokinetics make it more difficult to maintain an adequate anti-thrombotic effect without hemorrhagic complications.[23,24] Recommendations differ about the route, dose and duration of treatment.[25–30] A change to heparin has been advocated for the first trimester, for the entire pregnancy, or even before conception, and a report from the USA has included fertility testing of couples contemplating pregnancy to minimize the time of heparin exposure, although it is not practiced or even recommended generally.[31]

Intravenous administration using a heparin lock has been proposed so as to avoid painful subcutaneous injections and the inevitable bruising but this route provides a portal of entry for bacteria, and one case of staphylococcal endocarditis has been described. A much higher dose is needed to prevent prosthetic valve thrombosis or embolism than to prevent venous thromboembolism. The usual test is the activated partial thromboplastin time (APTT). A target APTT of 1.5, suggested in 1989, is clearly inadequate.[32] More recently, a minimum APTT of 2.0 was suggested, measured halfway between 12-hourly injections. The heparin dose required during pregnancy is higher and the half-life of heparin clearance increases with the dose. The consequence of this is that, as dosage increases toward the therapeutic range, even a small increment may bring about considerable prolongation of the APTT with risk of bleeding. Subtherapeutic anticoagulant doses are clearly undesirable and ineffective.[33–35] Stringent monitoring is required because of the narrow window of safety and in clinical practice increased bleeding has not been well documented.

Heparin treatment is arduous for the patient. Regular blood counts are required to detect thrombocytopenia, which brings a paradoxical risk of thrombosis because it is caused by platelet aggregation. Heparin induces osteopenia when used long term. This complication has been reported most often in pregnant women perhaps because they have been the group most often subjected to long-term treatment and also because of the pregnant woman's high calcium turnover. Other side effects include urticaria, bronchospasm and anaphylaxis.[31,37] However, careful use of intravenous heparin only during the 6–12 weeks of pregnancy with close monitoring of dosage is associated with very few complications.

Subcutaneous heparin

The recommendation for the use of subcutaneous heparin in pregnancy by Ginsberg et al. is based on: heparin's value in patients with angina and myocardial infarction and a study of 100 pregnancies in 77 women.[9,24] In 98 of 100 pregnancies, heparin therapy was given for prevention or treatment of thromboembolism, and in 2 of 100 pregnancies it was given for women with PHV. Therefore, Oakley has criticized this recommendation.[37]

Use of only subcutaneous heparin is inappropriate because of the following:

- The incidence of thromboembolism on subcutaneous heparin therapy during pregnancy in patients with mechanical prostheses is four times greater than in those treated with oral anticoagulants.[19]
- Two studies from the same institution documented mechanical PHV thrombosis with subcutaneous heparin.[9,10] In one of these studies, only 2 of 23 (8.7%) patients had mechanical valves: one had a cerebral embolus; three (14%) died, one from gastrointestinal bleeding and two with thrombosed PHV.
- Subcutaneous heparin does not improve fetal outcome and actually increases maternal mortality.[9,10]

Low-molecular-weight heparin

Presently, no good data exist documenting the benefits from the use of low-molecular-weight heparin (LMWH) in patients with PHV. Case reports of thrombosed PHV with the use of LMWH have been reported.[38,39] As a result, the Food and Drug Administration (FDA) in the USA has issued additions to the warning and precaution sections of the Lovenox (enoxaparin sodium) product labeling.[39] These warnings point out the following:

- This product (an LMWH) is not recommended for thrombotic prophylaxis in patients with PHV.
- Cases of PHV thrombosis and of maternal and fetal deaths have been reported with the use of this drug.
- Furthermore, in pregnant women who received this drug, both teratogenic and non-teratogenic effects have been reported.
- If LMWH is given in the first trimester because the mother requires >5 mg warfarin/day, the fetus will continue to be at increased risk from damage caused by bleeding as a result of the high warfarin dose, so if it turns out that LMWH

seems to provide safe and effective anticoagulation (supported or not by the results of future trials) it is likely to be continued right through pregnancy.

• The inability to reverse it quickly means that there would be less point in changing to it from 36 weeks and this adds to the advantages of elective CS at 36 weeks instead.

Despite these concerns, LMWH is increasingly being used in North America and Europe.[40–43] It has being strongly recommended, however, that routine dosing should be avoided and that there should be careful monitoring of anti-Xa levels. The American College of Chest Physicians guidelines suggest that if LMWH is utilized, anti-Xa levels of 1.0–1.2 units/mL should be achieved 4–6 hours after subcutaneous injection.[42] The precise efficacy of anti-Xa levels, however, remains unproven and, to date, no large series have been reported. One retrospective study reviewing published data between 1989 and 2004 reported 74 women with 81 pregnancies with mechanical prostheses, most of which were mitral.[43] Thromboemboli occurred in 10 of the 81 pregnancies (12%); all these patients had mitral valve prostheses. In 9 of these 10 patients, a fixed dose regimen of LMWH had been used and all 10 were on LMWH throughout the entire pregnancy. The authors recommended, therefore, that meticulous monitoring of anti-Xa levels is necessary if LMWH is utilized.

If LMWH is utilized in the first trimester because the mother needs >5 mg warfarin daily, the fetus continues to be at increased risk from bleeding complications from the high warfarin dose. In this situation, physicians may choose to continue LMWH throughout pregnancy, although based on the study noted above,[42] whether this is the safest approach remains to be determined. As this heparin is not rapidly reversible, it should be withdrawn at least 24 h before delivery and either changed to unfractionated heparin, which can be terminated abruptly, or elective cesarean section considered.

Direct thrombin inhibitors

Currently, there are no data for the use of direct thrombin inhibitors such as bivalirudin for adequate anticoagulation in patients with PHV.

Biological valves

Biological valves have limited durability because of structural valve deterioration (SVD), i.e. thickening, progressive calcification, mechanical wear and tear/rupture of the valve.[44] Planned obsolescence of biological valves, chosen to provide time for one or more safe pregnancies, is often readily accepted by the potential parents, but it should be carefully explained to the patient who must understand that replacement of PHVs may be needed within a few years of the first operation.[3,31] This second surgery carries an appreciable risk and comes at a time when the children are still small and dependent on their parents. Even though unpredictable individually, the highest mortality rate of reoperation is seen in patients in New York Heart Association (NYHA) functional class III/IV, in those with impaired left ventricular function or prosthetic valve endocarditis, or in an emergency, but it is probably still almost 5% when carried out electively for an initial PHV. The patient must also survive the repetition of the risk during the first postoperative year when paravalvular leaks, embolism and prosthetic valve endocarditis may occur.[31]

Bioprostheses

Two studies have shown that the operative mortality rate for initial PHV insertion was 4.3%.[44,45] At the present time in experienced and skilled centers, it may be as low as 1–2% for aortic valve replacement (AVR) and 3–4% for mitral valve replacement (MVR). The data of Badduke et al.[45] and Jamieson et al.[44] showed that, after porcine bioprosthetic PHV placement, the incidence of SVD at 10 years was 55 and 76%; the incidence of PHV-related reoperation was 60–80%[44,45] (Table 9.2). The incidence of SVD in those who were subsequently pregnant versus those who were not was 76.7 ± 14% versus 25.8 ± 8.5% ($P <$ 0.05; values are percentages ± the standard deviation or SD) in one study and 55.3 ± 8.2% versus 45.7 ± 4.8% ($P =$ NS or non-significant) in another. The important issue is **not** similar rates of SVD in women with or without subsequent pregnancy, but the very high rate of bioprosthetic SVD in people aged 16–39 years at the time of initial PHV implantation: about 50% at 10 years and 90% at 15 years (Figure 9.1).[46] Furthermore, SVD begins 2–3 years after PHV implantation in this age group. The mortality rate of reoperation was 3.8–8.7% (Table 9.2).[44,45] At 9 years, the rate of SVD of newer porcine valves and the stentless porcine valves is within the expected range of SVD exhibited with earlier stented porcine valves, indicating at present that all porcine valves have similar

Table 9.2 Bioprosthesis and pregnancy: late complications (10 years)

	Badduke et al.[45]	Jamieson et al.[44]
Actuarial (%)		
SVD	76.7 ± 14	55.3 ± 8.2
Valve-related complication	78.3 ± 12.7	—
Valve-related reoperation	79.7 ± 12.4	59.8 ± 7.8
Non-actuarial (%)		
SVD	47.1	50.9
PHV endocarditis	11.8	5.7
Thromboembolism	5.9	5.7
Non-SVD	—	1.9
Sudden death	—	1.9
Total	70.6	66.1
Mortality rate of reoperation (%)	8.7	3.8

Values are expressed as mean ± SD or percentage.

SVD, structural valve deterioration; PHV, prosthetic heart valve.

From Hung and Rahimtoola.[3]

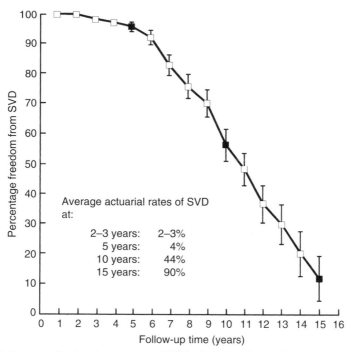

Figure 9.1 Structural valve deterioration (SVD) of aortic valve replacement porcine bioprosthesis (Stanford University): age 16–39 years at time of implantation. (Adapted from Yun et al.[46])

rates of SVD.[48] Although the rate of SVD at 10 and 15 years is usually pointed out to the patient as a reason for use of a bioprostheses, careful review of the data shows that after insertion of porcine bioprostheses in people aged 16–39 years SVD begins as early as 2 years and is about 10–15% at 5 years (Figure 9.1). Pregnancy by itself may be associated with SVD; the average rate was 24% (Table 9.3), which is partly accounted for by the expected early rate of SVD in young people[45] (Figure 9.1).

In addition, most women who have undergone an initial valve replacement for rheumatic valve disease have mitral valve disease and, thus, have mitral porcine bioprostheses, which have earlier onset of SVD and an overall incidence of SVD that is greater than with AVR. As a result, the incidence of SVD will be greater than cited above for AVR. Moreover, many are still in sinus rhythm when they have their children but may eventually develop atrial fibrillation, and will then require anticoagulant treatment. Patients with mitral valve disease have or develop left atrial enlargement and/or left atrial hypertension, which may result in thromboemboli, and also atrial fibrillation, which further increases the risks of thromboemboli.[31] Thus, use of a bioprosthesis is also associated with an incidence of emboli, which is similar in patients not taking anticoagulants to that in patients with mechanical prosthetic valves who are taking

Table 9.3 Bioprostheses and pregnancy: early structural valve deterioration (SVD)

References	No. of patients	No. of cases of early SVD	Percentage	Comments
Born et al.[17]	20	4	20	Needed reoperation during pregnancy or in puerperium
Bartolotti et al.[48]	7	2	29	<3 months after delivery
Salazar et al.[13]	5	3	60	During pregnancy and 7–12 months after pregnancy
Badduke et al.[45]	17	2	12	Reoperation 3–10 months after pregnancy
Hanania et al.[19]	42	5	12[a]	4–36 months after delivery
Sbarouni and Oakley[11]	49	17	35[b]	During pregnancy or soon after delivery
Total	**140**	**33**	**24**	

[a]Porcine valves

[b]Mainly porcine and few biological valves.

From Hung and Rahimtoola.[3]

Table 9.4 Reoperation for structural valve deterioration of biological valves

Bioprostheses/Homografts
- May be needed:
  - even before first pregnancy
  - during or soon after pregnancy
  - with increasing frequency up to 10–15 years
- Are associated with:
  - morbidity
  - mortality (babies/children will be without a biological mother)
- ≥ two to four reoperations may be needed over the woman's lifetime

anticoagulants. Increased risk of thromboembolism may be indicated by spontaneous echocardiographic contrast 'smoke' within the left atrium.[47,49]

In summary, three important issues need to be considered before a bioprosthetic PHV is implanted in a young woman before pregnancy (Table 9.4). Sbarouni and Oakley have asked: 'Why should young women be singled out for obligatory re-operation with this attendant risk?[11,31]

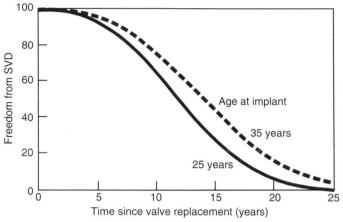

Figure 9.2 Structural valve deterioration (SVD) of homograft: aortic valve replacement by age at time of implant. (Adapted from Svensson et al.[51] and Takkenberg et al.[52])

Table 9.5 Key issues with regard to homograft valves

- More difficult to insert (requires reimplantation of coronary arteries)
- Perioperative myocardial infarction: about six % in those without associated coronary artery disease (CAD)
- Rate of structural valve deterioration (SVD) similar to bioprostheses
- More expensive than bioprostheses
- ≥ two to four reoperations may be needed over the woman's lifetime
- Reoperation(s) more difficult; requires repeat reimplantation(s) of coronary arteries. This is also true of reoperation on stentless bioprostheses

---

Pericardial bioprosthesis

There are limited data on pericardial bioprostheses in people aged 16–40 years at the time of the PHV. One non-peer-reviewed article probably shows somewhat lower rates of SVD than porcine bioprostheses.[51]

Homografts (allografts)

Homografts (allografts) have the same rate of SVD as porcine bioprostheses[50] (Figure 9.2). Data are not available for pregnant women and there are significant concerns with the use of homografts (Table 9.5 and see Table 9.4).

Autografts (pulmonary autograft for aortic valve replacement [Ross principle])

The Ross principle, first described by Donald Ross in 1967, involves two valve replacements for one valve disease.[53,54] It is a more complex and more difficult procedure, but does have some advantages, e.g. when inserted in children, the valve increases in size as the child grows. Of eight women who had fourteen pregnancies after receiving a pulmonary autograft, one woman developed dilated cardiomyopathy (?peripartum cardiomyopathy) 6 months after delivering, one developed obstruction of the unsupported fascial pulmonary valve and one developed acute endocarditis of the freeze-dried aortic homograft, which had been inserted in the pulmonary position. The remaining five patients were well at last follow-up.

A review of this procedure showed the following:

- Risk for thromboemboli was 0–1.2% per year.
- Risk of infective endocarditis was 0–1.2%.
- Reoperation within the first 6 months was 0, 1.5, 3.8 and 10% in four different studies.
- Late reoperation rates ranged from 0.4% to 1.5% per year.
- There is also a risk of rheumatic valvulitis in the autograft in those who have rheumatic heart valve disease.[55,56]

A recent study from Europe of patients, whose average age was 27 years at the time of the Ross principle operation, showed that the incidence of autograft dysfunction, defined as the development of moderate or severe aortic regurgitation, was 15% at 5 years and 25% at 7 years (Figure 9.3). In addition, associated aortic root dilatation in the young is about 58% at 7 years (Figure 9.4).

The only studies with a follow-up of >10 years are from Ross's group.[57,58–60] The freedom from autograft replacement ranged from 48.5 ± 13.7% at 19 years to 85% at 20 years;[3] the most likely explanation for this wide range is selection of patients reported in these four studies. In the series from the National Heart Hospital:[58]

- The operative mortality rate was 13%.
- In operative survivors (i.e. excluding operative mortality), late mortality rate was 40.5% and actuarially determined mortality rate at 15 and 20 years was 25% and 39%, respectively.
- Actuarially determined freedom from autograft replacement was 75% at 20 years.

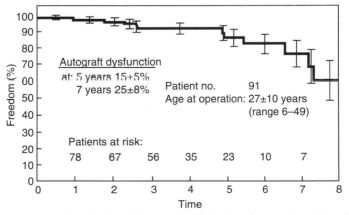

Figure 9.3 Ross principle: freedom from autograft dysfunction. (Adapted from Luciani et al.[61])

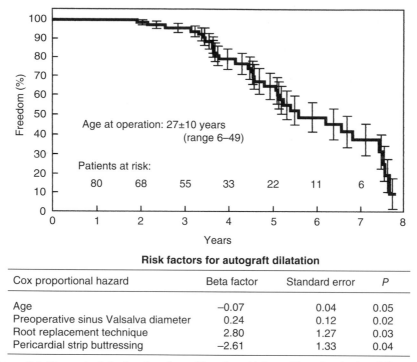

Risk factors for autograft dilatation

Cox proportional hazard	Beta factor	Standard error	P
Age	−0.07	0.04	0.05
Preoperative sinus Valsalva diameter	0.24	0.12	0.02
Root replacement technique	2.80	1.27	0.03
Pericardial strip buttressing	−2.61	1.33	0.04

Figure 9.4 Ross principle: freedom from dilatation. (Adapted from Luciani et al.[61])

From a patient's perspective, experience and skill in the performance of the Ross principle procedure is not as widely available when compared with that available for bioprostheses. In fact, Ross stated in an editorial from 2000 that the Ross procedure should be renamed the Ross principle because what is being performed today is very different from what he originally described.[54]

Reoperation to replace autografts may be more difficult (see Table 9.5). There is a need to replace the autograft as well as the aortic root and to repeat reimplantation of the coronary arteries. During the reoperation, homografts in the pulmonic position may also need to be replaced (Table 9.6).

Management strategies

The management of young women with valvular heart disease (VHD) who are contemplating a future pregnancy, the choice of PHV if one is necessary and the management of such patients during pregnancy were outlined by Hung and Rahimtoola in 2003 (Figure 9.5).[3] The choice of a PHV should be a joint decision by the patient, cardiologist and cardiac surgeon. In young women with a PHV, the importance of very early diagnosis of subsequent pregnancy needs to emphasized to the **patient** (Figure 9.6). It should be repeatedly emphasized to the patient that, if she misses a menstrual period and there is a possibility of a pregnancy, she should be tested immediately for pregnancy. If she is pregnant,

Table 9.6 Key issues concerning the Ross principle

- Two-valve replacements for one-valve disease
- Structural valve deterioration of homograft in the pulmonary position
- Rate of autograft dysfunction in young people about 25% at 7 years
- Rate of associated aortic root dilatation in young people about 58% at 7 years
- Very early autograft dysfunction in some patients (an incidence of up to 10%)
- Experience and skill not as widely available when compared with that available for bioprosthetic implantation
- Reoperation to replace autograft may be more difficult. Needs:
  - — replacement of autograft
  - — replacement of aortic root
  - — repeat reimplantation of coronary arteries
  - — homograft in pulmonary position may also need to be replaced

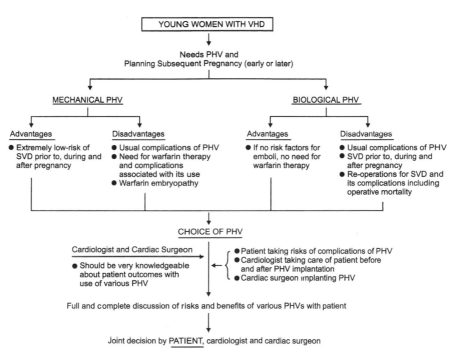

Figure 9.5 Young women with valvular heart disease (VHD) requiring prosthetic heart valve (PHV) and considering pregnancy. (Reproduced with permission from Hung and Rahimtoola.[3])

immediate consultation and joint care of the patient with a cardiologist and perinatologist should be sought.[31] If the woman has a mechanical prosthetic heart valve, then during weeks 6–12 of the pregnancy and before any type of delivery, warfarin should be discontinued and intravenous unfractionated heparin given. Warfarin crosses the placenta, the fetus is anticoagulated and there

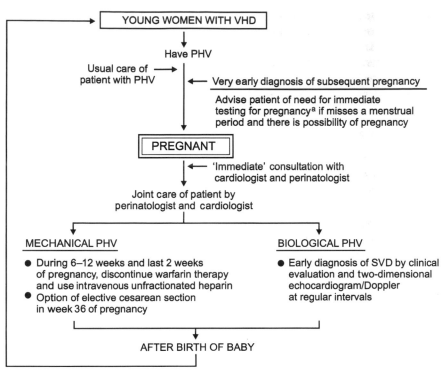

Figure 9.6 Young women with prosthetic valves and currently pregnant a Blood beta human chorionic gonadotropin. (Reproduced with permission from Hung and Rahimtoola.[3])

is a risk of intracranial hemorrhage during a vaginal delivery. Therefore, it is recommended to use intravenous unfractionated heparin in the last 4 weeks of pregnancy, which is discontinued before delivery.[33] Alternatively, there is the option for elective cesarean section.[16] If the patient has a biological PHV, there is a need for early diagnosis of SVD. Patients with aortic or mitral regurgitation (AR and MR, respectively) can cope with the volume load of pregnancy better than patients with severe valve stenosis, because the reduction of systemic vascular resistance during pregnancy favors a reduction in AR and MR. The volume load associated with pregnancy is not well tolerated in the presence of a severe valve stenosis (aortic stenosis defined as valve area $\leq 1.0\,cm^2$; $\leq 0.6\,cm^2/m^2$) or mitral stenosis (mitral valve area $\leq 1.5\,cm^2$).

Peripartum antimicrobial therapy

Prophylactic antibiotics

In patients with native VHD, the indications for antibiotic prophylaxis are the same as in the non-pregnant state to cover dental or other procedures or conditions likely to cause Gram-positive bacteraemia.[62]

The American Heart Association (AHA) position paper[62] and the subsequent American College of Cardiology (ACC)/AHA guidelines[63] do not recommend routine antibiotic prophylaxis in patients with VHD undergoing uncomplicated vaginal delivery, unless bleeding and tearing would occur, or with a Caesarean section, unless infection is suspected.[62] The AHA advises that antibiotics are indicated for high risk patients with PHVs, a previous history of endocarditis, complex congenital heart disease or a surgically constructed systemic-pulmonary conduit (Table 9.7).[62]

The Task Force on Infective Endocarditis of the European Society of Cardiology (ESC). Guidelines on Prevention, Diagnosis and Treatment recommends prophylaxis only in patients with high or moderate risk (so PHVs) undergoing gynaecological procedures in the presence of infection[64] but many practitioners routinely provide antibiotics.

The Task Force on Management of Cardiovascular Diseases During Pregnancy of the ESC advises that prophylaxis is indicated in patients with PHVs or previous endocarditis and may be chosen for anticipated normal delivery in other patients because complications are unpredictable. Antibiotics should be given before surgical delivery or cardiac surgery (Table 9.8).[65]

Table 9.7 American Heart Association recommendations for patients at high risk: cardiac conditions in which antimicrobial prophylaxis is indicated*

- Prosthetic heart valves
- Complex congenital cyanotic heart disease
- Previous infective endocarditis
- Surgically constructed systemic or pulmonary conduits
- Acquired valvular heart diseases
- Mitral valve prolapse with valvular regurgitation or severe valve thickening
- Non-cyanotic congenital heart diseases (except for secundum-type atrial septal defect) including bicuspid aortic valves
- Hypertrophic cardiomyopathy

*Adapted from Dajani et al.[62]

Table 9.8 The Task Force on the Management of Cardiovascular Diseases During Pregnancy of the ESC*

- Antibiotic prophylaxis is discretionary for anticipated normal delivery but should be given to patients with prosthetic heart valves or a history of endocarditis.
- Antibiotic prophylaxis may be chosen in other patients with anticipated normal delivery because complications are unpredictable.
- Antibiotics should be given to patients at risk of endocarditis before surgical intervention, cesarean delivery or cardiac surgery.

*Adapted from Oakley et al.[62]

The AHA official recommendations on prevention of infective endocarditis[62] advise antibiotic prophylaxis for normal delivery in patients with PHVs or previous endocarditis but The ACC/AHA Guidelines on management of VHD[63] state that antibiotics are optional in high risk patients (Eds.).

The incidence of bacteremia after normal delivery has been reported as between 0 and 5% and tends to include many different organisms.[30,62,63] Moreover, in clinical practice, it is not possible to guarantee that bleeding/tearing of the vagina/perineum will not occur and, therefore, we recommend routine antibiotic prophylaxis for delivery in all patients at risk of infective endocarditis.

Conclusions

Mechanical valves

- Patients with mechanical valves need close monitoring of warfarin therapy during pregnancy. Substitution of warfarin with intravenous unfractionated heparin in the first 6–12 weeks is associated with a low rate of warfarin embryopathy. The initiation of heparin therapy is clinically most feasible and practical at 4–6 weeks of pregnancy. Women who need <5 mg warfarin may be at low risk for fetal warfarin embryopathy and may receive warfarin throughout pregnancy, but more data are needed. Substitution of warfarin with intravenous unfractionated heparin in the last 2 weeks of pregnancy is associated with a reduced rate of bleeding in the baby during vaginal delivery and in the mother with vaginal delivery or with cesarean section.
- Subcutaneous heparin, LMWH and direct thrombin inhibitors cannot be recommended at the present time for use in these patients.
- If anticoagulation is needed, the use of LMWH is of concern because the FDA has cited the occurrence of both teratogenic and non-teratogenic effects with the use of LMWH. More data, including randomized trials, are needed.

Biological valves

- Both men and women aged 16–39 years at the time of bioprosthetic PHV implantation are at risk of SVD, which begins 2–3 years after valve replacement: at 10–15 years, the rate of SVD is very high (50–90%). Porcine bioprostheses have a risk of early SVD during or shortly after the end of pregnancy. Moreover, at 10 years there is a high rate of SVD (55%–77%) and valve-related reoperation (60–80%).
- One has to balance the risks of SVD and its consequences to the mother and family in those who receive a bioprosthetic PHV against the small risk of warfarin embryopathy in the fetus in those women who receive a mechanical PHV.
- There are limited data on the use of pericardial bioprostheses.
- There are limited data in patients who had received a homograft.
- More data are needed in patients who received a pulmonary autograft procedure according to the Ross principle.

references

1 DiSaia PJ. Pregnancy and delivery of a patient with a Starr–Edwards mitral valve prosthesis: report of a case. *Obstet Gynecol* 1966;**28**:469–72.
2 Hall JG. Embryopathy associated with oral anticoagulant therapy. *Birth Defects* 1965;**12**:133–40.

3 Hung L, Rahimtoola SH. Prosthetic heart valves and pregnancy. *Circulation* 2003;**107**:1240–6.

4 Hall JAG, Paul RM, Wilson KM. Maternal and fetal sequelae of anticoagulation during pregnancy. *Am J Med* 1980;**68**:122–40.

5 Sahul WL, Emery H, Hall JG. Chondrodysplasia punctata and maternal warfarin use during pregnancy. *Am J Dis Child* 1975;**129**:362.

6 Ben Ismail M, Abid F, Trabelsi S, Taktak M, Fekih M. Cardiac valve prostheses, anticoagulation and pregnancy. *Br Heart J* 1986;**55**:101–5.

7 Chen WWC, Chau CS, Lee PK et al. Pregnancy in patients with prosthetic heart-valves: an experience with 45 pregnancies. *Q J Med* 1982;**51**:358–65.

8 Larrea JL, Nunez L, Reque JA et al. Pregnancy and mechanical valve prosthesis: a high-risk situation for the mother and the fetus. *Ann Thorac Surg* 1983;**36**: 459–63.

9 Salazar E, Izaguirre R, Verdejo J et al. Failure of adjusted doses of subcutaneous heparin to prevent thrombo-embolic phenomena in pregnant patients with mechanical cardiac valve prosthesis. *J Am Coll Cardiol* 1996;**27**:1698–703.

10 Iturbe-Alessio I, del Carmen Fonseca M, Mutchinik O et al. Risks of anticoagulant therapy in pregnant women with artificial heart valves. *N Engl J Med* 1986;**315**: 1390–3.

11 Sbarouni E, Oakley CM. Outcome of pregnancy in women with valve prosthesis. *Br Heart J* 1994;**71**:196–201.

12 Chong MKB, Harvey D, Deswiet M. Follow-up study of children whose mothers were treated with warfarin during pregnancy. *Br J Obstet Gynaecol* 1984;**91**:1070–3.

13 Salazar E, Zajarias A, Gutierrez N et al. The problem of cardiac valve prosthesis, anticoagulant, and pregnancy. *Circulation* 1984;**70**(suppl 1):169–77.

14 Pavunkumar P, Venugopal P, Kaul U et al. Pregnancy in patients with prosthetic cardiac valve: a 10-year experience. *Scand J Thorac Cardiovasc Surg* 1988;**22**:9–22.

15 Sareli P, England MJ, Berk MR et al. Maternal and fetal sequelae of anticoagulation during pregnancy in patients with mechanical heart valve prostheses. *J Am Coll Cardiol* 1989;**63**:1462–5.

16 Cotrufo M, de Luca TSL, Calabro R et al. Coumadin anticoagulation during pregnancy in patients with mechanical valve prostheses. *Eur J Cardiothorac Surg* 1991;**5**:300–5.

17 Born D, Martinez EE, Almeida PAM et al. Pregnancy in patients with prosthetic heart valves: the effects of anticoagulation on mother, fetus, and neonate. *Am Heart J* 1992;**124**:413–17.

18 Wong V, Cheng CH, Chan KC. Fetal and neonatal outcome of exposure to anticoagulants during pregnancy. *Am J Med Genet* 1993;**45**:17–21.

19 Hanania G, Thomas D, Michel PL et al. Pregnancy in patients with valvular prostheses—retrospective cooperative study in France (155 cases). *J Arch Mal Coeur Vaiss* 1994;**87**:429–437.

20 Vitale N, Feo MD, DeSanto LS et al. Dose dependent fetal complications of warfarin in pregnant women with mechanical heart valves. *J Am Coll Cardiol* 1999;**33**:1637–41

21 LeSanto LS, Romano G, Corte AD et al. Mitral mechanical replacement in young rheumatic women: Analysis of long-term survival, valve-related complications, and pregnancy outcomes over a 3,707 patient-year follow-up. J Thorac Cardiovas Surg 2005;130:13–19.

22 Chan WC, Anand S, Ginsberg JS. Anticoagulation of pregnant women with mechanical valves: a systematic review of the literature. *Arch Intern Med* 2000;**160**:191–6.

23 Brill-Edwards P, Ginsberg JS, Johnston M, Hirsh J. Establishing a therapeutic range for heparin therapy. *Ann Intern Med* 1993; **119**:104–9.

24 Ginsberg JS, Kowalchuk G, Hirsh J et al. Heparin therapy during pregnancy—risks to the fetus and mother. *Arch Intern Med* 1989;**149**:2233–6.

25 Ginsberg JS, Barron WM. Pregnancy and prosthetic heart valves. *Lancet* 1994;**344**:1170–2.

26 Oakley CM. Anticoagulants in pregnancy.*Br Heart J* 1995;**74**:107–11.

27 Ginsberg JS, Hirsh J. Use of anticoagulants during pregnancy. *Chest* 1989;**95**: 156S–60S.

28 Ginsberg JS, Hirsh J. Anticoagulants during pregnancy. *Annu Rev Med* 1989;**40**:79–86.

29 Ginsberg JS, Barron WM. Pregnancy and prosthetic heart valves. *Lancet* 1994;**344**:1170–2.

30 Ginsberg JS, Greer I, Hirsh J. Use of anti-thrombotic agents during pregnancy. *Chest* 2001;**119**:122S–31S

31 Oakley C, ed. Artificial heart valves. In: *Heart Disease in Pregnancy.* London: BMJ Publishing Group, 1997: pp 135–46.

32 Ginsberg JS, Hirsh J. Use of anti-thrombotic agents during pregnancy. *Chest* 1998;**114**:524S–30S.

33 Salazar E, Zajarias A, Gutiarraz N, Iturbe I. The problem of cardiac valve prostheses: anticoagulants and pregnancy. *Circulation* 1984;**70**:169–77.

34 Whitfield LR, Lefe AS, Levy G. Effect of pregnancy on the relationship between concentration and anticoagulation action of heparin. *Clin Pharmacol Ther* 1983;**34**:23–8.

35 Bennett GG, Oakley CM. Pregnancy in a patient with mitral valve prosthesis. *Lancet* 1968;**i**:616–19.

36 Oakley CM. Clinical and pregnancy perspectives: anticoagulation. *Eur Heart J* 1995;**16**:1317–19.

37 Oakley CM. Anticoagulants in pregnancy. *Br Heart J* 1995;**74**:107–11.

38 Idir M, Madonna F, Rondant R. Collapse and massive pulmonary edema secondary to thrombosis of a mitral mechanical heart valve prosthesis during low-molecular weight heparin therapy. *J Heart Valve Dis* 1999;**8**:303–4.

39 FDA Med Watch. Available at: www.fda.gov/medwatch (accessed July 20, 2002).

40 Lee LH, Liauw PC, Ng AS. Low molecular weight heparin for thromboprophylaxis during pregnancy in 2 patients with mechanical mitral valve replacement. *Thromb Haemost* 1996;**76**:628–30.

41 Rowan JA, McCowan LM, Raudkivi PJ, North RA. Enoxaparin treatment in women with mechanical heart valves during pregnancy. *Am J Obstet Gynecol* 2001;**185**:633–7.

42 Bates SM, Greer IA, Hirsh J, Ginsberg JS. Use of antithrombotic agents during pregnancy: the Seventh ACCP Conference on Antithrombotic and Thrombolytic Therapy. *Chest* 2004;**126**(suppl 3):627S–44S.

43 Oran B, Lee-Parritz A, Ansell J. Low molecular weight heparin for the prophylaxis of thromboembolism in women with prosthetic mechanical heart valves during pregnancy. *Thromb Haemost* 2004;**92**:747–51.

44 Jamieson WRE, Miller DC, Akins CW et al. Pregnancy and bioprosthesis: influence on structural valve deterioration. *Ann Thorac Surg* 1995;**60**:S282–7.

45 Badduke ER, Jamieson RE, Miyashima RT et al. Pregnancy and childbearing in a population with biologic valvular prostheses. *J Thorac Cardiovasc Surg* 1991;**102**:179–86.

46 Yun KL, Miller DC, Moore KA et al. Durability of the Hancock MO bioprosthesis compared with the standard aortic valve bioprosthesis. *Ann Thorac Surg* 1995;**60**: 221–8.

47 Daniel WG, Nellessen U, Schroder E, Normast-Daniel B, Nikutta P, Lichtler PR. Left atrial spontaneous echo contrast in mitral valve disease: an indicator for increased thromboembolic risk. *J Am Coll Cardiol* 1988;**11**:1204–11.

48 Bartolotti U, Milano A, Massucco A et al. Pregnancy in patients with a porcine valve bioprosthesis. *Am J Cardiol* 1982;**50**:1051–4.

49 Butchart EG, Moreno de la Santa P, Rooney SJ, Lewis PA. The role of risk factors and trigger factors in cerebrovascular events after mitral valve replacement. *J Card Surg* 1994;9(suppl):228–36.

50 Grunkemeier GL, Li H-H, Naftel DC et al. Long-term performance of heart valve prosthesis. *Curr Probl in Cardiol* 2000;**25**:73–156.

51 Svensson LG, Blackstone EH, Cosgrove III OM. Surgical options in young adults with aortic valve disease. *G Curr Probl in Condiol* 2003;**28**:417–79.

52 Takkenberg JJ, van Herwerdeen LA, Eijkema NSMJ et al. Evolution of allograft aortic valve replacement over 13 years: Results of 275 procedures. *Eur J Cardio Thorac Surg* 2002;**21**:683–91.

53 Ross DN. Replacement of the aortic and mitral valves with a pulmonary autograft. *Lancet* 1967;**2**:956–81.

54 Ross DN. The pulmonary autograft: the Ross principle (or Ross procedural confusion). *J Heart Valve Dis* 2000;**9**:174–5.

55 Choudhary SK, Mather A, Chandler H et al. Aortic valve replacement with biological substitute. *J Cardiac Surg* 1998;**13**:1–8.

56 Pieters FAA, Al-Halees, Hade L et al. Results of the Ross operation in rheumatic versus non-rheumatic aortic valve disease. *J Heart Valve Dis* 2000;**9**:38–44.

57 Matsuki O, Oldta Y, Ahneida RS et al. Two decades experience with aortic valve replacement with pulmonary autograft. *J Thoracic Cardiovasc Surg* 1988;9••5:705–71.

58 Ross D, Jackson M, Davies J. Pulmonary autograft aortic valve replacement: long-term results. *J Cardiac Surg* 1991;**6**(suppl):529–33.

59 Ross D, Jackson M, Davies J. The pulmonary autograft: a permanent aortic valve. *Eur J Cardiothorac Surg* 1992;**6**:113–17.

60 Chambers JE, Somerville J, Stone S et al. Pulmonary autograft procedure for aortic valve disease: long-term results of the pioneer series. *Circulation* 1997;**96**:2206–14.

61 Luciani GB, Casali G, Favaro A et al. Fate of aortic not late after Ross operation. *Circulation* 2003;**108**(Suppl II):61–7.

62 Dajani AS, Taubert KA, Wilson W et al. Prevention of bacterial endocarditis: recommendations by the American Heart Association. *Circulation* 1997;**96**:358–66.

63 Bonow RD, Carabello B, Delern AC et al. ACC/AHA Guidelines for the management of patients with valvular heart disease. A report of the American college of Cardiology/American Heart Association Task Force on Practice Guidelines. *J Am Coll Cardiol* 1998;**32**:1486–588.

64 Horstkotte D, Follak F, Gutsehik E et al. The Task Force on Infective Endocarditis of the European Society of Cardiology. Guidelines on Prevention, Diagnosis and Treatment of Infective endocarditis. *Eur Heart J* 2004;**25**:267–76.

65 Oakley C, Child A, Iung B, Presbitero P, Tornos P, Expert Consensus Document on Management of Cardiovascular Diseases during Pregnancy, *Eur Heart J* 2003;**24**:761–81.

66 Baker TH, Hubbell R. Reappraisal of asymptomatic puerperal bacteremia. *Am J Obstet Gynecol* 1967;**97**:575–6.

CHAPTER 10

Management of pregnancy in Marfan syndrome, Ehlers–Danlos syndrome and other heritable connective tissue disorders

Lilian J Meijboom, Barbara JM Mulder

The major heritable disorders of connective tissue that may cause problems in obstetric management include Marfan syndrome, Ehlers–Danlos syndrome, osteogenesis imperfecta, pseudoxanthoma elasticum and achondroplasia.[1] Although individually rare, together they form an important group, requiring cooperative management by several specialists during pregnancy. Improved medical and surgical management permits affected women to reach childbearing age, but good advice should begin during family or individual counseling sessions, well before child bearing starts. The genetic risk, the possibilities of prenatal diagnosis and the obstetric risk to women should also be discussed later with the prospective parents and, if pregnancy is contraindicated, the alternatives of childlessness, adoption or ovum donation should be discussed.

Marfan syndrome

Marfan syndrome is an autosomal dominantly inherited connective tissue disorder with an estimated incidence of 1 in 5000. The syndrome involves many systems but the prominent manifestations are of skeletal, ocular and cardiovascular origin.[2] Aortic dilatation and dissection are the major causes of morbidity and mortality (Figure 10.1).[3,4] Marfan syndrome is the result of a mutation in the fibrillin gene on chromosome 15.[5] Genotype–phenotype correlations in Marfan syndrome have been complicated by the large number of unique mutations reported, as well as by clinical heterogeneity among individuals with the same mutation.[6,7] As a result of the intragenic heterogeneity, molecular genetic screening is hampered to a considerable extent, and the diagnosis of Marfan syndrome is still based mainly on clinical major and minor manifestations, as defined by a council of experts in the field, known as the Ghent nosology.[7,8] A

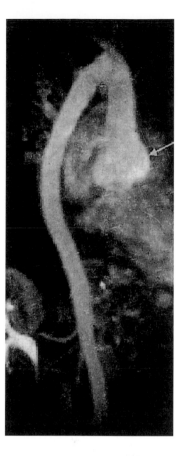

Figure 10.1 Magnetic resonance angiography of a dilated aortic root in a patient with Marfan syndrome.

definite diagnosis requires occurrence of major manifestations in two different categories, and involvement (presence of criteria) of a third category (Table 10.1). In clinical practice diagnosis should be established by a multidisciplinary team.

For women with Marfan syndrome, pregnancy presents a twofold problem: 50% risk of transmission of Marfan syndrome to the fetus and aortic dissection or progression of aortic dilatation in the mother.

Prenatal screening

If one parent has Marfan syndrome then there is a 50% chance in each pregnancy that the child (male or female) will inherit the dominant gene. In 25–30% of patients the syndrome arises as a spontaneous mutation in either the ovum or the sperm. If unaffected parents have such a child, the risk of recurrence in a subsequent pregnancy is the population prevalence (1 in 5000) and is negligible.

Currently pre-implantation diagnosis and prenatal diagnosis for Marfan syndrome are generally limited to those families in which the mutation in the

Table 10.1 Diagnostic criteria for Marfan syndrome

Category	Major criteria	Minor criteria
Family history	Independent diagnosis in parent, child, sibling	None
Genetics	Mutation *FBN-1*	None
Cardiovascular	Aortic root dilatation Dissection of ascending aorta	Mitral valve prolapse Calcification of the mitral valve (<40 years) Dilatation of pulmonary artery Dilatation/dissection of descending aorta
Ocular	Ectopia lentis	(Two needed): Flat cornea Myopia Elongated globe
Skeletal *	Pectus excavatum needing surgery Pectus carinatum Pes planus Wrist *and* thumb sign Scoliosis >20° or spondylolisthesis Arm span–height ratio >1.05 Protrusio acetabulae (radiograph, MRI) Diminished extension elbows (<170°)	Moderate pectus excavatum High narrowly arched palate Typical face Joint hypermobility
Pulmonary		Spontaneous pneumothorax Apical bullae
Skin		Unexplained stretch marks (striae) Recurrent or incisional herniae
Central nervous system	Lumbosacral dural ectasia (CT or MRI)	

*Presence of at least four of the manifestations listed under 'Major criteria' are necessary for the skeletal system to be classified as major feature. Presence of at least two of the manifestations listed under 'Major criteria' and at least two of the manifestations listed under 'Minor criteria' are necessary for the skeletal system to be involved (minor).

CT, computed tomography; MRI, magnetic resonance imaging.

FBN-1 gene is known. Mutation identification can be performed in individual cases but is time-consuming and, in about 20% of patients with a definite diagnosis of Marfan syndrome based on clinical findings, it is not possible to find a mutation.[9] On the other hand, polymorphism in the *FBN-1* gene can be found without any evidence of the disease.

The major advantage of pre-implantation diagnosis in comparison with prenatal diagnosis is the possibility of avoiding termination, which can be extremely distressing for the couples concerned. Another concern with respect to genetic counseling for prenatal diagnosis is the variability in phenotypic expressions, even within families. This wide clinical variability and the lack of clear-cut genotype–phenotype correlations make predictions about clinical severity difficult.[10] In a recent study two-thirds of patients expressed interest in using a prenatal test to determine whether their fetus would be affected with Marfan syndrome.[11] It is unknown in how many of these patients an elective abortion is performed.

Pregnancy and cardiovascular complications

During pregnancy important maternal cardiovascular changes occur, such as increases in blood volume, heart rate, stroke volume, cardiac output, left ventricular wall mass and end-diastolic dimensions.[12] In addition, hormonal changes occur, which lead to histological changes in the aorta. Fragmentation of the reticulum fibers, a diminished amount of acid mucopolysaccharides and loss of the normal corrugation of elastic fibers have been observed in the aortic wall of pregnant patients.[13] So, it has been suggested that both hemodynamic and hormonal mechanisms play an important role in the increased susceptibility to aortic dissection in women during pregnancy.

The aortic root diameter above which pregnancy should be discouraged in women with Marfan syndrome is still a matter of debate. The Canadian guidelines recommend that women with an aortic root diameter >44 mm should strongly be discouraged from becoming pregnant; the European guidelines discourage pregnancy above an aortic root diameter of 40 mm.[14,15] Both guidelines were based on three studies in which it became apparent that the risk for dissection was low in women with minimal cardiac involvement and an aortic root diameter <40 mm.[16–18] However, in these studies very few patients were included with aortic root diameters >40 mm.

In a recent prospective study no aortic dissections occurred in patients without previous aortic dissection and an aortic root diameter ≤45 mm.[19] Moreover, little to no change in aortic root diameter throughout pregnancy was observed. Only one woman known to have a previous type A dissection developed a type B dissection during her second pregnancy. So, pregnancy in women with Marfan syndrome seems to be relatively safe up to an aortic root diameter of 45 mm; however, a completely safe diameter does not exist. Also, in two studies it has been shown that pregnancy in women with Marfan syndrome has no negative effect on aortic root growth during long-term follow-up.[18,19]

In women with minimal cardiac involvement (aortic root diameter <45 mm, and no significant aortic or mitral regurgitation) pregnancy is relatively safe; however they should be told of a 1% risk of aortic dissection or other serious cardiac complications, such as endocarditis or congestive cardiac failure during pregnancy.[5,20] Family history and aortic growth should be taken into account when considering aortic surgery before pregnancy. Women with aortic root diameters >45 mm have an increased risk of developing aortic dissection during pregnancy; exact numbers are not known, however. We advocate that these women have an elective aortic root replacement before their pregnancy. Women with a previous dissection should be discouraged from becoming pregnant. In all women careful follow-up throughout pregnancy is mandatory. The third trimester of pregnancy, labour, delivery and the first month post partum carry the highest risk of aortic dissection.[17] Frequent echocardiographic imaging should be performed throughout pregnancy and the postpartum period to check for progressive aortic dilatation.

Dissection can occur without aortic dilatation. Severe chest or abdominal pain should be treated as possible aortic dissection and immediate ultrasound assessment of the entire aorta should be made. In a pregnant woman with a type A dissection, therapy should be aimed at saving two lives, and this is also determined by the gestational age of the fetus.[21] Before 28 weeks' gestation, aortic repair with the fetus kept *in situ* is recommended. If the fetus is truly viable (i.e. after 32 weeks' gestation) primary cesarean section followed by aortic repair, performed in one operative session, is the treatment of choice. Between 28 and 32 weeks' gestation, there is a dilemma, with the delivery strategy determined by the condition of the fetus. In the event of fetal distress, immediate delivery is mandatory. If aortic repair is well tolerated, treatment should be aimed at carrying the pregnancy as long as possible.[21] For type B dissection, medical treatment involving strict antihypertensive management is the preferred approach. Indications for surgery in pregnant women with type B dissection include leakage or rupture, progressive aortic dilatation, severe compromise of an arterial trunk, continued or recurrent pain, extension of the dissection while the patient is receiving adequate medical treatment or uncontrollable hypertension.[21,22]

In patients with Marfan syndrome, beta blockers should be started or continued during pregnancy, because it has been shown to slow down the rate of aortic dilatation and the occurrence of aortic complications in these patients.[23] Metoprolol, labetalol and atenolol are considered safe during pregnancy, but have been reported to cause some fetal problems when given early or mid-gestation.[24–26] In particular, atenolol has been linked with fetal growth retardation when given early in pregnancy. Clinical experience with labetalol is extensive and it is among the most widely used antihypertensive drugs in pregnancy.[27,28]

There is a lack of agreement as to the optimal treatment of pregnant women with prosthetic heart valves, much of which is based on the absence of adequate prospective controlled trials on this topic. Women should be informed fully about the importance of therapeutic anticoagulation throughout pregnancy and the maternal and fetal risk with each anticoagulant regimen, and should participate in the decision about which regimen to choose. In a pregnant woman with a mechanical prosthesis, the choice of anticoagulant therapy during the first trimester should take into account the greater thromboembolic risk with heparin and the risk of embryopathy with a vitamin K antagonist (warfarin). However, the use of vitamin K antagonist during the first trimester is the safest regimen for the mother. The current European recommendations are:[29]

either unfractionated heparin therapy until week 13, a change to warfarin until the middle of the third trimester, and then re-start unfractionated heparin therapy until delivery, or remain on warfarin and change to heparin only to cover elective cesarean section (see Chapter 9). Whatever the anticoagulation regimen, pregnancy in a patient with a mechanical prosthesis is associated with a maternal mortality rate of between 1 and 4%, mainly as a result of valve thrombosis while on heparin therapy, so this period should be as short as possible.

Outcome of pregnancy

Miscarriage under 20 weeks of pregnancy may be slightly more common in women with Marfan syndrome, mainly caused by a small group of women with Marfan syndrome who have habitual abortions.[17,30] It has been hypothesized that, as a result of genetic heterogeneity, certain patients may have a particular connective tissue abnormality associated with an increased risk of miscarriage.

An increased percentage of pre-term deliveries (15%) has been described mainly caused by pre-term premature rupture of the membranes (PPROM) and cervical incompetence. In a recent large study PPROM occurred in 5% of all pregnancies; in three other smaller Marfan studies the prevalence of PPROM varied between 0% and 2.5% in women with Marfan syndrome.[16,17,30,31] It is not yet known if there is a relationship present between PPROM and Marfan syndrome in the neonate, as has been described in Ehlers–Danlos syndrome. However, it is advisable not to take long journeys far from the intended center of delivery in the last month of pregnancy.

Presently, there has been no consensus about the optimal mode of delivery in women with Marfan syndrome. The concerns of vaginal delivery are the increase of systolic and diastolic blood pressure during each uterine contraction. The rise in systemic blood pressure depends on the magnitude and intensity of uterine contractions, position of the parturient, and the amount of pain and anxiety that the woman is feeling. It is unknown whether a cesarean section is safer in women with an enlarged aortic diameter. The concerns about cesarean delivery include:

- General anesthesia, if required, incurs blood pressure fluctuations associated with intubation and the anesthetic agent
- Increased blood loss, twice as great as with vaginal delivery
- Increased risk of wound and uterine infection
- Increased risk of thromboembolic complications.

Therefore, in every individual woman, especially in women with enlarged aortic diameters, the pros and cons of vaginal delivery and cesarean section should be given full consideration. Also, for patients with an enlarged aortic root diameter or previous elective Bentall operation, vaginal delivery with a short second stage of labour and a low threshold for assisted delivery (vacuum or forceps) is recommended. Women should preferably be placed in a left lateral recumbent position during labour in order to reduce volume shifts. Epidural anesthesia has been recommended for pain relief and thereby reduction of blood pressure and heart frequency. However, it should be noticed that in 95% of Marfan patients dural ectasia—one of the major criteria for Marfan syndrome—is present, which might result in considerable dilution of anesthetic medication.[32]

Endocarditis prophylaxis should be given in women with valve abnormalities in case of complicated delivery or cesarean section.[15,33]

In several studies the rate of neonatal death varied between 0% and 5%. In most of these children prematurity was the cause of death (making a cesarean section essential because the fetus will be anticoagulated and removing the option of a change to heparin before vaginal delivery in patients with mechanical valves). Fetal death occurred in about 2% of all pregnancies, which is slightly elevated compared with the general population.

Neonatal Marfan syndrome is rare and represents the most serious end of the spectrum of the disease. Presentation is characterized by massive mitral and tricuspid insufficiency, leading to congestive heart failure, failure to thrive, pulmonary hypertension and death shortly after birth.

Future pregnancies

Each woman with Marfan syndrome should be assessed cardiologically before starting a pregnancy. In our experience, couples who have an unaffected infant frequently go on to plan a second pregnancy. Those who have an affected infant often decide not to have further children. The wish to have children is a strong biological urge in some couples, but may not be as strong in others. For this reason, only the couples themselves, having taken expert advice from medical advisors, and after discussing the problem with their support team, including parents, brothers and sisters, and close friends, are capable of making the decision to have a child. Whatever the decision of the couple, the medical profession is always prepared to support the decision fully by providing the best medical and surgical care available to maximize the chance of a successful outcome of pregnancy for both the mother and the child.

Other options

Other reproductive options may be considered for two reasons: to minimize the cardiovascular risk for the mother and to avoid inheritance of the dominant gene in the child. Adoption of a child may be a good alternative. If the father has Marfan syndrome, artificial insemination by donor may be considered the genetic solution. The infant is then 50% genetically the offspring of the couple, and 100% the environmental child of the couple. For affected mothers with serious heart disease, a further possibility is to find a surrogate mother. Ovum donation would virtually eliminate the genetic risk. In vitro fertilization with pre-implantation diagnosis is a good possibility, with an average success rate (live births per transfer) of 30%.[34] Transferring more than one embryo increases the chance for a pregnancy, but also increases the risk of multiple gestation and the risk of dissection in women with Marfan syndrome.

Ehlers–Danlos syndrome

Ehlers–Danlos syndrome is a heterogeneous group of heritable disorders of connective tissue, characterized by skin extensibility, joint hypermobility and tissue fragility. The incidence is estimated at 1 in 5000 newborns.[35] In 1997 a new classification of Ehlers–Danlos syndrome in six major types has been proposed: classic (types I and II), hypermobility (type III), vascular (type IV), kyphoscoliosis (type VI), arthrochalasia (type VIIA and VIIB) and dermatosparaxis (type VIIC).[35] Most of the cases concern the classic type (60%), hypermobility type (30%) and vascular type (10%) and the remaining types are rare. Only the kyphoscoliosis and dermatosparaxis types inherit as autosomal recessive; the other types are autosomal dominant.

Pregnancy

Pregnancy is generally well tolerated in the classic and hypermobility types, with a favorable maternal and neonatal outcome.[36] During pregnancy the incidence of pelvic pain and instability is increased in women with Ehlers–Danlos syndrome (except for Ehlers–Danlos type 1). In all types, delivery may cause separation of the symphysis pubis and postpartum hemorrhage may be severe. Pre-term delivery occurs in about 20% of pregnancies in women with Ehlers–Danlos syndrome, preceded in most cases by PPROM. It has been shown that the membranes of fetuses with connective tissue disease have abnormal collagen content and are weaker than normal membranes.[37] Episiotomy and laparotomy incisions heal slowly, and perineal hematoma may occur despite an episiotomy. It is suggested that retention sutures should be used and that they should not be removed for at least 14 days, to avoid wound dehiscence. Affected infants tend to be hyperextensible and may have congenitally dislocated hips. Neonates may even be misdiagnosed as having neurological problems because of floppiness and bleeding disorders.

Vascular Ehlers–Danlos syndrome

Women with vascular Ehlers–Danlos syndrome (previous type IV) have an increased risk of complications of pregnancy as well as a 50% risk of having an affected child. Vascular Ehlers–Danlos syndrome, an autosomal dominant disorder caused by a mutation in the *COL3A1* gene, is of particular importance because this is the only form associated with a high risk of early death as a result of arterial, intestinal and uterine rupture.[38,39] Arterial complications are the leading cause of death in all patients with vascular Ehlers–Danlos syndrome because they are unpredictable and surgical repair is difficult as a result of tissue fragility. The medial survival in a recent series was 48 years.[38] Pepin et al. studied, retrospectively, 183 pregnancies in 81 women with vascular Ehlers–Danlos syndrome.[38] Twelve women died during the peripartum period or within 2 weeks of delivery (five of uterine rupture during labour, two of vessel rupture at delivery and five in the postpartum period after vessel rupture). Although several women died of uterus rupture at term, it is not yet known if elective cesarean section would decrease mortality. Pregnancy in women affected with vascular Ehlers–Danlos syndrome should be considered as high risk and followed at specialized centers. Special attention should be given during labour, delivery and the postpartum period. In theory, prenatal molecular diagnosis is possible for families with known mutations. In practice, however, this procedure can be risky if the affected parent is the mother, because of the need to perform obstetric procedures (chorionic villous sampling or amniocentesis).

Osteogenesis imperfecta

Osteogenesis imperfecta is a group of inherited connective tissue disorders in which the synthesis or structure of type 1 collagen, the major protein constituent of bone and many other connective tissues, is defective and causes osseous fragility. Other clinical features of these disorders may include joint laxity, dentinogenesis imperfecta, deafness and increased fragility of connective tissue. Severity varies widely, ranging from intrauterine fractures and perinatal lethality to very mild forms without fractures.[40] The clinical heterogeneity apparent in osteogenesis imperfecta is largely explained by different mutations in one of the two genes (*COL1A1* and *COL1A2*) that encode the two alpha chains of collagen type 1. Based on the pattern of inheritance, age at presentation, radiological features and natural history, Sillence et al. described four types of osteogenesis imperfecta, which provide the clinical framework for the diagnosis.[41] Type I is an autosomal dominant form with blue sclerae, normal height or mild short stature; type II is caused by a new mutation or parental mosaicism and results in death *in utero* or a few days after birth; type III is autosomal recessive (rare) or inherited as a result of parental mosaicism, with patients being very short with grayish sclerae, and having limb and spine deformities secondary to multiple fractures, which can lead to respiratory difficulties—identified as a leading cause of death in this patient group; and type IV is an autosomal dominant variety with mild-to-moderate bone deformity with grayish or white sclerae and variable short stature.

The prevalence of osteogenesis imperfecta as a group is about 1 in 10 000–12 000, whereas the incidence of each specific type is between 1 in 28 500 and 1 in 60 000.[39,42] Although prenatal diagnosis is possible with chorionic villous sampling, amniocentesis and detailed anomaly scan, it is known that expressivity of the autosomal dominant forms may vary greatly among family members and therefore does not reflect the fetal severity.[43]

Pregnancy and osteogenesis imperfecta

Women with osteogenesis imperfecta in pregnancy present a challenge to clinicians because there are potentially two patients with the disease. In addition to the mother with osteogenesis imperfecta, her baby has about a 25–50% chance of being affected.[44] Pregnancy can increase joint laxity, thereby affecting mobility in some patients besides exacerbating any pre-existing complications.

Complications during pregnancy include increasing respiratory compromise, especially in women with short stature and kyphoscoliosis, cephalopelvic disproportion as a result of previous pelvic fractures, uterine rupture, and separation of the symphysis pubis.[45] Severe back pain is a common complication (13%) during and after pregnancy in women with osteogenesis imperfecta. In many of these cases the back pain could be related to crush fractures of vertebrae.[46]

Few evidence-based guidelines exist for obstetric management of fetuses affected with any form of osteogenesis imperfecta. Recently, neonatal outcome was studied for 167 pregnancies in which the diagnosis of osteogenesis imperfecta was made perinatally.[47] cesarean delivery did not decrease fracture rates at birth in infants with non-lethal forms of osteogenesis imperfecta, but nor did it prolong survival for those with lethal forms. Although there is only one study with regard to the best mode of delivery, vaginal delivery is to be anticipated with cesarean section reserved for the usual maternal and fetal indications. Cephalopelvic disproportion resulting from maternal pelvic fractures indicates that there is a need for assessment of the maternal pelvis before and during pregnancy and this may be the indication for cesarean delivery.

If vaginal delivery is chosen, instrumentation should be minimized with the most severely affected fetuses to avoid intracranial trauma. Delivery in a tertiary center is recommended, if a severe but non-lethal form of osteogenesis imperfecta is suspected. Mothers are prone to accelerated bone loss after pregnancy and breast-feeding, so it may be appropriate to advise the avoidance of long periods of breast-feeding.[48] General anesthesia is associated with an increased risk of malignant hyperthermia, and spinal or epidural anesthesia may lead to fracture of osteoporotic vertebrae.[49] Endotracheal intubation may be difficult because of limited cervical spine movement, brittle teeth and receding mandible.[46] If technically possible, epidural anesthesia may be preferable. An arterial line can be inserted for blood pressure monitoring if arterial blood gas analysis is also required. Otherwise, digital blood pressure monitoring is adequate. Temperature should be monitored continuously, and a cooling blanket and cold intravenous fluids be available.

Pseudoxanthoma elasticum

Pseudoxanthoma elasticum is a genetic multisystem disorder characterized by calcified dystrophic elastic fibers in the skin, retina and arteries. The underlying defect is a mutation in the *ABCC6* gene on chromosome 16 that encodes an ATP-binding cassette transporter.[50,51] The incidence has been estimated at 1 in 25000–50000. Clinically pseudoxanthoma elasticum is characterized by yellowish papules and plaques, with or without cutaneous laxity, on flexural areas such as the side of the neck, elbow crease and armpit. Vascular complications include intermittent claudication, premature coronary and cerebral vascular disease, and gastrointestinal hemorrhage.[52] The retina demonstrates angioid streaks (thin cracks in the retina caused by calcified elastic fibers) that may be associated with subretinal neovascularization, hemorrhage and central visual loss. The heart may be affected by endomyocardial fibrosis so a full cardiovascular appraisal with echocardiography and magnetic resonance imaging (MRI) is advisable.

Pregnancy and pseudoxanthoma elasticum

In a recent large study of 795 pregnancies in 407 women with pseudoxanthoma elasticum, 83% ended in live births and 1% in stillbirths.[53] Hypertension occurred in 10% of pregnancies, and gastric bleeding and retinal complications in <1%. Although 12% of pregnancies were associated with worsening of skin manifestations, there was no correlation of either gravidity or ever having been pregnant with ultimate severity of skin, ocular or cardiovascular manifestations. There is no basis for advising women with pseudoxanthoma elasticum to avoid becoming pregnant, because most pregnancies in such women are uncomplicated. Pseudoxanthoma elasticum is mostly inherited as an autosomal recessive trait. Therefore the risk of a woman with pseudoxanthoma elasticum having affected offspring is very low unless the father is a carrier of a pseudoxanthoma elasticum mutation.

Achondroplasia

Achondroplasia is the most common cause of dwarfism, with an estimated prevalence between 1 in 15 000 and 1 in 40 000.[39] It is inherited as an autosomal dominant trait with complete penetrance, but about 80% of cases represent spontaneous mutations. All women with achondroplasia should be delivered by cesarean section because the maternal pelvis is invariably small and contracted, resulting in cephalopelvic disproportion. Pregnancy may cause cardiorespiratory problems (resulting from the small chest cavity). General anesthesia should be used because spinal stenosis, osteophytes, short pedicles or a small epidural space makes conduction anesthesia difficult. This increases the risk of dural puncture, and may limit the spread of local anesthetic. If epidural anesthetic is necessary, attempting puncture above the lordotic lumbar spine may permit easier location and catheterization of the epidural space. A low dose of epidural anesthetic is usually sufficient. Cervical spine instability can lead to increased difficulty with tracheal intubation, necessitating the use of a small tracheal tube.[54 58]

References

1 Royce PM, Steinmann B, eds. *Connective Tissue and Its Heritable Disorders*. New York: Wiley-Liss, 1993.
2 Pyeritz RE, McKusick VA. The Marfan syndrome: diagnosis and management. *N Engl J Med* 1979;**300**:772–7.
3 Groenink M, Lohuis TA, Tijssen JG et al. Survival and complication free survival in Marfan's syndrome: implications of current guidelines. *Heart* 1999;**82**:499–504.

4 Silverman DI, Burton KJ, Gray J et al. Life expectancy in the Marfan syndrome. *Am J Cardiol* 1995;**75**(2):157–60.

5 Dietz HC, Cutting GR, Pyeritz RE et al. Marfan syndrome caused by a recurrent de novo missense mutation in the fibrillin gene. *Nature* 1991;**352**:337–9.

6 Collod-Béroud G, Le Bourdelles S, Ades L et al. Update of the UMD-FBN1 mutation database and creation of an FBN1 polymorphism database. *Hum Mutat* 2003;**22**: 199–208.

7 De Paepe A, Devereux RB, Dietz HC, Hennekam RC, Pyeritz RE. Revised diagnostic criteria for the Marfan syndrome. *Am J Med Genet* 1996;**62**:417–26.

8 Dietz HC, Pyeritz RE. Mutations in the human gene for fibrillin-1 (FBN1) in the Marfan syndrome and related disorders. *Hum Mol Genet* 1995;**4**(Spec):1799–809.

9 Loeys B, Nuytinck L, Delvaux I, De Bie S, De Paepe A. Genotype and phenotype analysis of 171 patients referred for molecular study of the fibrillin-1 gene FBN1 because of suspected Marfan syndrome. *Arch Intern Med* 2001;**161**:2447–54.

10 Loeys B, Nuytinck L, Van Acker P et al. Strategies for prenatal and preimplantation genetic diagnosis in Marfan syndrome (MFS). *Prenat Diagn* 2002;**22**(1):22–8.

11 Peters KF, Kong F, Hanslo M, Biesecker BB. Living with Marfan syndrome III. Quality of life and reproductive planning. *Clin Genet* 2002;**62**:110–20.

12 Robson SC, Hunter S, Boys RJ et al. Serial study of factors influencing changes in cardiac output during human pregnancy. *Am J Physiol* 1989;**256**:H1060–5.

13 Manalo-Estrella P, Barker AE. Histopathologic findings in human aortic media associated with pregnancy. *Arch Pathol* 1967;**83**:336–41.

14 Expert Consensus Document on management of cardiovascular diseases during pregnancy. *Eur Heart J* 2003;**24**:761–81.

15 Therrien J, Gatzoulis M, Graham T et al. Canadian Cardiovascular Society Consensus Conference 2001 update: Recommendations for the Management of Adults with Congenital Heart Disease—Part II. *Can J Cardiol* 2001;**17**:1029–50.

16 Lipscomb KJ, Smith JC, Clarke B, Donnai P, Harris R. Outcome of pregnancy in women with Marfan's syndrome. *Br J Obstet Gynaecol* 1997;**104**:201–6.

17 Pyeritz RE. Maternal and fetal complications of pregnancy in the Marfan syndrome. *Am J Med* 1981;**71**:784–90.

18 Rossiter JP, Repke JT, Morales AJ, Murphy EA, Pyeritz RE. A prospective longitudinal evaluation of pregnancy in the Marfan syndrome. *Am J Obstet Gynecol* 1995;**173**: 1599–606.

19 Meijboom LJ, Vos FD, Timmermans J, Boers F, Zwinderman AH, Mulder BJM. Pregnancy and aortic growth in the Marfan syndrome; a prospective study. *Eur Heart J* 2005;**26**:914–20.

20 De Bie S, De Paepe A, Delvaux I, Davies S, Hennekam RC. Marfan syndrome in Europe. *Community Genet* 2004;**7**:216–25.

21 Zeebregts CJ, Schepens MA, Hameeteman TM, Morshuis WJ, de la Riviere AB. Acute aortic dissection complicating pregnancy. *Ann Thorac Surg* 1997;**64**:1345–8.

22 Borst HG, Heineman MK, Stone CD. *Surgical Treatment of Aortic Dissection*. New York: Churchill Livingstone, 1996: pp 47–54, 282.

23 Shores J, Berger KR, Murphy EA, Pyeritz RE. Progression of aortic dilatation and the benefit of long-term beta-adrenergic blockade in Marfan's syndrome. *N Engl J Med* 1994;**330**:1335–41.

24 Butters L, Kennedy S, Rubin PC. Atenolol in essential hypertension during pregnancy. *BMJ* 1990;**301**:587–9.

25 Lip GY, Beevers M, Churchill D, Shaffer LM, Beevers DG. Effect of atenolol on birth weight. *Am J Cardiol* 1997;**79**:1436–8.

26 Rosenthal T, Oparil S. The effect of antihypertensive drugs on the fetus. *J Hum Hypertens* 2002;**16**:293–8.

27 Pickles CJ, Broughton PF, Symonds EM. A randomised placebo controlled trial of labetalol in the treatment of mild to moderate pregnancy induced hypertension. *Br J Obstet Gynaecol* 1992;**99**:964–8.

28 Sibai BM, Mabie WC, Shamsa F, Villar MA, Anderson GD. A comparison of no medication versus methyldopa or labetalol in chronic hypertension during pregnancy. *Am J Obstet Gynecol* 1990;**162**:960–6.

29 Expert Consensus Document on management of cardiovascular disease during pregnancy. *Eur Heart J* 2003;**24**:761–81

30 Meijboom LJ, Drenthen W, Pieper PG et al., on behalf of the ZAHARA investigators. Obstetric complications in the Marfan syndrome. *Int J Cardiol* 2006;**110**:53–9.

31 Lind J, Wallenburg HC. The Marfan syndrome and pregnancy: a retrospective study in a Dutch population. *Eur J Obstet Gynecol Reprod Biol* 2001;**98**:28–35.

32 Oosterhof T, Groenink M, Hulsmans FJ et al. Quantitative assessment of dural ectasia as a marker for Marfan syndrome. *Radiology* 2001;**220**:514–18.

33 American Heart Association. Guidelines for endocarditis prophylaxis. *JAMA* 1997;**227**:1794–801.

34 Nyboe Andersen A, Gianaroli L, Nygren KG. Assisted reproductive technology in Europe, 2000. Results generated from European registers by ESHRE. *Hum Reprod* 2004;**19**:490.

35 Beighton P, De Paepe A, Steinman B, Tsipouras P, Wenstrup RJ. Ehlers–Danlos syndromes: revised nosology, Villefranche 1997. *Am J Med Genet* 1998;**77**:31–7.

36 Lind J, Wallenburg IISC. Pregnancy and Ehlers–Danlos syndrome: a retrospective study in a Dutch population. *Acta Obstet Gynaecol Scand* 2002;**81**:293–300.

37 Parry S, Strauss JF 3rd. Premature rupture of the fetal membranes. *N Engl J Med* 1998;**338**:663–70.

38 Pepin M, Schwarze U, Superti-Furga A, Byers PH. Clinical and genetic features of Ehlers–Danlos syndrome type IV, the vascular type. *N Engl J Med* 2000;**342**:673–80.

39 Orioli IM, Castilla EE, Barbosa-Neto JG. The birth prevalence rates for the skeletal dysplasias. *J Med Genet* 1986;**23**:328–32.

40 Shapiro JR, Stover ML, Burn VE et al. An osteopenic nonfracture syndrome with features of mild osteogenesis imperfecta associated with the substitution of a cysteine for glycine at triple helix position 43 in the pro alpha 1(I) chain of type I collagen. *J Clin Invest* 1992;**89**:567–73.

41 Sillence DO, Senn A, Danks DM. Genetic heterogeneity in osteogenesis imperfecta. *J Med Genet* 1979; **16**:101–16.

42 Andersen PE Jr, Hauge M. Osteogenesis imperfecta: a genetic, radiological, and epidemiological study. *Clin Genet* 1989;**36**:250–5.

43 Carlson JW, Harlass FE. Management of osteogenesis imperfecta in pregnancy. A case report. *J Reprod Med* 1993;**38**:228–32.

44 Sharma A, George L, Erskin K. Osteogenesis imperfecta in pregnancy: two case reports and review of literature. *Obstet Gynecol Surv* 2001;**56**:563–6.

45 Young BK, Gorstein F. Maternal osteogenesis imperfecta. *Obstet Gynecol* 1968;**31**:461.

46 Mcallion SJ, Paterson CR. Musculo-skeletal problems associated with pregnancy in women with osteogenesis imperfecta. *J Obstet Gynecol* 2002;**22**:169–72.

47 Cubert R, Cheng EY, Mack S, Pepin MG, Byers PH. Osteogenesis imperfecta: mode of delivery and neonatal outcome. *Obstet Gynecol* 2001;**97**:66–9.

48 Smith R, Phillips AJ. Osteoporosis during pregnancy and its management. *Scand J Rheumatol Suppl* 1998;**107**:66–7.

49 Solomons CC, Myers DN. Hyperthermia of osteogenesis imperfecta and its relationship to malignant hyperthermia. In: Gordon RA, Gritt BA, Kalow W (eds), *International Symposium on Malignant Hyperthermia*. Springfield, III: Thomas 1971: p 319.

50 Le Saux O, Urban Z, Tschuch C et al. Mutations in a gene encoding an ABC transporter cause pseudoxanthoma elasticum. *Nat Genet* 2000;**25**:223.

51 Bergen AA, Plomp AS, Schuurman EJ et al. Mutations in ABCC6 cause pseudoxanthoma elasticum. *Nat Genet* 2000;**25**:228.

52 Neldner K. Pseudoxanthoma elasticum. *Clin Dermatol* 1988;**6**:1–156.

53 Bercovitch L, Leroux T, Terry S, Weinstock MA. Pregnancy and obstetrical outcomes in pseudoxanthoma elasticum. *Br J Dermatol* 2004;**151**:1011–18.

54 Kuczkowski KM. Labour analgesia for the parturient with an uncommon disorder: a common dilemma in the delivery suite. *Obstet Gynecol Surv* 2003;**58**:800–3.

55 Monedero P, Garcia-Pedrajas F, Coca I, Fernandez-Liesa JI, Panadero A, de los Rios J. Is management of anesthesia in achondroplastic dwarfs really a challenge? *J Clin Anesth* 1997;**9**:208–12.

56 Wardall GJ, Frame WT. Extradural anaesthesia for caesarean section in achondroplasia. *Br J Anaesth* 1990;**64**:367–70.

57 Carstoniu J, Yee I, Halpern S. Epidural anaesthesia for caesarean section in an achondroplastic dwarf. *Can J Anaesth* 1992;**33**:708–11.

58 Lattanzi DR, Harger JH. Achondroplasia and pregnancy. *J Reprod Med* 1982;**27**:363–6.

Note: This chapter is based on Chapter 12 by Anne Child in the first edition of Heart Disease in Pregnancy.

CHAPTER 11

Heart disease, pregnancy and systemic autoimmune diseases

Guillermo Ruiz-Irastorza, Munther A Khamashta,
Graham RV Hughes

The heart can be involved during the course of many systemic autoimmune diseases. Specific manifestations include pericardial disease, myocarditis/cardiomyopathy, valve disease, heart block, aortitis, systemic or pulmonary hypertension, and myocardial infarction.

Many patients who have this group of diseases are women in their childbearing years. Pregnancy can modify the clinical course of the disease and itself be greatly influenced by the development of a number of complications in these high-risk patients. Heart disease can be a major problem in pregnant women with systemic autoimmune diseases, with a definite influence on the prognosis of both the mother and the baby. This chapter reviews the cardiac manifestations associated with the different systemic autoimmune diseases, as well as the mutual influence of these conditions on pregnancy. Several specific, high-risk situations will be analyzed from the clinical management point of view.

Systemic autoimmune diseases and the heart (Table 11.1)

Systemic lupus erythematosus and anti-phospholipid syndrome

Systemic lupus erythematosus (SLE) is a disease with a wide spectrum of clinical manifestations. The skin and the musculoskeletal system are most frequently involved, although lupus can affect virtually any organ of the body. Lupus nephritis, interstitial lung disease, hemolytic anemia, thrombocytopenia and psychosis are examples of visceral involvement in SLE.[1] A number of autoantibodies are frequently found in lupus patients. Antinuclear antibodies (ANAs) are almost universal. Among them, antibodies with specificity, such as anti-DNA, anti-Ro, anti-La, anti-Sm and anti-U_1RNP, appear with variable frequency, and correlate with specific clinical features (e.g. nephritis, sicca syndrome or Raynaud's disease). Being a disease with a wide spectrum of manifestations, the diagnosis of lupus relies mostly on clinical judgment and the presence of these serologic markers. The widely used classification criteria of the American College of Rheumatology (ACR), updated in 1997,[2,3] were not meant for clinical diagnosis but have become useful tools for the correct inclusion of lupus patients

Table 11.1 Cardiac complications in systemic autoimmune diseases

Condition	Cardiac manifestations
Systemic lupus erythematosus	Pericarditis
	Myocarditis (rare)
	Valvular disease
	Arterial (coronary thrombosis)
	Systemic hypertension
	Pulmonary hypertension
	Congenital heart block
Anti-phospholipid syndrome	Valvular disease
	Arterial (coronary thrombosis)
	Systemic hypertension
	Pulmonary hypertension
Systemic sclerosis	Pericarditis (rare)
	Myocarditis
	Myocardial fibrosis
	Conduction defects
	Coronary artery disease
	Pulmonary hypertension
Inflammatory myopathies	Heart failure
	Arrhythmias
	Vasospastic angina
	Pericarditis (rare)
Mixed connective tissue disease	Pericarditis
	Pulmonary hypertension
	Myocarditis
	Conduction defects
Vasculitis	Coronary aneurysms
	Myocardial ischemia
	Heart failure
	Large vessel inflammation
	Thrombosis
	Aneurysm of the sinus of Valsalva

in research projects. However, clinical features within the ACR list, as well as others such as history of glandular fever, recurrent miscarriage, oral and/or ocular dryness, or childhood 'rheumatism'[4] should alert the clinician to the diagnosis of SLE.

Anti-phospholipid antibodies (aPLs), including anticardiolipin antibodies (aCLs) and lupus anticoagulant (LA), appear in about 40% of lupus patients. These antibodies correlate with recurrent thrombosis and obstetric complications, such as miscarriage, fetal loss and prematurity.[5] The development of such clinical features in the presence of persistently positive aPLs constitutes the anti-phospholipid syndrome (APS), which can occur in the context of SLE, other autoimmune diseases or as primary APS.[6]

The heart is often involved in SLE.[7] Pericarditis is the most frequent cardiac manifestation of lupus and is indistinguishable from other forms of acute pericarditis. It is usually recurrent, associated with pleural disease and characteristically shows low complement levels in the pericardial fluid. Lupus serositis usually responds well to steroids and antimalarials.

Valvular disease has a strong association with the presence of aPLs. The mitral and aortic valves are the most frequently involved, regurgitation being more common than stenosis. The severity of valve disease is variable, sometimes leading to frank hemodynamic compromise that requires a surgical approach. Systemic emboli are another potential complication of valve lesions in SLE and APS. Medical management is not well established because neither corticosteroids nor anti-thrombotic/anticoagulant drugs have shown clear efficacy in preventing progression.[8] Many patients experience eventual hemodynamic deterioration that requires surgical valve replacement.[9] Cardiac surgery may be particularly complicated in these patients, with an increased frequency of thromboembolic complications and late structural deterioration of the prosthetic valves.[10]

Lupus patients are at increased risk of coronary artery thrombosis.[11] Atherosclerosis is more prevalent in this group[12] and coronary thrombosis has been described in the context of APS.[8] Strict control of vascular risk factors, along with anti-thrombotic therapy in aPL-positive lupus patients and anticoagulation in those with APS and any form of thrombosis, is recommended.[13] Recent data point to a protective effect of antimalarials against thrombosis.[14]

Pulmonary hypertension (PHT) is a rare but potentially lethal complication of SLE and APS.[15] The exact prevalence in both conditions is not well defined; however, severe symptomatic forms are fortunately infrequent. Risk factors for the development of PHT in patients with SLE are controversial, some studies showing an increased risk for PHT among patients with Raynaud's disease, anti-U_1RNP and aPLs.[16,17]

Congenital heart block (CHB) is a rare complication suffered by babies born to mothers with anti-Ro and anti-La antibodies, in a unique model of passive autoimmunity.[18] Incomplete forms of CHB can be seen. However, complete heart block is the most frequent form of presentation.[19,20]

Systemic sclerosis

Systemic sclerosis is a condition with a hallmark of the proliferation of cutaneous fibroblasts leading to tightening of the skin (scleroderma, or 'hard skin' in Greek). Raynaud's disease is almost universal in patients with systemic sclerosis. Visceral involvement is frequent. Diffuse forms of the disease (i.e. those affecting the skin of the trunk as well as of the face and extremities) tend to involve the esophagus, kidney (malignant hypertension) and lungs (interstitial disease), and express antibodies against topoisomerase 1 (anti-Scl-70). Limited forms (i.e. those sparing the skin of the trunk) do not usually affect the kidney or the lung parenchyma. Instead, patients with limited systemic sclerosis develop PHT at a higher frequency, as well as **c**alcinosis, **R**aynaud's disease, **e**sophageal disease, **s**clerodactyly and **t**elangiectasias (CREST syndrome). Anticentromere antibodies are the marker of this form of scleroderma.[21]

The heart can be involved during the course of systemic sclerosis in several forms.[22] Pericardial disease is not as common as in other connective tissue diseases, such as SLE. Clinically silent conduction defects or arrhythmias are frequent, although overt tachybradycardia is rare. The myocardium can be affected by the fibrotic process that takes place in systemic sclerosis; systolic and diastolic dysfunction are seen in late phases of the disease.

PHT is the most severe organic complication of both limited and diffuse systemic sclerosis.[21] The usual clinical patterns are two: limited scleroderma–anticentromere antibodies–vascular arterial PHT and diffuse scleroderma–anti-Scl70 antibodies–secondary (to lung fibrosis) PHT. However, a minority of patients with limited forms can develop pulmonary fibrosis, and some patients with diffuse systemic sclerosis can suffer vascular PHT, usually in the presence of nucleolar antinuclear antibodies.[21] Transthoracic Doppler echocardiography has a good correlation with right-sided catheterization,[23] an estimated pulmonary arterial systolic pressure ≥30 mmHg being the usual threshold for the definition of PHT. In addition, a decreasing diffusing capacity for carbon monoxide (D_{LCO}) in the absence of significant interstitial involvement of the lungs is a good predictor of the presence of PHT and can be used together with echocardiography.

Cardiopulmonary complications are nowadays the leading causes of death in patients with both forms of systemic sclerosis.[24] Therefore, early detection and treatment of these conditions are a major issue in the management of patients with scleroderma.

Inflammatory myopathies

Inflammatory myopathies include polymyositis (PM), dermatomyositis (DM) and inclusion body myositis. The last type, usually refractory to immunosuppressive treatment, affects older patients, so pregnancy is an infrequent event in this group. PM and DM share common features in terms of muscle involvement; however, they are completely different diseases from the clinical (cutaneous involvement in DM), pathologic (perimysial inflammatory infiltration in DM, endomysial in PM) and pathogenetic points of view (humoral, or T-helper 2 or Th2 autoimmune response in DM, cellular or Th1 in PM). Both PM and DM can be complicated by pulmonary involvement, usually interstitial disease associated with the presence of anti-tRNA synthetase antibodies, the most common of which are anti-histidyl-tRNA synthetase (anti-Jo1) antibodies.[25]

Despite the muscular myocardium, clinically evident heart involvement seems to be infrequent in the context of systemic inflammatory myopathies.[26] Systolic dysfunction is not a major issue, except for a small subgroup of patients with antibodies against signal recognition particle (anti-SRP), who develop a form of severe PM with associated cardiomyopathy.[25] Conduction defects and pericardial involvement have occasionally been described.[26] PHT secondary to extensive pulmonary fibrosis is a rare event.

Mixed connective tissue disease

Mixed connective tissue disease (MCTD) shares features of SLE, systemic sclerosis and inflammatory myopathies, with Raynaud's disease as a prominent symptom. The serological markers of this condition are anti-U_1RNP antibodies.

Cardiovascular manifestations in MCTD include pericarditis, mitral valve prolapse and, more rarely, myocarditis and conduction defects.[26] The most feared cardiovascular complication is PHT. From a clinical and pathological point of view, PHT seen in patients with MCTD is similar to that seen in patients with SLE and CREST.[27]

Systemic vasculitis

Cardiac involvement is not frequent in systemic vasculitis.[28] The most characteristic condition is Kawasaki's disease, which is typically complicated by coronary artery aneurysms, usually in children. Myocardial ischemia can be a feature of polyarteritis nodosa and Churg–Strauss syndrome, often presenting as heart failure.[29] It is less common in ANCA-positive small-vessel vasculitis (Wegener's granulomatosis and micropolyangiitis). Involvement of the large vessels is typical of temporal arteritis, which almost invariably occurs in patients aged over 50, and Takayasu's arteritis, affecting young women.

Thrombosis, usually venous, is one of the possible complications of Behçet's disease, a condition characterized by recurrent oral and genital ulcers, and recurrent uveitis.[30] Aneurysms, endomyocardial fibrosis and conduction defects have also been reported.[31]

Pregnancy and systemic autoimmune diseases

Pregnancy is a critical period for many women with autoimmune diseases. Effects are reciprocal, i.e. pregnancy can modify the course of the disease and the latter can also influence the prognosis of pregnancy, both for the mother and for the baby. An additional problem centers on the correct pharmacological management of pregnant women with autoimmune diseases, because many of the usual drugs are contraindicated during this period (Table 11.2). In general terms, inflammatory activity is best controlled with oral steroids (bearing in mind that high doses increase the risk of hypertension, diabetes, infection and premature rupture of membranes, among others).[5] Hydroxychloroquine (which is not useful for acute situations) and, in severe cases, intravenous pulses of methylprednisolone and azathioprine are used. Prophylaxis or treatment of thromboembolic complications is best achieved with heparin, preferably the low-molecular-weight (LMW) variety, as a result of easy self-administration, safety profile and lower risk of osteoporosis.[32,33]

Table 11.2 Summary of drugs permitted and contraindicated during pregnancy

Permitted	Contraindicated
Immunosuppressive drugs	
Azathioprine	Cyclophosphamide
Ciclosporin	Methotrexate
	Mycophenolate mofetil
Corticosteroids	
Prednisolone[a]	Dexamethasone[b]
Methylprednisolone	
Antimalarials	
Hydroxychloroquine[a]	Chloroquine
Antihypertensive drugs	
Methyldopa[a]	ACE inhibitors[a]
Labetalol[a]	Diuretics
Nifedipine[a]	
Anticoagulant and anti-aggregant drugs	
Heparin and LMWH[a]	Warfarin[a]
Aspirin (low dose)[a]	
Other	
Immunoglobulins[a]	NSAIDs (third trimester)
Vitamin D[a]	

[a]Drugs allowed during breast-feeding.

[b]Except for *in utero* treatment of fetal myocarditis, hydrops fetalis or immature babies.

ACE, angiotensin-converting enzyme; LMWH, low-molecular-weight heparin; NSAIDs, non-steroidal anti-inflammatory drugs.

SLE and APS

The influence of pregnancy on the course of SLE is debated.[34] However, consistent data point to increased lupus activity during and shortly after pregnancy.[35,36] APS patients are at increased risk of having recurrent miscarriage (both early and late), prematurity and low birthweight babies, maternal thrombosis and severe pre-eclampsia.[5] CHB constitutes a complication of SLE unique to pregnant patients (see below). Valve disease related to SLE/APS may be difficult to manage during pregnancy, as a result of hemodynamic and anticoagulation issues (see below).

Systemic sclerosis and inflammatory myopathies

Systemic sclerosis is not usually affected by pregnancy. Experience is limited, because this is an infrequent condition. Many pregnancies in women with scleroderma progress uneventfully. The proportion of mothers who experience a worsening of their disease is below 25%.[37,38] Arthralgia and gastroesophageal reflux tend to be exacerbated during pregnancy.[39] On the other hand, Raynaud's disease usually improves.[39] Those women with early diffuse forms are at highest risk of a renal crisis during pregnancy.[39] Patients with systemic sclerosis and PHT usually have a complicated course during pregnancy, including life-threatening situations (see below). Thus, this condition should be considered a contraindication for pregnancy.

Experience of PM and DM in pregnancy is scarce. A recent review has been published, summarizing 47 pregnancies in 37 patients.[40] In general, maternal and fetal prognoses are conditioned by disease activity at conception and maternal pharmacological treatment. Serious complications seem unusual.

Mixed connective tissue disease

There is little experience of pregnant women with MCTD.[41] In general, the course of pregnancy in women with this condition is variable. Potential complications include pre-eclampsia, renal disease and PHT. Sporadic cases of neonatal lupus in babies born to mothers with MCTD have been reported.[41]

Systemic vasculitis

Analysis of small series and case reports points to different pregnancy courses depending on the specific type of vasculitis and the degree of activity. Longstanding quiescent patients are more likely to experience uneventful pregnancies.[42] Women with renal involvement are more prone to suffer hypertension.[42,43] Pre-eclampsia is a major issue in pregnant women with Takayasu's arteritis.[44] Thromboses are a potential complication of pregnancy in women with Behçet's disease;[42] however, many pregnancies do not develop significant complications.[45]

Specific clinical situations

Congenital heart block

Neonatal lupus is a rare complication affecting children born to mothers with lupus, Sjögren syndrome and, less often, other autoimmune diseases, with the most serious form of presentation being CHB. This syndrome is closely related to the presence of maternal anti-Ro and anti-La antibodies. These antibodies gain access to the fetal circulation during the active transport of IgG across the placenta, which happens between weeks 16 and 30 of gestation. The prevalence of CHB among newborns of anti-Ro-positive women with known connective tissue diseases is around 2%.[18] However, this risk increases to 15% in younger siblings of an infant with CHB.[46] The actual prevalence may be even higher, because incomplete forms of CHB have been described, including first-degree heart block that can progress during childhood.[46] Up to 60% of children affected by CHB need a permanent pacemaker and around 20% may die in the perinatal period.[20]

Serial fetal echocardiograms must be performed between weeks 16 and 34 of pregnancy to all women with anti-Ro and/or anti-La antibodies.[46] If incomplete heart block is identified, therapy with fluorinated steroids—dexamethasone or betamethasone, which cross the placental barrier—is recommended because there is a chance of reversibility (total or partial).[47] Likewise, children with myocarditis, ascites or hydrops must be treated. The response of established complete heart block is poor, so some authors advocate no therapy in these cases, whereas others recommend a trial of steroids in cases of recent-onset heart block. With regard to the specific drug to be chosen, preferences are shifting towards betamethasone, as a result of recent studies that link neurological complications in the neonate with the use of multiple-dose dexamethasone.[48,49]

As a result of the high risk of recurrent CHB in women with previously affected children, prophylactic treatment with intravenous immunoglobulins during the period of transplacental active transport of IgG, with the aim of blocking pathogenic antibodies, has been proposed for a multicenter research project.[50]

Pulmonary hypertension

According to the last consensus classification criteria during the conference held in Venice 2003,[51] connective tissue diseases, particularly systemic sclerosis, mixed connective tissue disease and SLE,[52] can be a direct cause of PHT (class 1.3.1). In addition, chronic thromboembolic disease (classes 4.1 and 4.2) can be the consequence of hypercoagulable states, one of the most prevalent acquired thrombophilias being APS.[52]

The prognosis of PHT used to be grim, with median survival below 3 years after diagnosis.[52] Fortunately, the development of several effective therapies, including prostacyclin analogues, endothelin-receptor antagonists, phosphodiesterase inhibitors and nitric oxide, have improved the quality of life, and even the survival of patients with PHT.[53] However, the prognosis of connective tissue disorder-associated PHT seems to be worse than in idiopathic forms and response to treatment not so apparent.[52]

Pregnancy, and particularly labour, increase the cardiac burden substantially.[54] The pregnancy-related mortality rate has been estimated as up to 50%, usually within the early postpartum period.[55] Therefore, PHT is considered a major contraindication for pregnancy and effective contraception is recommended to affected fertile women.[53]

Recent case reports stress the successful management of pregnancy in individual women with primary PHT, using novel vasodilators such as inhaled nitric oxide[56,57] and epoprostenol, both intravenous and inhaled.[58] However, a recent retrospective review of 15 pregnancies—from 1992 to 2002—in a referral center for PHT has shown a 36% maternal mortality rate.[59] Mortality in pregnant women with SLE/APS-related PHT was also high in a series from Birmingham University—two of three patients—despite use of nitric oxide and prostacyclin analogues.[60]

In conclusion, PHT continues to be a very high-risk condition in pregnant women, despite important advances in medical management. High maternal mortality justifies the contraindication of pregnancy in all women with all forms of PHT.[59,60] However, if pregnancy occurs, these patients must be managed by a combined team, including physicians with experience in PHT, in a center with fully equipped intensive care and neonatal units. Inhaled nitric oxide and intravenous, as well as inhaled prostacyclin analogues, can be used with close monitoring of hemodynamic parameters.[59] The choice between vaginal and cesarean delivery is not straightforward, and the decision must be taken by all the involved team (obstetric, medical and anesthetic). In general terms, regional anesthesia is preferred. In addition, intensive care monitoring of the mother in the postpartum period, with full anticoagulation with heparin, is indicated.[59]

Hypertensive disorders

Hypertension is a cause of major complications in both the mother and the baby.[61] This is defined as a systolic/diastolic blood pressure of 140/90 mmHg or higher, which can be present before pregnancy or develop as a complication of pregnancy, usually after 20 weeks' gestation.[61] Pre-eclampsia is defined as the presence of pregnancy-induced hypertension plus proteinuria of at least 300 mg/day.[62]

Pre-existing hypertension, obesity, multiple pregnancy and maternal age over 40 years are considered risk factors for the development of pre-eclampsia.[63] Among autoimmune diseases, positivity for aPLs has been shown to be one of the most significant risk factors for pre-eclampsia in a recent systematic review.[63] In fact, similar changes in placental arteries have been observed in women with APS and with pre-eclampsia.[64] The aPLs may be particularly linked with severe forms of pre-eclampsia;[65] a complication of severe pre-eclampsia with renal failure, hemolysis, thrombocytopenia and liver involvement (the so-called HELLP syndrome) has been observed in patients with APS.[66,67]

Renal involvement also increases the risk for hypertension. Thus, women with SLE and previous nephritis,[68] and those with diffuse forms of systemic sclerosis, especially during the early active phases of the disease,[39] should be considered at an increased risk for all forms of pregnancy-induced hypertension. In women with SLE, pre-eclampsia may mimic a flare of lupus nephritis. The finding of other clinical (i.e. arthritis, rash, fever) or biochemical (i.e. raised anti-DNA levels, low C3 or C4) signs of SLE activity or the presence of urinary red cell casts support a diagnosis of SLE renal involvement, whereas elevation of serum uric acid or liver enzymes suggests pre-eclampsia.[69]

Women at high risk for the development of pre-eclampsia must be subject to close follow-up during pregnancy, including frequent monitoring of blood pressure and proteinuria. Doppler studies of the uterine arteries may identify those women more prone to suffer toxemia: the presence of bilateral prediastolic notches correlates with an increased risk for pre-eclampsia.[70] Thus, regular uterine artery Doppler around 22–24 weeks should be included in the antenatal care plan of women with SLE, aPLs and systemic sclerosis.

Medical management of pregnancy-induced hypertension includes alpha-methyldopa as first-line therapy, with calcium-channel antagonists (such as nifedipine) and beta blockers (such as labetalol) as second-line agents.[69] Angiotensin-converting enzyme (ACE) inhibitors are contraindicated during pregnancy, because of the risk of oligohydramnios and renal failure in the fetus.[69] The exception is the occurrence of a scleroderma renal crisis, a medical emergency in which response to other antihypertensive drugs is poor.[39] In cases of severe pre-eclampsia, intensive care unit management and early delivery must be considered.[69] Low-dose aspirin has been shown to decrease the risk of pre-eclampsia and related adverse fetal outcomes; however, the magnitude of this effect is modest in unselected populations.[71] Despite the lack of data in women with autoimmune diseases, it seems prudent to offer aspirin to all patients with aPLs and diffuse systemic sclerosis, as well as to those with SLE and previous renal involvement.

Thrombosis

Pregnancy combines a procoagulant state, meant to avoid massive maternal bleeding during delivery, and venous stasis caused by venous dilatation and compression by the gravid uterus.[72] Thus, pregnant women are at an increased risk of thromboembolic complications. This risk is obviously higher among women with any prothrombotic condition, such as the presence of aPLs.

APS is one of the few thrombophilias that produce arterial and venous thrombosis with similar frequency.[73] Arterial events have a predilection for the brain; however, coronary and peripheral artery thrombosis can occur.[73] Stroke is also a marker of high-risk pregnancies.[74] Several studies have shown the high risk of thrombotic recurrences when secondary prophylaxis is not initiated or withdrawn.[75–78] Therefore, women with APS and previous thrombosis—or whose first event occurs during pregnancy—should maintain anti-thrombotic treatment throughout their whole pregnancy and also during the postpartum period.[79]

There is less experience of asymptomatic women with aPLs, with or without SLE. It is common practice to offer them low-dose aspirin and recommend stronger thromboprophylaxis during the postpartum period.[32]

Management of women with APS and previous thrombosis is largely empirical, because this group of patients has been systematically excluded from clinical trials.[80] Recent guidelines recommend that women with APS and previous thrombotic events should receive anti-thrombotic therapy with heparin throughout the whole pregnancy, with oral anticoagulants being reinstituted as soon as possible after delivery.[32,81] Specific proposed schedules range from adjusted doses of calcium heparin according to APTT or anti-Xa activity, or full therapeutic doses of LMW heparin (dalteparin 200 U/kg per day, or enoxaparin 1 mg/kg every 12 h or 1.5 mg/kg per day, or nadroparin 171 U/kg per day) to prophylactic doses of LMWH (dalteparin 5000 U or enoxaparin 40 mg once daily until 16 weeks' gestation, doubling the dose every 12 h onwards). Concomitant treatment with low-dose aspirin is generally recommended whatever heparin regimen is prescribed.[32]

A special situation includes those women with SLE/APS-related valvular disease with prosthetic valves. Warfarin is more effective than either unfractionated heparin or LMWH in preventing thromboembolic complications; however, it is relatively contraindicated during early pregnancy as a result of the risk of associated embryopathy.[81] Current recommendations include unfractionated heparin between weeks 6 and 12 and close to delivery, maintaining warfarin during the rest of pregnancy[81] (see Chapter 9). Low-dose aspirin can be used in association with LMWH (82) and is recommended in all women with APS except in those with mechanical prosthetic valves, who, in addition, should retain an intensity of anticoagulation high enough to prevent thrombotic complications.[32]

Thromboprophylaxis may represent a risk during labour, particularly if epidural anesthesia is administered. Stopping heparin at least 12 h before any interventional procedure is generally considered safe. Many anesthesiologists also require a minimum of 7 days without aspirin to perform a spinal tap.[83] Even under these circumstances, some feel more comfortable using general anesthesia in this group of patients.

Conclusion

Systemic autoimmune diseases frequently affect the cardiovascular system. The most clinically relevant associations are: SLE and Sjögren syndrome (with anti-Ro and anti-La antibodies), CHB; APS–thrombosis; and systemic sclerosis–pulmonary hypertension. Pregnancy is a very special period that can influence and be influenced by autoimmune diseases. Serial fetal echocardiograms must be performed between weeks 16 and 34 of pregnancy to all women with anti-Ro and/or anti-La antibodies, although CHB can be treated only if detected at very early stages. Women with APS must receive adequate thromboprophylaxis throughout their pregnancy and the puerperium. Pulmonary hypertension is a major contraindication for pregnancy as a result of the high maternal mortality. Women with APS, systemic sclerosis, previous hypertension or previous or active renal involvement (e.g. in SLE) are at risk of developing hypertensive complications during pregnancy. In these women, hypertension should be controlled and special surveillance for the development of pre-eclampsia taken, with frequent checking of the urine for proteinuria. Women at risk of pre-eclampsia should receive prophylactic treatment with low-dose aspirin.

With correct medical–obstetrical management, most women with systemic autoimmune diseases, including those with cardiovascular manifestations, can complete successful pregnancies.

References

1 Cervera R, Khamashta MA, Font J et al. Morbidity and mortality in systemic lupus erythematosus during a 5-year period. A multicenter prospective study of 1000 patients. *Medicine (Baltimore)* 1999;**78**:167–75.

2 Tan EM, Cohen AS, Fries JF et al. The 1982 revised criteria for the classification of systemic lupus erythematosus. *Arthritis Rheum* 1982;**25**:1271–7.

3 Hochberg MC. Updating the American College of Rheumatology revised criteria for the classification of systemic lupus erythematosus. *Arthritis Rheum* 1997;**40**:1725.

4 Hughes GRV. Is it lupus? The St. Thomas' Hospital 'alternative' criteria. *Clin Exp Rheumatol* 1998;**16**:250–2.

5 Ruiz-Irastorza G, Khamashta MA, Nelson-Piercy C, Hughes GRV. Effects of lupus and antiphospholipid syndrome on pregnancy. *Yearbook Obstet Gynaecol* 2002;**10**:105–19.

6 Hughes GRV. The antiphospholipid syndrome: ten years on. *Lancet* 1993;**342**:341–4.

7 Doria A, Iaccarino L, Sarzi-Puttini P, Atzeni F, Turriel M, Petri M. Cardiac involvement in systemic lupus erythematosus. *Lupus* 2005;**14**:683–6.

8 Lockshin M, Tenedios F, Petri M et al. Cardiac disease in the antiphospholipid syndrome: recommendations for treatment. Committee consensus report. *Lupus* 2003;**12**:518–23.

9 Tenedios F, Erkan D, Lockshin MD. Cardiac involvement in the antiphospholipid syndrome. *Lupus* 2005;**14**:691–6.

10 Berkun Y, Elami A, Meir K, Mevorach D, Naparstek Y. Increased morbidity and mortality in patients with antiphospholipid syndrome undergoing valve replacement surgery. *J Thorac Cardiovasc Surg* 2004;**127**:414–20.

11 Manzi S, Meilhn EN, Rairie JE et al. Age specific incidence rates of myocardial infarction and angina in women with SLE: comparison with the Framingham study. *Am J Epidemiol* 1997;**145**:408–15.

12 Roman MJ, Shanker BA, Davis A et al. Prevalence and correlates of accelerated atherosclerosis in systemic lupus erythematosus. *N Engl J Med* 2003;**349**:2399–406.

13 Ruiz-Irastorza G, Khamashta MA, Hunt BJ, Escudero A, Cuadrado MJ, Hughes GRV. Bleeding and recurrent thrombosis in definite antiphospholipid syndrome: analysis of a series of 66 patients treated with oral anticoagulation to a target INR of 3.5. *Arch Intern Med* 2002;**162**:1164–9.

14 Erkan D, Yazici Y, Peterson MG, Sammaritano L, Lockshin MD. A cross-section study of clinical thrombotic risk factors and preventive treatments in antiphospholipid syndrome. *Rheumatology* 2002;**41**:924–9.

15 McGoon M, Gutterman D, Steen V et al. Screening, early detection and diagnosis of pulmonary arterial hypertension. ACCP evidence-based clinical practice guidelines. *Chest* 2004;**126**:14S–34S.

16 Li EK, Tam LS. Pulmonary hypertension in systemic lupus erythematosus: clinical association and survival in 18 patients. *J Rheumatol* 1999;**26**:1923–9.

17 Asherson RA, Higenbottam TW, Xuan ATD, Khamashta MA, Hughes GRV. Pulmonary hypertension in a lupus clinic: experience with twenty-four patients. *J Rheumatol* 1990;**17**:1292–8.

18 Brucato A, Frassi M, Franceschini F et al. Risk of congenital complete heart block in newborns of mothers with anti-Ro/SSA antibodies detected by counterimmunoelectrophoresis: a prospective study of 100 women. *Arthritis Rheum* 2001;**44**:1832–5.

19 Buyon JP, Kim MY, Copel JA, Friedman DM. Anti-Ro/SSA antibodies and congenital heart block: necessary but not sufficient. *Arthritis Rheum* 2001;**44**:1723–7.

20 Tseng CE, Buyon JP. Neonatal lupus syndromes. *Rheum Dis Clin North Am* 1997;23:31–54.

21 Wigley FM, Hummers LK. Clinical features of systemic sclerosis. In: Hochberg MC, Silman AJ, Smolen JS, Weinblatt ME, Weisman MH (eds), *Rheumatology*, 3rd edn. Edinburgh: Mosby, 2003: pp 1463–79.

22 Ferri C, Giuggioli D, Sebastiani M, Colaci M, Emdin M. Heart involvement in systemic sclerosis. *Lupus* 2005;**14**:702–7.
23 Denton CP, Cailes JB, Phillips GD, Wells AU, Black CM, Du Bois RM. Comparison of Doppler echocardiography and right heart catheterization to assess pulmonary hypertension in systemic sclerosis. *Br J Rheumatol* 1997;**36**:239–43.
24 Ferri C, Valentini G, Cozzi F et al. Systemic sclerosis. Demographic, clinical and serological features and survival in 1012 Italian patients. *Medicine* 2002;**81**:139–53.
25 Oddis CV, Medsger TA Jr. Inflammatory muscle disease: clinical features. In: Hochberg MC, Silman AJ, Smolen JS, Weinblatt ME, Weisman MH (eds), *Rheumatology*, 3rd edn. Edinburgh: Mosby, 2003: pp 1537–54.
26 Lundberg IE. Cardiac involvement in autoimmune myositis and mixed connective tissue disease. *Lupus* 2005;**14**:708–12.
27 Bull TM, Fagan KA, Badesch DB. Pulmonary vascular manifestations of mixed connective tissue disease. *Rheum Dis Clin N Am* 2005;**31**:451–64.
28 Savage CO, Harper L, Cockwell DA, Howie AJ. Vasculitis. *BMJ* 2000;**320**:1325–8.
29 Pagnoux C, Guillevin L. Cardiac involvement in small and medium-sized vessel vasculitis. *Lupus* 2005;**14**:718–22.
30 Marshall S. Behçet disease. *Best Pract Res Clin Rheumatol* 2004;**18**:291–311.
31 Atzeni F, Sarzi-Puttini P, Doria A, Boiardi L, Pipitone N, Salvarini C. Behçet disease and cardiovascular involvement. *Lupus* 2005;**14**:723–6.
32 Ruiz-Irastorza G, Khamashta MA. Management of thrombosis in antiphospholipid syndrome and systemic lupus erythematosus in pregnancy. *Ann N Y Acad Sci* 2005; **1051**:606–12.
33 Ruiz-Irastorza G, Khamashta MA, Nelson-Piercy C, Hughes GR. Lupus pregnancy: is heparin a risk factor for osteoporosis? *Lupus* 2001;**10**:597–600.
34 Ruiz-Irastorza G, Khamashta MA. Evaluation of systemic lupus erythematosus activity during pregnancy. *Lupus* 2004;**13**:679–82.
35 Petri M, Howard D, Repke J. Frequency of lupus flare in pregnancy. The Hopkins Lupus Pregnancy Center experience. *Arthritis Rheum* 1991;**34**:1538–45.
36 Ruiz-Irastorza G, Lima F, Alves J et al. Increased rate of lupus flare during pregnancy and the puerperium: a prospective study of 78 pregnancies. *Br J Rheumatol* 1996;**35**:133–8.
37 Steen VD, Conte C, Day N, Ramsey-Goldman R, Medsger TA. Pregnancy in women with systemic sclerosis. *Arthritis Rheum* 1989;**32**:151–7.
38 Steen VD, Brodeur M, Conte C. Prospective pregnancy study in women with systemic sclerosis (SSc). *Arthritis Rheum* 1996;**39**:S151.
39 Steen VD. Scleroderma and pregnancy. *Rheum Dis Clin North Am* 1997;**23**:133–47.
40 Silva CA, Sultan SM, Isenberg DA. Pregnancy outcome in adult-onset idiopathic inflammatory myopathy. *Rheumatology (Oxford)* 2003;**42**:1168–72.
41 Kitridou RC. Pregnancy in mixed connective tissue disease. *Rheum Dis Clin N Am* 2005;**31**:497–508.
42 Gordon C. Pregnancy and autoimmune disease. *Best Pract Res Clin Rheumatol* 2004;**18**:359–79.
43 Lima F, Buchanan NMM, Froes L, Kerslake S, Khamashta MA, Hughes GRV. Pregnancy in granulomatous vasculitis. *Ann Rheum Dis* 1995;**54**:604–6.
44 Sharma BK, Jain S, Vasishta K. Outcome of pregnancy in Takayasu arteritis. *Int J Cardiol* 2000;**75**:S159–62.
45 Marsal S, Falga C, Simeon CP, Vilardell M, Bosch JA. Behçet disease and pregnancy relationship study. *Br J Rheumatol* 1997;**36**:234–8.

46 Buyon JP, Rupel A, Clancy RM. Neonatal lupus syndromes. *Lupus* 2004;**13**:705–12.

47 Saaleb S, Copel J, Friedman D, Buyon JP. Comparison of treatment with fluorinated glucocorticoids to the natural history of autoantibody-associated congenital heart block. *Arthritis Rheum* 1999;**42**:2335–45.

48 Whitelaw A, Thoresen M. Antenatal steroids and the developing brain. *Arch Dis Child Neonatal* 2000;**83**:F154–7.

49 Baud O, Foix-L'Helias L, Kamisnski M et al. Antenatal glucocorticoid treatment and cystic periventricular leukomalacia in very premature infants. *N Engl J Med* 1999;**341**:1190–6.

50 Hughes G. The eradication of congenital heart block. *Lupus* 2004;**13**:489.

51 Simonneau G, Galie N, Rubin L et al. Clinical classification of pulmonary arterial hypertension. *J Am Coll Cardiol* 2004;**43**:S5–S12.

52 Galie N, Manes A, Farahani KV et al. Pulmonary arterial hypertension associated to connective tissue diseases. *Lupus* 2005;**14**:713–17.

53 Humbert M, Sitbon O, Simonneau G. Treatment of pulmonary arterial hypertension. *N Engl J Med* 2004;**351**:1425–36.

54 Monnery L, Nanson J, Charlton G. Primary pulmonary hypertension in pregnancy: a role for novel vasodilators. *Br J Anaesth* 2001;**87**:295–8.

55 Lupton M, Oteng-Ntim E, Ayida G, Steer PJ. Cardiac disease in pregnancy. *Curr Opin Obstet Gynecol* 2002;**14**:137–43.

56 Decoene C, Bourzoufi K, Moreau D, Narducci F, Crepin F, Krivosic-Horber R. Use of inhaled nitric oxide for emergency cesarean section in a woman with unexpected primary pulmonary hypertension. *Can J Anaesth* 2001;**48**:584–7.

57 Lam GK, Stafford RE, Thorp J, Moise KJ Jr, Cairns BA. Inhaled nitric oxide for primary pulmonary hypertension in pregnancy. *Obstet Gynecol* 2001;**98**:895–8.

58 Bildirici I, Shumway JB. Intravenous and inhaled epoprostenol for primary pulmonary hypertension during pregnancy. *Am J Obstet Gynecol* 2004;**103**:1102–5.

59 Bonnin M, Mercier FJ, Sitbob O et al. Severe pulmonary hypertension during pregnancy. Mode of delivery and anesthetic management of 15 consecutive cases. *Anesthesiology* 2005;**102**:1133–7.

60 McMillan E, Martin WL, Waugh J et al. Management of pregnancy in women with pulmonary hypertension secondary to SLE and anti-phospholipid syndrome. *Lupus* 2002;**11**:392–8.

61 Milne F, Redman C, Walker J et al. The pre-eclampsia community guideline (PRE-COG): how to screen for and detect onset of pre-eclampsia in the community. *BMJ* 2005;**330**:576–80.

62 Johnson MJ. Obstetric complications and rheumatic disease. *Rheum Dis Clin North Am* 1997;**23**:169–82.

63 Duckitt K, Harrington D. Risk factors for pre-eclampsia at antenatal booking: systematic review of controlled studies. *BMJ* 2005;**330**:565.

64 Stone S, Khamashta MA, Poston L. Placentation, antiphospholipid syndrome and pregnancy outcome. *Lupus* 2001;**10**:67–74.

65 Dekker GA, de Vries JI, Doelitzsch PM et al. Underlying disorders associated with severe early onset pre-eclampsia. *Am J Obstet Gynecol* 1995;**173**:1042–8.

66 Petri M. Hopkins Lupus Pregnancy Center: 1987 to 1996. *Rheum Dis Clin North Am* 1997;**23**:1–13.

67 Ornstein MH, Rand JH. An association between refractory HELLP syndrome and antiphospholipid antibodies during pregnancy: a report of 2 cases. *J Rheumatol* 1994;**21**:1360–4.

68 Packham DK, Lam SS, Nichols K et al. Lupus nephritis and pregnancy. *Q J Med* 1992;**83**:315–24.

69 Nelson-Piercy C. Hypertension and pre-eclampsia. In: Nelson-Piercy C (ed.), *Handbook of Obstetric Medicine*. Isis Medical Media, Oxford, 1997: pp 1–16.

70 Papageorghiou AT, Roberts N. Uterine artery Doppler screening for adverse pregnancy outcome. *Curr Op Obstet Gynecol* 2005;**17**:584–90.

71 Duley L, Henderson-Smart D, Knight M, King J. Antiplatelet drugs for prevention of pre-eclampsia and its consequences: systematic review. *BMJ* 2001;**322**:329–33.

72 Bazaan M, Donvito V. Low-molecular-weight heparin during pregnancy. *Thromb Res* 2001;**101**:V175–86.

73 Ruiz-Irastorza G, Khamashta MA, Hughes GRV. Hughes syndrome crosses boundaries. *Autoimmun Rev* 2002;**1**:43–8.

74 Cuadrado MJ, Mendonça LLF, Khamashta MA et al. Maternal and fetal outcome in antiphospholipid syndrome pregnancies with a history of previous cerebral ischemia (abstract). *Arthritis Rheum* 1999;**42**:S265.

75 Khamashta MA, Cuadrado MJ, Mujic F, Taub NA, Hunt BJ, Hughes GRV. The management of thrombosis in the antiphospholipid-antibody syndrome. *N Engl J Med* 1995;**332**:993–7.

76 Rosove MH, Brewer PMC. Antiphospholipid thrombosis: clinical course after the first thrombotic event in 70 patients. *Ann Intern Med* 1992;**117**:303–8.

77 Schulman S, Svenungsson E, Granqvist S and the Duration of Anticoagulation Study Group. Anticardiolipin antibodies predict early recurrence in thromboembolism and death among patients with venous thromboembolism following anticoagulant therapy. *Am J Med* 1998;**104**:332–8.

78 Kearon C, Gent M, Hirsh J et al. A comparison of three months of anticoagulation with extended anticoagulation for a first episode of idiopathic venous thromboembolism. *N Engl J Med* 1999;**340**:901–7.

79 Derksen RHWM, Khamashta MA, Branch DW. Management of the obstetric antiphospholipid syndrome. *Arthritis Rheum* 2004;**50**:1028–39.

80 Ruiz-Irastorza G, Khamashta MA, Hughes GRV. Treatment of pregnancy loss in Hughes syndrome: a critical update. *Autoimmunity Rev* 2002;**1**:298–304.

81 Bates S, Greer IA, Hirsh J, Ginsberg JS. Use of antithrombotic agents during pregnancy. The seventh ACCP conference on antithrombotic and thrombolytic therapy. *Chest* 2004;**126**:627S–44S.

82 Lupton M, Oteng-Ntim E, Ayida G, Steer PJ. Cardiac disease in pregnancy. *Curr Opin Obstet Gynecol* 2002;**14**:137–43.

83 Wetzl RG. Anesthesiological aspects of pregnancy in patients with rheumatic diseases. *Lupus* 2004;**13**:699–702.

CHAPTER 12

Pulmonary disease and cor pulmonale

Claire L Shovlin, Anita K Simonds, JMB Hughes

In this chapter, we focus on diffuse lung diseases and extrapulmonary disease that cause secondary pulmonary hypertension (PHT) as a consequence of destructive bronchial or alveolar pathology and/or alveolar hypoxia, rather than primary pathology of the heart or pulmonary vessels. We also discuss pulmonary arteriovenous malformations in which there is severe arterial hypoxaemia but no secondary PHT. The effects of asthma, tuberculosis and bacterial and viral pneumonias on pregnancy are covered elsewhere.[1]

Effects of pregnancy on the normal lung

The effects of pregnancy on lung mechanics, pulmonary gas exchange and control of ventilation have been extensively studied and reviewed.[1,2] The most important physiological changes in the respiratory system during pregnancy, summarized in Table 12.1, and described in detail below, are:
• An increase in minute ventilation (mostly hormonally induced) leading to hypocapnia
• A low end-expiratory lung volume related to the enlarging uterus.
Apart from causing dyspnea, these pregnancy-induced changes do not significantly compromise the normal respiratory system.

No change in vital capacity or diffusing capacity

Lung mechanics
The lung volume is not affected until the second half of pregnancy when the uterus enlarges, raising intra-abdominal pressure and altering the configuration of the diaphragm and chest wall. Although the vital capacity (VC) is unchanged in pregnancy (erect and supine), there is a 20% reduction in the functional residual capacity (FRC). As a result, breathing at rest takes place closer to residual volume than normal. This may lead to an increase in the closing capacity, such that small bronchi in the dependent lung zones collapse at lower lung volumes, including those reached during tidal breathing, and mild hypoxemia may ensue, particularly in the supine position.[3] Total lung capacity (TLC) (and therefore residual volume or RV) are unchanged in pregnancy.

Table 12.1 Cardiorespiratory changes in pregnancy

Factor	Change
Minute ventilation (%)	10–40
Functional residual capacity (%)	−20
Oxygen consumption (%)	5–20
PaO_2 (kPa)	1.07–1.73
$PaCO_2$ (kPa)	0.93–1.6
Cardiac output (%)	+20–40
Pulmonary artery pressure (mmHg)	−3
Pulmonary vascular resistance (%)	−33

Airway resistance at resting lung volume is reduced by 50%,[2] probably because the hormonal changes in pregnancy causing smooth muscle relaxation of the bronchi offset the airway narrowing and higher resistance that should result from the low FRC. Lung compliance is normal. The oxygen cost of breathing is increased in pregnancy by about 25%, probably as a result of the extra work needed to displace the chest wall and abdominal contents. Respiratory muscle function, including that of the diaphragm, is unaltered.[1]

Resting minute ventilation ($\dot{V}E$) increases in pregnancy by 10% at 3 months, 30% at 6 months and 45% near term as a result of an increase in tidal volume, not respiratory frequency. Oxygen consumption ($\dot{V}O_2$) also increases in a linear fashion throughout pregnancy (+20% near term) but to a lesser extent so that the ventilatory equivalent ($\dot{V}E/\dot{V}CO_2$) increases.[1] The $\dot{V}E/\dot{V}O_2$ ratio also increases, so that arterial PCO_2 falls progressively to 3.6–4.3 kPa (27–32 mmHg).[4] This hyperventilation of pregnancy raises alveolar and arterial PO_2 especially in the erect posture.[5] Although this normally has little effect on arterial oxygen saturation (SaO_2) at sea level, it plays an important part in raising SaO_2 at altitude (see below) or in the presence of lung disease at sea level. The increase in $\dot{V}O_2$ in the first two trimesters reflects the extra renal and cardiac work in pregnancy, although there must be additional causes of increases in oxygen consumption. In the last trimester, the uterus, placenta and fetus account for 50% of the additional $\dot{V}O_2$.[1]

In the most definitive study involving 21 pregnant women, there was no difference in pulmonary diffusing capacity ($DLCO$) in the second and third trimesters of pregnancy compared with 3–5 months post partum, but there was a significant increase (10%) in the first trimester. This is probably because expansion of the pulmonary capillary bed, secondary to the increase in cardiac output (which rises early in pregnancy [by 1.5–2.0 L/min] and reaches a steady level[6]) leads to an increase in $DLCO$ in the first trimester. This is offset in the second and third trimesters by a fall in lung volume[7] and alveolar surface area or D_L/V_A, because of the enlarging uterus.[8] The explanation for these changes is complex.

Control of breathing

The increase in minute ventilation that begins early in pregnancy is greater than the increased metabolic demands require. Increased progesterone levels are the main factor driving ventilation; $Paco_2$ is linearly and inversely related to the log of serum progesterone concentration, during both the menstrual cycle and pregnancy, and there is a reduction in resting ventilation in postmenopausal and amenorrheic women.[9] Estrogen and its receptors act synergistically with progesterone at central (hypothalamus) and peripheral (carotid body) sites to stimulate ventilation. Both hypoxic and hypercapnic ventilatory responsiveness increase during pregnancy.[5,9]

Pregnancy and the pulmonary circulation

The rise in cardiac output throughout pregnancy is associated with a fall in pulmonary vascular resistance: 0.51 mmHg/L per min in 11 healthy women at 16 weeks of pregnancy compared with 0.76 mmHg/L per min in 15 non-pregnant controls. There was no change in pulmonary blood volume, but a fall in mean pulmonary artery pressure from 13 mmHg to 10 mmHg. Moore, in an extensive review, pointed out that in animals there is a reduced vascular reactivity in pregnancy to alveolar hypoxia, prostaglandin-$F_{2\alpha}$, norepinephrine and angiotensin II.[10] Chronic infusion of estradiol-17β in sheep reproduces many of the cardiovascular responses associated with pregnancy, such as systemic vasodilatation and a blunted pressure response to angiotensin II.[11]

Effect of high altitude

• *Physiological changes of pregnancy compensate to some extent for the hypoxemia.*
The increase in Pao_2 during a normal pregnancy at sea level (1.07–1.73 kPa or 8–13 mmHg) is unimportant in terms of increasing arterial oxygen content because of the flatness of the oxygen dissociation curve.[5] In Leadville, Colorado, at an altitude of 3100 m, Sao_2 was only 92% in the non-pregnant state (normal 97–98%) in 33 women, but increased to 94% during pregnancy as a result of the accompanying hyperventilation.[12] In a further study in the Andes at 4300 m, Sao_2 was 83% in the non-pregnant state and 87% in week 36 of pregnancy.[13] In spite of a fall in hemoglobin concentration ([Hb]) in pregnancy, arterial oxygen content remained the same as before pregnancy. There was a 25% increase in resting ventilation and a fourfold increase in hypoxic ventilatory responsiveness (HVR) (because of chronic altitude exposure, a blunted response was present in the non-pregnant state). Compared with sea level the pregnancy-induced increase in cardiac output was reduced (+13%), possibly as a result of pulmonary hypertension (pulmonary pressures were not measured). There was a fair correlation ($r = 0.44$, $p < 0.05$) between HVR and infant birthweight. These studies show that the hyperventilation of pregnancy can compensate to some extent for the hypoxemia of altitude and, by extrapolation, lung disease at sea level. It is also possible that the higher Pao_2 and low $Paco_2$ in the pregnant state increases O_2 and CO_2 tension gradients across the placenta to the benefit of the fetus. The

fetus also benefits at altitude from a persistence of fetal hemoglobin and a left-ward shift in the oxygen dissociation curve.

Pulmonary disorders associated with ventilatory insufficiency and cor pulmonale in pregnancy

Pregnancy and reduced lung volumes

• *Pregnancy well tolerated if women are not dyspnoeic at rest.*

In a review by Gaensler et al.[14] women after pneumonectomy underwent pregnancies without any increase in complications. Women with extensive resections, provided that they are not breathless at rest, tolerate pregnancy without difficulty. Emphysema from α_1-antitrypsin deficiency was associated with a successful outcome in a single case report.[15]

Pregnancy and cystic fibrosis

• *Outcome of pregnancy influenced by maternal respiratory function pre-pregnancy*
• *Maternal fertility and life expectancy issues.*

Cystic fibrosis (CF) is an autosomal recessive disease associated with defective production of the cystic fibrosis transmembrane conductance regulator (CFTR) protein, which regulates chloride (and, indirectly, sodium and water) passage across luminal cell membranes. The most prominent effects are malnutrition from pancreatic insufficiency and malabsorption, and disseminated bronchiectasis with recurrent pulmonary infections, leading to airflow obstruction, loss of lung tissue, pulmonary hypertension and, ultimately, cor pulmonale and death in the third or fourth decade of life. Thanks to dedicated CF teams and clinics offering 'best practice' in the treatment of recurrent chest infections and malabsorption, the median survival has improved (US figures) from 14 years in 1969 to 32 years in 2000.

Fertility in women with CF may be reduced by inspissated cervical mucus plugs and by failure of ovulation (amenorrhea), which is itself associated with malnutrition (<17% body fat composition) and poor respiratory function (forced expiratory volume in 1 second or FEV_1 <50% predicted). Nevertheless, the outlook for those who become pregnant is good. Two recent reports have analyzed data from the UK Cystic Fibrosis Database[16] and the US Cystic Fibrosis National Patient Registry.[17] For the UK, a cohort of all CF women who became pregnant from 1995 to 2001 was studied. Of 1143 CF women of reproductive age, 65 (5.7%) achieved a pregnancy (about half the expected rate for the general population); there were 85 pregnancies in total. The outcomes were good (74% full-term and 17% pre-term pregnancies, 8% spontaneous and 0% therapeutic abortions, no maternal deaths). These results mirrored those in other countries (Canada, France, Scandinavia). By contrast, in an earlier UK study,[18] spanning the years 1977–1996, only 36% of 72 pregnancies went to full term, and 20% ended with a therapeutic abortion.

The US study[17], focusing more on pre- and post-pregnancy pulmonary function, was particularly upbeat, saying that pregnancy was not associated with decrease in survival (either short or long term), or a greater rate of decline in lung function, in relation to non-pregnant CF controls, after adjustment for age, height, weight, number of respiratory exacerbations per year, pulmonary function or diabetes mellitus (often associated with severe pancreatic insufficiency). As a cautionary note, the authors pointed out that 20% of mothers with CF will be dead before their child's tenth birthday (40% if the mother's FEV_1 <40%).

Edenborough's review[19] concludes that 'healthy' CF patients with FEV_1 >75% predicted and normal nutrition can expect a normal pregnancy, producing a live healthy baby at term, and with no more deterioration in lung function than if they had not been pregnant. With poorer lung function, FEV_1 <60%, there is a greater likelihood of the delivery of a pre-term baby, by cesarean section, with increased maternal and infant complications and reduced likelihood of breast-feeding. Pulmonary function seems to be a better predictor of pregnancy outcomes than body weight or body mass index (BMI). Edenborough's recommendations[19] are, in brief: for FEV_1 >50%, the outcome in terms of the infant is likely to be good. With FEV_1 <50%, only half the pregnancies will result in a live delivery and maternal survival will be poor. The rate of decline of FEV_1 may be more important than the absolute level. Evidence of pulmonary hypertension, with a low diffusing capacity/transfer factor (D_{LCO}/T_{LCO}) (< 50% predicted), coupled with cor pulmonale (low Pao_2 and high $Paco_2$) is an absolute contraindication to pregnancy. FEV_1 <50% is a relative contraindication. Increasing numbers of double lung transplantations are being reported in CF. Although there appears to be little extra risk of rejection, organ failure or fetal anomalies, Edenborough recommends[19] that pregnancy should be delayed for at least 2 years after a transplantation.

Table 12.2 lists the extrapulmonary disorders that may be associated with ventilatory insufficiency and cor pulmonale in pregnancy. Chest wall disorders, including scoliosis and kyphosis, neuromuscular diseases affecting the respiratory muscles and central drive disorders can progress to ventilatory failure, and ultimately cor pulmonale, if the load placed on the respiratory system exceeds the capacity to accommodate this, or if the ventilatory drive is inadequate. In chest wall disease and respiratory muscle weakness, a restrictive ventilatory defect characterized by reduced forced vital capacity, FEV_1 and TLC, with normal FEV_1/FVC ratio, is seen. Many neuromuscular disorders are complicated by scoliosis.

Overview of pregnancy issues in extrapulmonary disorders

Patients with adolescent-onset scoliosis are generally at low risk of cardiorespiratory problems in pregnancy. In early onset scoliosis and stable mild respiratory muscle weakness, a successful outcome may be achieved if vital capacity

Table 12.2 Extrapulmonary conditions that may be associated with ventilatory insufficiency during pregnancy

---

Chest wall disorders
- Scoliosis: idiopathic (majority), neuromuscular, osteogenic, associated with inherited disorders, e.g. neurofibromatosis, Marfan syndrome
- Kyphosis: spinal TB, idiopathic

Neuromuscular disorders
- Muscular dystrophies
    Limb girdle muscular dystrophy
    Congenital muscular dystrophy
    Facioscapulohumeral muscular dystrophy
- Myopathies
    Congenital
        Nemaline acid maltase deficiency (Pompe's disease)
        Mitochondrial central core
    Acquired: polymyositis myasthenia gravis
- Spinal muscular atrophy: anterior horn cell disease
- Combined muscle weakness and ventilatory drive disorder: myotonic dystrophy

Ventilatory drive disorders
- Primary alveolar hypoventilation
- Central sleep apnea

Obstructive sleep apnea

---

is in excess of about 0.80–1.25 L and there is no evidence of pulmonary hypertension.[20]

If hypercapnic respiratory failure or cor pulmonale develop in pregnancy or the postpartum period, the woman may benefit from non-invasive nasal intermittent positive-pressure ventilation or negative-pressure ventilation.

Nasal intermittent ventilation (NIV) should be considered in women with even a mild degree of sleep-disordered breathing. Continuous airway pressure therapy is effective in obstructive sleep apnea.

In high-risk cases it is essential to use a multidisciplinary approach with the early involvement of a respiratory team familiar with NIV support, together with close monitoring of nocturnal and diurnal oxygenation.[21]

Scoliosis

- *Relatively good outcome of pregnancy if modest (<50°) thoracic scoliosis; temporary mechanical ventilation may be required for more severe cases.*

Scoliosis is the most common of the chest wall disorders, and lateral curves of more than 70° affect 0.01% of the population. Of thoracic scolioses 80% are idiopathic, the remainder being the result of neuromuscular disease, osteogenic causes or thoracic surgery, or associated with congenital disease. Adolescent-onset curves occur more commonly in women, whereas early-onset curves show no sex preference. The presence of a scoliosis has important implications in pregnancy, because a substantial thoracic curvature can cause ventilatory insufficiency and cor pulmonale, and lumbar curves can cause obstetric complications. Menarche tends to be delayed in girls with scoliosis.[22]

The frequency of pregnancy in patients with chest wall disorders has been variously reported. In a series from Johannesburg, 50 women with chest wall disease (predominantly Pott's kyphosis) were identified in a total of 119 678 deliveries.[23] This high figure (1 : 2394) reflects the prevalence of TB in South Africa. Other studies have recorded an incidence of kyphoscoliosis in pregnancy varying from 1 : 1471 to 1 : 12 000, an average figure being 1 : 5253.[23] From a different perspective, Siegler and Zorab reported pregnancies in 64 patients with thoracic scoliosis among 205 women with scoliosis who were attending a respiratory clinic.[24] The outcome of pregnancy differs between groups with previously identified respiratory problems and those presenting anew in pregnancy.

More recent work confirms a relatively good outcome of pregnancy in chest wall disorders.[25] This is probably because most affected women have a modest (<50°) thoracic scoliosis, which is unlikely to cause cardiopulmonary or obstetric problems. Some patients are, however, at high risk of cardiorespiratory decompensation during pregnancy, labour and the postpartum period.[20,26]

Although women with a thoracic spinal curvature of less than 50° experience minimal effects on chest wall mechanics, a reduction in chest wall compliance is seen in those with more pronounced curves.[27] Ventilatory insufficiency is exacerbated during sleep. This is because, in rapid eye movement (REM) sleep, intercostal inhibition occurs leading to a reliance on the diaphragm to generate tidal volume. Ventilatory drive is also reduced in both non-REM and REM sleep. As a consequence, marked hypoventilation can occur during sleep if diaphragm function is limited. This causes hypoxemia with potential adverse effects on maternal and fetal health. Monitoring of respiration during sleep is therefore important when ventilatory insufficiency is suspected. If untreated, severe nocturnal hypoventilation progresses to daytime hypoxemia and hypercapnia, pulmonary hypertension and right heart failure.

In scoliotic patients with a vital capacity of less than a liter, pulmonary artery pressure may rise on exercise in the absence of hypoxemia.[28] This rise is the result of the increased cardiac output passing through a low capacity pulmonary vascular bed. It is not known if the increased cardiac output in pregnant women with scoliosis can provoke pulmonary hypertension by a similar mechanism, or whether estrogenic effects on the pulmonary vasculature in pregnancy can offset this process.

Longitudinal studies have shown that patients with idiopathic scoliosis who are at risk of cardiopulmonary decompensation have a VC <50% of predicted.[29] This risk is enhanced if VC is less than about 1 L. Early-onset scoliosis (age of onset <5 years) is associated with an increased incidence of cardiorespiratory failure and high mortality. This is thought to be caused by the onset of chest wall deformity inhibiting alveolar duplication and growth of the pulmonary vasculature.

The converse of these observations is that women with adolescent-onset scoliosis and VC > 50% of predicted can be reassured that they are unlikely to experience respiratory difficulties.

Outcome of pregnancy in scoliosis

Phelan et al.[26] estimated that the maternal mortality rate was 2.6% and the perinatal mortality rate 3.8% in scoliotic patients. However, these statistics depend on patient selection and the underlying disease.

In a series of 50 pregnant women with kyphoscoliosis presenting to Baragwanath Hospital in South Africa over a 9-year period, 42 had spinal TB, 3 had previously had poliomyelitis, 1 a spinal tumor, and the cause of the deformity was unknown in 4.[23] There were two maternal deaths from cardiorespiratory failure, three patients survived cardiac or respiratory failure, and two developed bronchitis postpartum. There were five perinatal deaths, although malpresentation was uncommon. Lung function data were unavailable, but the most important prognostic factors were the severity of the deformity and a thoracic site.

By contrast, in European and American series scoliosis is usually idiopathic. A UK survey of the outcome of 35 pregnancies in 14 patients with marked idiopathic thoracic scoliosis (Cobb angle > 90°), meaning that vital capacity was 1365 mL (range 33–61% of predicted), showed no maternal complications or fetal loss.

Subsequent data on 118 pregnancies in 64 patients with thoracic scoliosis (mainly idiopathic) were reported from the Royal Brompton Hospital, in the UK:[24] 42 patients had curves that exceeded 60° and 12 had a VC < 1 L. Disproportionate breathlessness occurred during pregnancy in 17% of patients, but none developed cardiorespiratory decompensation. Vaginal delivery was successful in 83%. A deficiency of this retrospective postal questionnaire survey addressed to the patients is that maternal deaths are missed. However, the authors thought that continued follow-up excluded this possibility in non-responders.

Several workers have confirmed that stable mild-to-moderate thoracolumbar curves are unlikely to progress during or after pregnancy.[30,31] Neurogenic or myopathic scolioses, particularly if unstable, may be adversely affected.

The factors that contribute to respiratory insufficiency in pregnancy have been examined by Sawicka et al. in a study of six patients with chest wall diseases.[20] Four had idiopathic scoliosis and two previous poliomyelitis. All had developed scoliosis before the age of 8 years. Mean VC was 920 mL (33% of predicted). One woman also had asthma. Five developed progressive dyspnea in the second or third trimester. Four progressed to respiratory failure and cor pulmonale before term; two were managed with negative pressure ventilation, one with non-invasive positive-pressure support, and the fourth with controlled oxygen therapy. Early elective cesarean section was carried out in four patients. Three experienced acute cardiopulmonary distress post partum, requiring mechanical ventilation. All patients survived and there was no neonatal loss, but five mothers have subsequently required non-invasive respiratory support at night.

Although negative pressure ventilation using the iron lung was successful in the above study, the newer non-invasive technique of NIV is more widely available and easier to apply. NIV has been used effectively in this unit (Box 12.1 and Figure 12.1) and elsewhere to maintain arterial blood gases in pregnant women with scoliosis with or without neuromuscular disease.

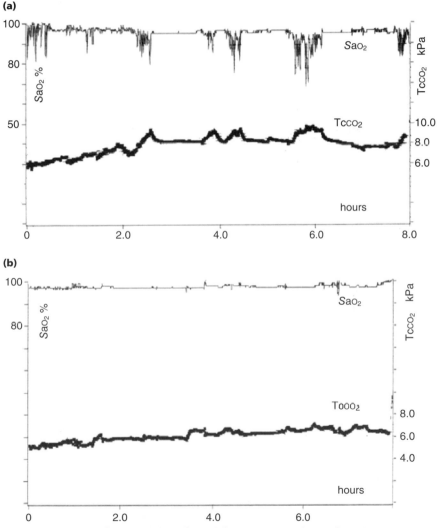

Figure 12.1 Overnight monitoring of arterial oxygen saturation and transcutaneous CO_2 in patient with congenital muscular dystrophy: (a) before treatment with NIV and (b) 24 weeks' pregnant using NIV overnight (see Box 12.1).

Box 12.1 Case of pregnancy in patient with rigid spine syndrome and congenital muscular dystrophy

Born with bilateral foot contractures. No family history of neuromuscular disease. Treated with surgery and plaster casting for contractures as infant
   Delayed motor milestones
Age 11 years: development of lordoscoliosis. Noted to be breathless on walking 50 m, with ineffective cough
Age 16 years: delayed puberty, poor weight gain. Training as a hairdresser but difficulty holding hair dryer for long period. Referred for further assessment

Investigations
Thin build, rigid spine with thoracolumbar lordoscoliosis. Mild weakness particularly of neck flexion, elbow flexion and extension, and finger extension. Normal reflexes. FVC 1.35 L (43% predicted by span) in sitting position and 1.05 L (34% predicted) in supine position: representing a fall in absolute FVC of 22%

Respiratory muscle strength measurements: maximum inspiratory mouth pressure of 36.7 cmH$_2$O (normal >80 cmH$_2$O), maximum expiratory mouth pressure 52.2 cmH$_2$O (normal >100 cmH$_2$O), with sniff trans-diaphragmatic pressure 46.7 cmH$_2$O (normal >80 cmH$_2$O) and cough gastric pressure 99 cmH$_2$O (normal >120 cmH$_2$O). Bilateral phrenic nerve conduction times were normal

Echocardiogram: normal left ventricular and right ventricular size and function. Weight 31 kg.

Muscle biopsy: consistent with merosin-positive congenital muscular dystrophy and associated rigid spine syndrome

Overnight monitoring of respiration was carried out (Figure 12.1a). This showed a normal baseline awake Sao_2 of 96% with dips to a minimum of between 70 and 70% in REM sleep. Transcutaneous $Paco_2$ ($Tcco_2$) rose from 6.29 to peaks of 9.7 kPa

Management: as the patient had symptoms of morning headache, daytime fatigue with confirmed nocturnal hypoventilation on sleep study and failure to thrive, she started nocturnal NIV using a pressure preset ventilator. After several weeks she noticed improved exercise tolerance and resolution of morning headaches, especially after parties the night before. Weight increased to 34.1 kg over several months, followed by onset of menstruation

Age 17 years: now able to work as part-time hairdresser and in burger bar. Using NIV each night, even on dancing holidays with friends in Ibiza
Age 19 years: stable FEV$_1$/FVC = 990/1250 mL
Age 23 years: pregnant. Genetic counseling: felt to be low risk of fetus being affected. Orthopedic assessment: spinal curvature stable.

Continued

Normal pregnancy and weight gain. Fetal ultrasound scans: normal development

Repeat sleep study (Figure 12.1b). NIV settings adjusted in attempt to mimic normal control of CO_2 during pregnancy and achieve normal Sao_2 levels overnight

Daytime arterial blood gas tensions at 24 weeks pregnancy: Pao_2 14.2 kPa, $Paco_2$ 2.41 kPa, FEV_1/FVC 1.1/1.25 L. Continued to use NIV at night and for short rest period during day in third trimester. Close liaison of medical, anesthetic and obstetric teams. Elective cesarean section at 36 weeks under epidural anesthesia. Used NIV during delivery and in recovery period. Normal female infant: weight 4 lb 8 oz. Discharged after 48 hours

Post partum: FEV_1/FVC 1.05/1.28 L, Pao_2 14.7 kPa, $Paco_2$ 3.9 kPa. No progression of scoliosis during pregnancy. Continues to use NIV at night

Child: normal motor milestones

Outcome of pregnancy in neuromuscular disease

• *Careful monitoring, early delivery, may require ventilatory support.*

Although neuromuscular disorders are relatively uncommon it is estimated that at least 200 000 individuals in Europe have inherited or acquired neuromuscular disease.

Alterations in chest wall properties may also occur in patients with respiratory muscle weakness in the absence of spinal or rib cage deformity. Estenne et al. showed that chest wall compliance was reduced in 75% of patients without scoliosis and with a vital capacity between 50 and 60% of predicted. Pulmonary compliance may also be reduced as a result of a low tidal volume pattern of respiration and shift in the pulmonary pressure–volume curve.[32] In chest wall disorders the respiratory muscles work at a mechanical disadvantage, thereby increasing the work of breathing. Although there is no evidence that respiratory muscle function is impaired during pregnancy, weak inspiratory muscles may be unable to sustain the additional workload of increased thoracic impedance that occurs in pregnancy.[33] Patients with respiratory muscle weakness, particularly if the diaphragm is involved, are liable to develop hypercapnia if respiratory muscle strength is <30% predicted.

Microatelectasis and more generalized atelectasis with a tendency to recurrent chest infections occur in individuals with low inspiratory muscle strength, and poor ability to cough results from expiratory muscle weakness. Basal atelectasis may be exacerbated by a low FRC which becomes lower as the uterus enlarges. Bulbar insufficiency increases the risk of chest infections from aspiration.

Despite the suggestion that patients with scoliosis secondary to muscular dystrophy, resulting in a VC < 1.0 L, may have a poor maternal and fetal outcome,[34] recent work has shown that this is not the case, particularly if ventilatory support is provided. There are an increasing number of reports of successful outcome of pregnancy in spinal muscular atrophy (SMA),[35] and other neuromuscular conditions in patients with minimal respiratory reserve[36]—indeed the VC was as low as 5% predicted in some individuals. In all, careful monitoring of maternal arterial blood gas tensions was carried out with early elective delivery. Respiratory support was provided using NIV.

Primary alveolar hypoventilation and pregnancy

• *Limited experience*

This condition (also known as Ondine's curse) is characterized by absent or reduced ventilatory responses to hypercapnia, hypoxia or both. Lung volumes are normal. Without intervention, gross hypoventilation occurs during sleep, as the voluntary control of breathing is removed. Affected people progress to decompensated hypercapnic failure and cor pulmonale. The condition may be present at birth or acquired (for unknown reasons) in later life. Pieters et al. reported a woman who developed primary alveolar hypoventilation in her 20s, presenting with hypercapnic respiratory failure, polycythemia and pulmonary hypertension (pulmonary arterial pressure 100 mmHg).[37] Respiratory failure was controlled with NIV and cardiac findings reverted to normal after several months of nocturnal ventilatory support. The patient subsequently became pregnant and continued to use nocturnal NIV throughout the pregnancy. No change in ventilatory settings was required. Fetal growth was normal. Labour was induced at 39 weeks and uncomplicated delivery was achieved by vacuum extraction. At 27-month follow-up both infant and mother were in good health.

Obstructive sleep apnea and pregnancy

• *OSA may be exacerbated by pregnancy*
• *NIV should be considered in females with even a mild degree of sleep disordered breathing.*

Obstructive sleep apnea (OSA) has recently been recognized as a major cause of respiratory insufficiency during sleep. Initially thought to be uncommon in premenopausal women, OSA complicating pregnancy has been reported and is probably under-recognized.

Overnight monitoring shows multiple dips in Sao_2 as a result of recurrent periods of upper airway obstruction during sleep. The fall in FRC that accompanies late pregnancy is likely to result in a greater degree of desaturation during apneas or periods of hypoventilation when compared with the non-pregnant state, because alveolar oxygen stores are more rapidly depleted.[38] Each apnea is terminated by arousal that results in sleep fragmentation and somnolence during the day. Arousals are associated with increased sympathetic outflow, which causes swings in systemic blood pressure.[39,40]

High levels of progesterone in pregnancy do not prevent sleep-disordered breathing in women with moderate or severe OSA. The incidence of OSA in pregnancy is not known, although many women report snoring and poor sleep quality.[41] A reduction in pharyngeal dimensions and reduced nasal patency in pregnancy are likely to contribute.[42] Monitoring of respiration during sleep is essential to diagnose OSA,[43] which can be successfully managed, as described below.

A 32-year-old woman presented with severe OSA (apnea/hypopnea index 159/h) in the last trimester.[44] The patient was obese (weight 155 kg, BMI 55) and gained 12 kg during pregnancy. There was a past history of heavy snoring, with daytime somnolence getting worse in the first two trimesters. A sleep study at 36 weeks showed that apneas provoked marked maternal desaturation to a minimum level of 40%, and bradycardia during REM sleep. Cardiotocography showed normal fetal heart rate during the apneas. The patient was treated with continuous positive airway pressure (CPAP) at $15 \, cmH_2O$ during sleep, and delivered electively at 39 weeks. The infant survived but showed signs of growth retardation, suggesting that earlier intervention with CPAP might have been helpful. A repeat maternal sleep study 2 months post partum (weight loss 10 kg) showed persistent apneas with a slightly reduced apnea/hypopnea index (122/h). In this case OSA clearly preceded pregnancy, but was probably exacerbated by weight gain, and increased thoracic and upper airway impedance. Weight gain may precipitate OSA and it is possible that mild-to-moderate OSA may present afresh in pregnancy, triggered at least in part by these mechanisms.

It is probable that there is an association between sleep-disordered breathing/OSA and hypertension in pregnancy, but a causal link and/or association between sleep apnea and pre-eclampsia has not yet been established.[42]

Assessment and management of extrapulmonary ventilatory insufficiency in pregnancy

Pre-pregnancy genetic counseling and discussion of potential medical and obstetric risks are of great importance in patients with restrictive disorders. Prenatal diagnosis is available in an increasing number of inherited neuromuscular conditions. Clinical examination of a woman with chest wall disease should establish the extent of the deformity, degree of respiratory muscle involvement and pulmonary function. Global respiratory muscle strength can be measured with a simple mouth pressure meter. A significant fall in VC on assuming the supine position is seen in patients with diaphragmatic weakness.

A VC of 1 L or less indicates a high risk of respiratory insufficiency during pregnancy. Arterial blood gases should be checked, together with monitoring of overnight Sao_2 and $Paco_2$, and breathing pattern. A sleep study should also be carried out in women with snoring, disturbed sleep, witnessed apneas or daytime somnolence. The risk of OSA is likely to be increased in obese people.

Severe pulmonary hypertension from whatever cause is a major contraindication to pregnancy.[1] The loudness of the pulmonary component of the second heart sound (P2) may be unreliable in scoliosis because of rotation of the heart, but if P2 is louder than the aortic component, pulmonary hypertension is likely.[45] Any suspicion of pulmonary hypertension should be confirmed by ECG and echocardiogram. It should be remembered that congenital heart disease is more common in patients with congenital scoliosis than in the rest of the population.[46,47]

Labour or cesarean section may be managed best by spinal epidural because this reduces the risks of atelectasis.[1] Surprisingly, spinal epidural does not appear to be less effective or associated with more complications in patients who have had previous spinal surgery. The successful use of a spinal microcatheter to provide anesthesia for cesarean section in a patient with cervical deformity and scoliosis caused by Klippel–Feil syndrome has been described.[48] Lumbar and lumbar–sacral scoliosis were associated with a comparatively low rate of obstetric complications in one series.[25] However, in a review of 77 cases with spinal deformity, 71% of deliveries required cesarean section or forceps assistance.[26] As expected, caudal deformities were associated with a higher rate of pelvic disproportion.

The case history in Box 12.1 outlines the clinical course in a young woman with congenital muscular dystrophy associated with rigid spine syndrome. She presented with nocturnal hypoventilation, failure to thrive and delayed puberty. Use of NIV resulted in weight gain, menarche and subsequent successful pregnancy.

Pulmonary arteriovenous malformations and pregnancy

- *Dangerous even when asymptomatic*
- *Pregnancy related growth and maternal deaths due to massive haemoptysis*
- *Patient also likely to have hereditary haemorrhagic telangiectasia.*

Pulmonary arteriovenous malformations (PAVMs) are thin-walled abnormal vessels that replace normal capillaries between the pulmonary arterial and venous circulations.[49] They provide a direct capillary-free communication between the pulmonary and systemic circulations with three main consequences:

1 Pulmonary arterial blood passing through these right-to-left shunts cannot be oxygenated, leading to hypoxemia.
2 The fragile vessels may hemorrhage into a bronchus or the pleural cavity.
3 The absence of a filtering capillary bed leads to paradoxical embolic stroke and brain abscess.

In addition, as over 90% of patients with PAVMs have underlying hereditary hemorrhagic telangiectasia (HHT, Osler–Weber–Rendu syndrome), additional HHT-related risks are a concern.

Of these, the most important risk for pregnant patients is life-threatening hemoptysis, which may be prevented if PAVMs are diagnosed and treated. Embolization offers the safest method of treatment and may be safely undertaken in late pregnancy if required.

However, unless chest radiographs or respiratory investigations have been performed, the obstetrician and patient are likely to be unaware that the patient has PAVMs because of the paucity of PAVM-associated signs and symptoms.

Data amalgamated from all case series reported between 1948 and 1998 revealed that, although a third of patients were cyanosed or clubbed, barely 50% of patients had any respiratory symptoms[50] and breathlessness may not be appreciated until after the condition has been treated because PAVM patients tolerate worsening hypoxemia on exercise, as a result of their low pulmonary vascular resistance and ability to generate a supranormal cardiac output, which may increase further on exercise.

How to recognize PAVM patients

HHT: a clue to the presence of PAVMs
- *'Do you, or anyone in your family, have nosebleeds?'*
Although PAVMs do occur sporadically, in our series about 90% are the result of underlying HHT. HHT is classically recognized by familial nose bleeds, chronic gastrointestinal bleeding and the characteristic mucocutaneous telangiectasia[51] and, as a result, many patients will have family members or themselves under review by ENT surgeons, dermatologists, gastroenterologists or other specialists. In addition to pulmonary AVMs (>30%), the condition also causes cerebral (10%), hepatic (30%) and spinal (<1%) AVMs. International consensus diagnostic criteria require the presence of three of the four criteria of HHT for a definitive diagnosis, the four criteria being spontaneous recurrent nosebleeds, mucocutaneous telangiectasia, visceral involvement and an affected first-degree relative.

However, although features of HHT were recorded in 229 of our PAVM patients, only 83 of these (36%) had required specialist medical care for other aspects of HHT. Furthermore, as HHT is a disorder of late-onset penetrance, during their child-bearing years, an apparently unaffected child of an HHT patient still has a 5–20% chance of actually carrying the HHT disease gene.[51] Thus the affected pregnant HHT patient may not have an existing diagnosis of HHT.

As most patients with HHT do not know their diagnosis, the most important clinical question is 'Do you, or anyone in your family, have nosebleeds?'. PAVMs will be present in 30–50% of HHT patients, may be suspected if oxygen saturation levels are low , but cannot be excluded by normal Sao_2, or chest radiographs. As the fetal radiation risks from further imaging are difficult to justify, our practice is to advise all individuals with suspected HHT of the potential pregnancy-related hazards of PAVMs.

Pregnancy and PAVMs

Pregnancy well tolerated even with substantial hypoxemia
In our first retrospective series of HHT patients and their first-degree relatives,[52] there were 23 pregnancies in 12 women (from 8 different HHT families) with known PAVMs. Of these, 6 demonstrated evidence of PAVM growth during pregnancy, including the case described in Figure 12.2. This is an individual in whom PAVMs were diagnosed at 13 years as a result of cyanosis and dyspnea.

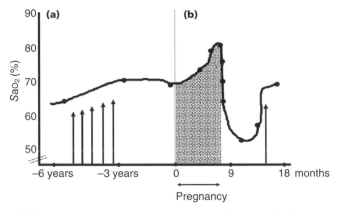

Figure 12.2 PAVMs and pregnancy: oxygen saturation (Sao_2): (a) before pregnancy (years) and (b) during and after pregnancy (months). Stippled area indicates pregnancy; arrows indicate times of embolization.

(HHT was also diagnosed in view of nosebleeds, telangiectasia and a positive family history.) Initial investigations revealed extensive PAVMs, Sao_2 65% erect, and a right-to-left shunt of 48%. After five embolization sessions over 6 years, Sao_2 remained very low (73% erect) with right-to-left shunt 38%. The woman became pregnant aged 19 years and decided to proceed with the pregnancy, after being counseled of the hazards to her health. She attended an antenatal clinic every week from 22 weeks' gestation, and arterial oxygen saturations were measured on each occasion. Her Sao_2 in the sitting or erect posture actually increased somewhat during her pregnancy (from 67–73% to 80–82%), but fell to low levels in the postpartum period (71–65% to 53%, subsequently 58%) with an increase in right-to-left shunt from 38% to 50%. There was some recovery at 9 months post partum. The baby was perfectly healthy and had a normal weight for his gestational age.

This case illustrates that a normal pregnancy and delivery of a normal baby can occur in the presence of severe arterial hypoxaemia. We knew from previous studies that this patient had a good cardiovascular response to exercise, the cardiac output at 30 watts being 12.8–16.5 L/min (140–180% of predicted) at an Sao_2 of 61–67%. Thus, she could respond to the cardiovascular stress of pregnancy in the same manner and maintain a normal oxygen delivery to her tissues, including the placenta.

Risk of PAVM growth

In six of our cases in our first series, pregnancy-related PAVM growth or increased right-to-left shunt was noted, including the case illustrated in Figure 12.2. Two other similar cases have been reported in the literature. To assess the frequency of pregnancy-related PAVM growth, we recently reviewed data on the 121 female PAVM patients reviewed at our institution between May 1999

Table 12.3 Oxygen saturation (Sao_2) before, during and after pregnancy in 10 women with PAVMs

Position	Comparison	Median difference in Sao_2 (IQ range)	P
Standing	Before vs during	1.8 (0.00, 6.0)	0.05
	Before vs after	−2.0 (−4.4, −0.9)	0.02
Lying	Before vs during	1.3 (0.0, 2.5)	0.09
	Before vs after	−2.5 (−3.4, −0.3)	0.03

Arterial oxygen saturation (Sao_2) was measured in all clinic patients lying and standing for 10 min, with measurements made each minute. − indicates a fall in Sao_2 between the earlier and later measurements.

and February 2004.[53] Excluding early miscarriages, 10 women had pregnancies, and all delivered healthy babies. The summary of these data are in Table 12.3. Overall, there was a significant decrease in Sao_2 from before to after pregnancy in both positions ($n = 9$), supported by radiological evidence of PAVM growth in most cases, some associated with recanalization of existing feeding arteries in previously treated patients. The cause of the growth or remodeling remains unclear.

Importantly, these data, as in the case in Figure 12.2, suggest an improvement in Sao_2 during pregnancy, which may mask the presence or growth of PAVMs. Potential causes include the increase in mixed venous oxygen resulting from pregnancy-induced changes in minute ventilation, and cardiac output and direct compression of the lower lobe PAVMs by the gravid uterus.

Risk of hemoptysis

In our first retrospective series of HHT patients and their first-degree relatives,[52] two first-degree relatives died in the last trimester of pregnancy as a result of fatal pulmonary hemorrhages. There are other case reports of pulmonary hemorrhage from PAVMs during pregnancy—in the report by Ference et al., three of the seven women were pregnant at the time.[54]

In our more recent series of consecutive PAVM patients,[53] 3 of 10 (30%) had substantial hemoptysis during pregnancy necessitating induction of labour (×1) or emergency embolizations. All three had normal pulmonary artery pressures (mean ≤12 mmHg) and two had relatively limited PAVM disease ($Sao_2 \geq 96\%$, right-to-left shunt ≤5%).

Issues in labour management

PAVM related

In view of the risk of paradoxical emboli, particular care should be taken to avoid embolization of air or microbes. Thus delivery should be covered by antibiotic prophylaxis as for other surgical interventions. General anesthesia with positive-pressure ventilation risks a temporary increase in shunt flow. These features have led some in the past to favor vaginal deliveries. However, the other aspects of HHT that will affect most women with PAVMs need to be considered.

HHT related
Spinal AVMs are thought to affect 1% of HHT patients, and are often asymptomatic.[55] Paraplegia caused by spinal hemorrhage is a very rare but recognized complication of spinal or epidural insertion.[56] Although there are no reports linking such spinal hemorrhage from spinal AVMs induced by regional anesthesia to PAVM/HHT patients, in view of the potentially catastrophic consequences, our current practice is to suggest that epidurals are avoided unless spinal AVMs have been excluded by appropriate imaging.

Cerebral AVMs (CAVMs) affect up to 10% of HHT patients and are usually asymptomatic, and thus often undiagnosed because screening for asymptomatic cerebral AVMs in HHT patients is not recommended in the UK and Europe. In a series of 32 cases, the risk of intracranial hemorrhage from cerebral AVM appeared to be higher during the second and third trimester of pregnancy than during delivery,[57] and higher if there had been a previous cerebral AVM bleed[57] in keeping with data from the non-pregnant cerebral AVM population.

Conclusion
An experienced obstetric and obstetric anesthetic team should be involved to discuss the risks associated with the various delivery modes and anesthetic options. Although some have advocated assisted vaginal delivery, concern about epidural safety and the possibility of spinal AVMs leads us to favor elective cesarean section in our practice, recognizing that cesarean delivery may increase the hazard of paradoxical air embolism.

Advice for patients with PAVMs who are pregnant or wish to become pregnant
We advise patients and their families (via a written patient information leaflet), their obstetricians and other medical practitioners that
- PAVMs, even if associated with severe arterial hypoxemia, should not harm the baby *in utero*.
- For the majority of PAVM patients, pregnancy is uneventful, but pregnancy poses a risk to a small proportion of women with PAVMs, and individual patients may need to be cautioned against pregnancy on a case-by-case basis.
- Women with PAVMs should be treated maximally pre-pregnancy if possible.
- PAVMs are likely to enlarge during pregnancy.
- Fatal maternal hemorrhage has been described, and therefore any hemoptysis should be seen as a medical emergency and prompt immediate admission for consideration of embolization and/or early delivery.

- The patient should also be aware that she is likely to have HHT, any offspring would then have a 50% risk of inheriting HHT, and the possibility of spinal or cerebral AVMs may influence labour management (as above). If HHT is symptomatic, they may be reassured by the anecdotal data that any deterioration in nosebleeds or skin telangiectasia is likely to be temporary, with no firm data about effects on hepatic and cerebral AVMs.

General conclusions

- A normal pregnancy stresses the respiratory system less than the cardiovascular system.
- The pulmonary hypertension of respiratory disease is more of a hazard to the pregnant woman than a reduction in ventilatory capacity. The development of cor pulmonale in pregnancy is a possibility in any mother whose pulmonary function is <50% predicted, or whose respiratory muscle power or gas exchange is severely compromised.
- The risk of cor pulmonale in pregnancy is probably linked to the level of pulmonary arterial pressure, with a watershed at 40 mmHg systolic, fortunately only rarely exceeded by the pulmonary hypertension associated with residence at altitude, cystic fibrosis, and neuromuscular and chest wall disorders.
- The standard medical treatment for cor pulmonale comprises: control of respiratory infection with antibiotics and physiotherapy; avoidance of fluid retention; relief of deteriorating hypoxemia with additional inspired oxygen; support of ventilatory failure with nasal positive-pressure ventilation; and relief of airflow obstruction with nebulized bronchodilators. There is no indication for additional vasodilator drugs because the PHT of primary respiratory disease is not particularly severe, and because beta-agonist bronchodilator preparations are also pulmonary vasodilators. Patients with cystic fibrosis should be managed jointly with a cystic fibrosis clinic.
- Pulmonary arteriovenous malformations with right-to-left shunting, usually associated with hereditary hemorrhagic telangiectasia, are a special case, because pulmonary artery pressures are normal or low, even though arterial hypoxemia may be severe. Cardiac output increases to supernormal levels to compensate for the arterial hypoxemia, and the fetus develops normally. But the mother runs the risks of pulmonary hemorrhage, an increase in the right-to left shunt or paradoxical emboli.

References

1 de Swiet M, ed. Diseases of the respiratory system. In: *Medical Disorders in Obstetric Practice*. Oxford: Blackwell, 2002: pp 1–23.
2 Gee JBL, Packer BS, Millen JE et al. Pulmonary mechanics during pregnancy. *J Clin Invest* 1967;**46**:945–52.
3 Awe RJ, Nicotra MB, Newson TD et al. Arterial oxygenation and alveolar–arterial gradients in term pregnancy. *Obstet Gynecol* 1979;**53**:182–6.
4 Weinberger SE, Weiss ST, Cohen WR et al. Pregnancy and the lung. *Am Rev Respir Dis* 1980;**121**:559–81.

5 Templeton A, Kelman GR. Maternal blood gases (PaO_2–PaO_2), physiological shunt and VD/VT in pregnancy. *Br J Anaesth* 1976;**48**:1001–4.

6 Lees MM, Taylor SH, Scott DB et al. A study of cardiac output at rest during pregnancy. *J Obstet Gynaecol Br Commonw* 1967;**74**:319–28.

7 Milne JA, Mills RJ, Coutts JRT et al. The effect of human pregnancy on the pulmonary transfer factor for carbon monoxide as measured by the single breath method. *Clin Sci Mol Med* 1977;**53**:271–6.

8 Gazioglu K, Kaltreider NL, Rosen M et al. Pulmonary function during pregnancy in normal women and in patients with cardiopulmonary disease. *Thorax* 1970;**25**: 445–50.

9 Tatsumi K, Hannhart B, Moore LG. Influences of sex steroids on ventilation and ventilatory control. In: Dempsey JA, Pack AI (eds), *Regulation of Breathing*. New York: Marcel Dekker, 1994: pp 829–64.

10 Moore LG. Circulation in the pregnant and non pregnant state. In: Weir EK, Reeves JT (eds), *Pulmonary Vascular Physiology and Pathophysiology*. New York: Marcel Dekker, 1989:135–72.

11 Magness RR, Parker CR, Rosenfeld CR. Systemic and uterine responses to chronic infusion of estradiol-17β. *Am J Physiol* 1993;**265**:E690–8.

12 Moore LG, Jahniggen D, Rounds SS et al. Maternal hyperventilation helps preserve arterial oxygenation during high-altitude pregnancy. *J Appl Physiol* 1982;**52**:690–4.

13 Moore LG, Brodeur P, Clunbe O et al. Maternal hypoxic ventilatory response, ventilation, and infant birth weight at 4300 m. *J Appl Physiol* 1986;**60**:1401–6.

14 Gaensler EA, Patton WE, Verstraeten JM et al. Pulmonary function in pregnancy. III. Serial observations in patients with pulmonary insufficiency. *Am Rev Tuber Pulmon Dis* 1953;**67**:779–97.

15 Giesler CF, Buehler JH, Depp R. Alpha 1-antitrypsin deficiency. Severe obstructive disease and pregnancy. *Obstet Gynecol* 1977;**49**:31–4.

16 Boyd JM, Mehta A, Murphy DJ. Fertility and pregnancy outcomes in men and women with cystic fibrosis in the United Kingdom. *Human Repr* 2004;**19**:2238–43.

17 Goss CH, Rubenfeld GD, Otto K et al. The effect of pregnancy on survival in women with cystic fibrosis. *Chest* 2003;**124**:1460–8.

18 Edenborough FP, Mackenzie WE, Stableforth DE. The outcome of 75 pregnancies in 55 women with cystic fibrosis in the United Kingdom 1977–1996; *Br J Obstet Gynaecol* 2000;**107**:254–261.

19 Edenborough FP. Women with cystic fibrosis and their potential for reproduction. *Thorax* 2001;**56**:649–55.

20 Sawicka EH, Spencer GT, Branthwaite MA. Management of respiratory failure complicating pregnancy in severe kyphoscoliosis: a new use for an old technique? *Br J Dis Chest* 1986;**80**:191–6.

21 Simonds AK. Domiciliary non-invasive ventilation in restrictive disorders and stable neuromuscular disease. In: Simonds AK (ed.), *Non-invasive Respiratory Support. A practical handbook*. London: Arnold, 2001: pp 131–45.

22 King TE. Restrictive lung disease in pregnancy. *Clin Chest Med* 1992;**13**:607–22.

23 Kopenhager T, Kopenhager T. A review of 50 pregnant patients with kyphoscoliosis. *Br J Obstet Gynaecol* 1977;**84**:585–7.

24 Siegler D, Zorab PA. Pregnancy in thoracic scoliosis. *Br J Dis Chest* 1981;**75**:367–70.

25 To WW, Wong MW. Kyphoscoliosis complicating pregnancy. *Int J Gynecol Obstet* 1996;**55**:123.

26 Phelan JP, Dainer MJ, Cowherd DW. Pregnancy complicated by thoracolumbar scoliosis. *South Med J* 1978;**71**:76–8.

27 Bergofsky EH. Respiratory failure in disorders of the thoracic cage. *Am Rev Respir Dis* 1979;**119**:643–69.

28 Shneerson JM. Pulmonary artery pressure in thoracic scoliosis during and after exercise while breathing air and pure oxygen. *Thorax* 1978;**33**:747–54.

29 Branthwaite MA. Cardiorespiratory consequences of unfused idiopathic scoliosis. *Br J Dis Chest* 1986;**80**:360–9.

30 Blount WP, Mellencamp DD. The effect of pregnancy on idiopathic scoliosis. *J Bone Joint Surg* 1980;**62A**:1083–7.

31 Betz RR, Bunnell WP, Lambrecht-Mulier E et al. Scoliosis and pregnancy. *J Bone Joint Surg* 1987;**69A**:90–5.

32 Gibson GJ, Pride NB, Newsom-Davis JN et al. Pulmonary mechanics in patients with respiratory muscle weakness. *Am Rev Respir Dis* 1977;**115**:389–95.

33 Contreras G, Gutierrez M, Beroiza T et al. Ventilatory drive and respiratory muscle function in pregnancy. *Am Rev Respir Dis* 1995;**144**:837–41.

34 Gamzu R, Shenhav M, Fainaru O et al. Impact of pregnancy on respiratory capacity in women with muscular dystrophy and kyphoscoliosis. *J Reprod Med* 2002;**47**:53–6.

35 Yim R, Kirschner K, Murphy E et al. Successful pregnancy in a patient with spinal muscular atrophy and severe kyphoscoliosis. *Am J Phys Med* 2003;**82**:222–5.

36 Bach JR. Successful pregnancies for ventilator users. *Am J Phys Med* 2003;**82**:226–9.

37 Pieters TH, Amy JJ, Burrini D et al. Normal pregnancy in primary alveolar hypoventilation treated with nocturnal nasal intermittent positive pressure ventilation. *Eur Respir J* 1995;**8**:1424–7.

38 Cheun JK, Choi KT. Arterial oxygen desaturation rate following obstructive apnea in parturients. *J Korean Med Sci* 1992;**7**:6–10.

39 Noda A, Okada T, Hayashi H et al. 24 hour ambulatory blood pressure variability in obstructive sleep apnea syndrome. *Chest* 1993;**103**:1343–7.

40 Davies RJO, Vardi-Visy K, Clarke M et al. Identification of sleep disruption and sleep disordered breathing profile from systolic blood pressure profile. *Thorax* 1993;**48**:1242–7.

41 Feinsilver SH, Hertz G. Respiration during sleep in pregnancy. *Clin Chest Med* 1992;**13**:637–44.

42 Edwards N, Middleton PG, Blyton DM et al. Sleep disordered breathing and pregnancy. *Thorax* 2002;**57**:555–8.

43 Simonds AK. Sleep studies of respiratory function and home respiratory support. *BMJ* 1994;**309**:35–40.

44 Charbonneau M, Falcone T, Cosio MG et al. Obstructive sleep apnea during pregnancy. Therapy and implications for fetal health. *Am Rev Respir Dis* 1991;**144**:461–3.

45 Shneerson KM. Deformities of the thoracic cage. II. Acquired deformities. In: Emerson P (ed.), *Thoracic Medicine*. London: Butterworths, 1981: pp 363–4.

46 Reckles LN, Peterson HA, Bianco AJ et al. The association of scoliosis and congenital heart disease. *J Bone Joint Surg* 1975;**57A**:449–55.

47 Simonds AK, Carroll N, Branthwaite MA. Kyphoscoliosis as a cause of cardiorespiratory failure: pitfalls of diagnosis. *Respir Med* 1989;**83**:149–50.

48 Dresner MR, Maclean AR. Anaesthesia for caesarean section in a patient with Klippel–Feil syndrome. *Anaesthesia* 1995;**50**:807–9.

49 Shovlin C, Jackson J. Pulmonary arteriovenous malformations. In: Peacock A, Rubin L (eds), *Pulmonary Circulation*, 2nd edn. London: Arnold, 2004.

50 Shovlin CL, Letarte M. Hereditary haemorrhagic telangiectasia and pulmonary arteriovenous malformations: issues in clinical management and review of pathogenic mechanisms. *Thorax* 1999;**54**:714–29.

51 Begbie ME, Wallace G, Shovlin CL. Hereditary haemorrhagic telangiectasia (Osler–Weber–Rendu syndrome): a view from the 21st century. *Postgrad Med J* 2003;**79**:18–24.

52 Shovlin CL, Winstock AR, Peters AM et al. Medical complications of pregnancy in hereditary haemorrhagic telangiectasia. *Q J Med* 1995;**88**:879–87.

53 Macedo P, Jackson JE, McCarthy A et al. Maternal risks of pregnancy in patients with pulmonary arteriovenous malformations. *Thorax* 2004;**59**:ii87.

54 Ference BA, Shannon TM, White RI et al. Life threatening pulmonary hemorrhage with pulmonary arteriovenous malformations and hereditary hemorrhagic telangiectasia. *Chest* 1994;**106**:1387–92.

55 Guttmacher AE, Marchuk DA, White RI. Hereditary hemorrhagic telangiectasia. *N Engl J Med* 1995;**333**:918–24.

56 Sage DJ. Epidurals, spinals and bleeding disorders in pregnancy: a review. *Anaesth Intensive Care* 1990;**18**:319–26.

57 Velut S, Vinikoff L, Destrieux C et al. Cerebro-meningeal hemorrhage secondary to ruptured vascular malformation during pregnancy and post-partum. *Neurochirurgie* 2000;**46**:95–104.

CHAPTER 13

Hypertrophic cardiomyopathy and pregnancy

Jorge R Alegria, Rick A Nishimura

Hypertrophic cardiomyopathy is a unique disease entity that is characterized by a primary hypertrophy of a non-dilated ventricle with underlying myocyte and myofibrillar disarray.[1-3] It has fascinated cardiologists ever since the disorder was rediscovered as a clinical entity after Donald Teare described an autopsy series of eight patients who had died suddenly,[4] and Sir Russell Brock encountered 'subaortic stenosis' at an operation for presumed valvular aortic stenosis.[5] Hypertrophic cardiomyopathy has subsequently been found to be a relatively common genetic disorder, seen in about 1 in 500 of the adult population. It is usually caused by a missense mutation in 1 of at least 10 genes that encode the proteins of the cardiac sarcomere.[6,7]

The clinical diagnosis of hypertrophic cardiomyopathy is established with two-dimensional echocardiography demonstrating marked left ventricular hypertrophy, which is typically asymmetric in distribution in the absence of other diseases that could produce a secondary hypertrophy.[6] The World Health Association has supported the term 'hypertrophic cardiomyopathy' to describe the spectrum of this disease entity.[8] Most patients with hypertrophic cardiomyopathy are asymptomatic but a subset will present with symptoms of exertional chest pain, dyspnea, fatigue, palpitations and syncope. Sudden death may be the initial manifestation of the disease. The pathophysiology is complex and consists of a combination of dynamic outflow tract obstruction, diastolic dysfunction, myocardial ischemia, mitral regurgitation and arrhythmias. It is now recognized that there is a wide spectrum of morphologic and phenotypic abnormalities in patients with hypertrophic cardiomyopathy, which exists not only between individuals at different ages but within families. In the past, hypertrophic cardiomyopathy was considered to be a rare disorder with a grave prognosis. Subsequent studies from non-referral centers have shown that hypertrophic cardiomyopathy is not uncommon and the overall prognosis of a large population of patients with hypertrophic cardiomyopathy is relatively benign.[6,9] There is a subset of patients, however, who are at high risk of sudden death or heart failure and require aggressive risk stratification. Thus, although most patients with hypertrophic cardiomyopathy can safely have a pregnancy, it is important to have an understanding of the disease and identify those at risk when managing these patients.

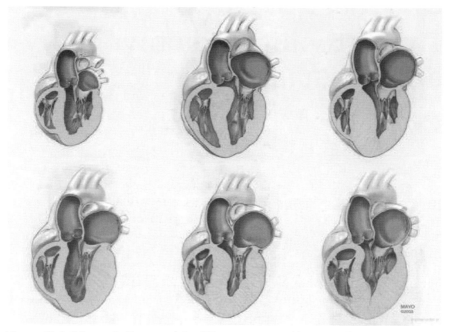

Figure 13.1 Schematic diagram of the different variants of hypertrophic cardiomyopathy. Upper left is the normal heart. Shown are variants of the location and degree of hypertrophy. By permission of the Mayo Foundation for Medical Education and Research.

Anatomy and pathophysiology

The indispensable finding in hypertrophic cardiomyopathy is hypertrophy of the myocardium in the absence of a secondary etiology such as hypertension, infiltrative or glycogen storage disorders. Although initially the hypertrophy was described as primarily involving the ventricular septum, this hypertrophy can be localized to the basal septum, free wall or ventricular apex (Figure 13.1). Concentric hypertrophy of all walls can also be seen in patients with hypertrophic cardiomyopathy. There is now also evidence that some patients may have a gene mutation associated with familial hypertrophic cardiomyopathy, and yet may not necessarily have hypertrophy at initial screening as a result of incomplete penetrance.[10] The hypertrophy may be a late manifestation of the disease and not show itself until later decades of life. Sophisticated analysis of myocardial function using Doppler tissue imaging may be able to detect this pre-clinical stage.[11–13]

Although most patients are asymptomatic, there is a subset of patients who have severe limiting symptoms from hypertrophic cardiomyopathy. This can be caused by one or more of several pathophysiologic processes. Diastolic dysfunction resulting from abnormal ventricular relaxation and poor ventricular compliance plays a major role in producing these symptoms. Myocardial ischemia from oxygen supply–demand mismatch, intraluminal thickening of the intra-

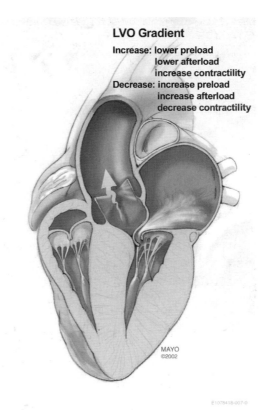

Figure 13.2 Schematic diagram of the left ventricle in hypertrophic cardiomyopathy during systole. There is projection of the basal septum into the outflow tract with systolic anterior motion of the mitral valve, which results in left ventricular outflow tract obstruction. The obstruction is dynamic, dependent on the preload, afterload and contractility of the heart. By permission of the Mayo Foundation for Medical Education and Research.

arterial bed and decreased coronary flow reserve may contribute to these symptoms. Autonomic dysfunction may also occur, resulting in inappropriate vasodilatation.

A subset of patients have dynamic left ventricular outflow tract obstruction, which may be responsible for symptoms[3,14] (Figure 13.2). This is caused by severe hypertrophy of the basal septum projecting into the left ventricular outflow tract and secondary systolic anterior motion of the mitral valve. The abnormal mitral valve motion is produced either by a 'Venturi effect' from an increase in velocity sucking the mitral valve into the outflow tract or by 'drag forces' pushing redundant mitral valve leaflets into the outflow tract.[15] Secondary mitral regurgitation may be present from distortion of the mitral valve apparatus and contribute further to symptoms. The mitral valve apparatus is almost always abnormal in these patients, with anterior displacement of the papillary muscles, which position the mitral valve leaflets so as to contribute further to this outflow tract obstruction.[16] It is the young patients with severe outflow tract obstruction who are at highest risk for hemodynamic deterioration during pregnancy.

Diagnosis of hypertrophic cardiomyopathy in patients of child-bearing age

As young patients with hypertrophic cardiomyopathy are symptom free, the diagnosis of hypertrophic cardiomyopathy is primarily made through family screening or after a routine medical examination when a murmur is heard on auscultation or an abnormal ECG is found. Hypertrophic cardiomyopathy is sometimes first recognized during pregnancy when systolic murmurs lead to cardiologic referral. As the murmur of left ventricular outflow tract obstruction is dynamic, maneuvers such as squat to stand should be performed. In patients with hypertrophic cardiomyopathy, the length and intensity of a late systolic ejection murmur should significantly increase upon assuming the standing position.

The ECG is almost always abnormal in patients beyond the first decade of life with hypertrophic cardiomyopathy (Figure 13.3).[17,18] It often shows features of atrial and ventricular hypertrophy that are associated with marked ST- and T-wave abnormalities. Echocardiography should always be performed in pa-

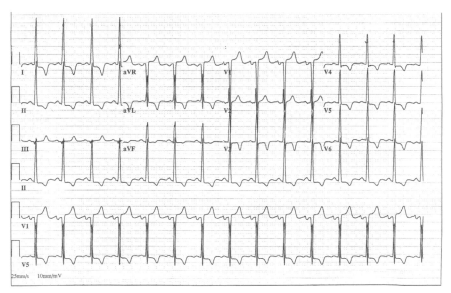

Figure 13.3 A 12-lead ECG from a patient with hypertrophic cardiomyopathy. There is left ventricular hypertrophy present. There is high voltage as well as secondary ST–T-wave abnormalities. There is left atrial enlargement.

tients with an abnormal ECG to look for the increase in left ventricular wall thickening that is considered the 'gold standard' of diagnosis when present (Figure 13.4). However, in some patients with an abnormal ECG, it may not identify hypertrophy, especially if it is localized to an abnormal location such as the apex. In a situation where there is significant unexplained abnormality of the ECG, repeat echocardiography with contrast enhancement or magnetic resonance imaging (MRI) should be performed.

The presence or absence of left ventricular outflow tract obstruction should be documented both by examination and by echocardiography. Systolic anterior motion of the mitral valve with a late peaking, high-velocity Doppler signal in the left ventricular outflow tract is diagnostic of dynamic left ventricular outflow tract obstruction (Figure 13.5). The magnitude of the obstruction is determined by the peak Doppler velocity (Figure 13.5 shows a velocity of more than 6 m/sec) and should be measured at rest and during provocation (after a premature ventricular contraction, during the strain phase of the Valsalva maneuver or during inhalation of amyl nitrite). Secondary mitral regurgitation, characterized by a posteriorly directed jet, should be identified and semi-quantified.

Genetics and family screening

Hypertrophic cardiomyopathy is usually the result of a missense mutation in the sarcomeric protein genes and transmitted in an autosomal dominant manner. There are over 200 mutations that have been identified in 10 different sarcomeric genes.[19] Thus, once the diagnosis of hypertrophic cardiomyopathy has been made, all patients should undergo genetic counseling and family screening. This should be performed even if the patient is completely asymptomatic. All first-degree relatives of the proband should be screened with physical examination, an ECG and echocardiography. In adolescence, screening should be performed every year throughout their growth spurt. In adults, screening should be performed every 5 years because hypertrophy may appear late in patients with certain gene mutations. In the future, genetic analysis should aid in helping screen the presence or absence of hypertrophic disease in first-degree relatives of patients with documented hypertrophic cardiomyopathy. Although initial data suggested that certain specific mutations may predispose to sudden death or have a benign course,[20] the accuracy of this prediction has been challenged with studies of unrelated hypertrophic cardiomyopathy patients that demonstrated that specific malignant or benign mutations are rare and clinical outcomes cannot be successfully predicted.[21,22]

In women who wish to become pregnant, genetic counseling is essential. There is a 50% chance that the child may have hypertrophic cardiomyopathy. If hypertrophic cardiomyopathy becomes manifest in the very early childhood years, severe disease occurs and the prognosis may be dismal.[23] The utility of prenatal ultrasound screening is controversial. In the future prenatal molecular diagnosis may be performed.[24]

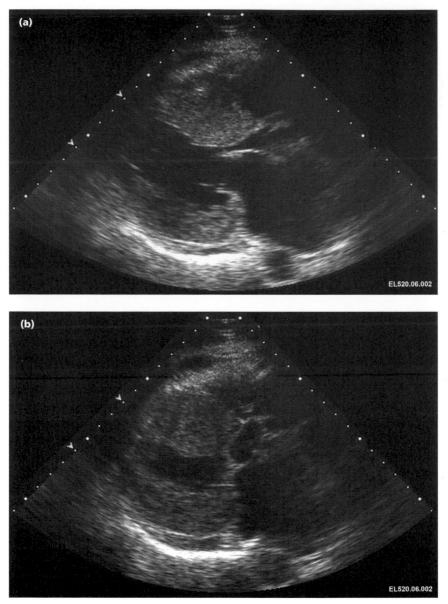

Figure 13.4 A two-dimensional echocardiogram from a patient with hypertrophic cardiomyopathy. There is an increase in left ventricular wall thickness, with a greater increase in thickness of the ventricular septum. (a): parasternal long-axis view during diastole. (b): parasternal long-axis view during systole.

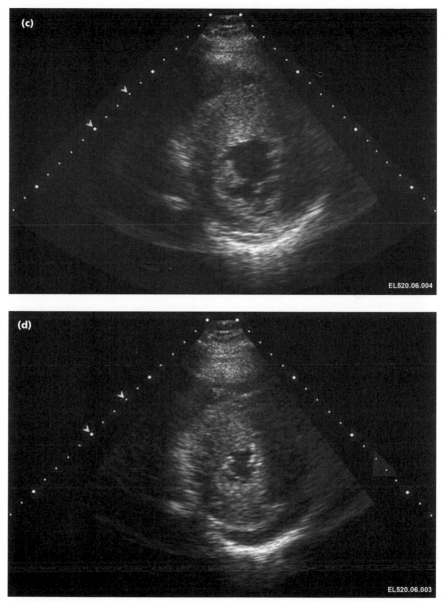

Figure 13.4 *Continued* (c): short axis, diastole. (d): short axis, systole. There is systolic anterior motion of the mitral valve causing left ventricular outflow tract obstruction.

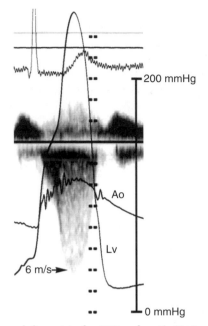

Figure 13.5 Simultaneous left ventricular (LV) and aortic (Ao) pressure from catheterization with continuous wave Doppler of the LV outflow tract. The peak velocity of 6 m/sec by Doppler corresponds to the gradient of 150 mmHg by catheterization.

Risks in pregnancy

The risks in pregnancy are related either to hemodynamic deterioration or arrhythmias and sudden death. Most young woman with hypertrophic cardiomyopathy will go through pregnancy without difficulty.[25–29] The increased blood volume and stroke volume of pregnancy are beneficial for the dynamic left ventricular outflow tract obstruction. Most women who have no or mild symptoms before the pregnancy will not develop more symptoms during the pregnancy course. There are some who become more dyspneic as a result of the larger blood volume but this can be controlled with low-dose diuretics.

In patients who have moderate to severe symptoms before the pregnancy, symptoms will worsen in 10–30% of patients, especially if there is pre-existing left ventricular outflow tract obstruction. The higher the left ventricular outflow tract gradient, the more likely that there will be progressive symptoms.[25] It is the subset of patients with very severe obstruction (gradient >100 mmHg) who are at highest risk of hemodynamic deterioration during pregnancy and delivery.

Sudden death or resuscitated ventricular fibrillation is unusual but has been reported to occur in patients with hypertrophic cardiomyopathy during pregnancy.[25,30–33] In an Italian series of 100 women with hypertrophic cardiomyopathy, there were two pregnancy-related arrhythmic deaths.[25] The maternal mortality rate was 10 per 1000 live births and was higher than the expected mortality rate in the Italian population (relative risk 17.1, 95% CI 2.0–61.8). However, the absolute risk of death was low and each of the two patients who died had significant risk factors for sudden cardiac death: one had severe hypertrophy and severe outflow tract obstruction (>115 mmHg) and the other a highly malignant family history of hypertrophic cardiomyopathy (five young relatives died suddenly).

Management in pregnancy

Even though the outcome is usually favorable, some patients will develop symptoms for the first time during pregnancy, or pre-existing symptoms will get worse. When symptoms are present, beta blockade should be started Table 13.1. The dosage of beta blocker should be titrated to attain a resting heart rate less than 70 beats/min (bpm). Beta blockers have the potential to cause growth retardation, low Apgar scores or neonatal hypoglycemia in the infants but this is rare.[21,34] Breast-feeding is not contraindicated but atenolol, acebutolol, nadolol and sotalol are secreted in breast milk in larger amounts than the other beta blockers. Verapamil is also safe for use in pregnancy if beta blockers are not tolerated, but can cause hemodynamic deterioration and sudden death if started in a patient with a severe resting left ventricular outflow tract obstruction. When verapamil is initiated in patients with severe left ventricular obstruction, this should be done under monitored conditions in hospital.

Low-dose diuretics may be useful if patients develop pulmonary congestive symptoms during the pregnancy as a result of the volume overload. However, care must be taken not to cause too much of a reduction in preload because this may exacerbate the left ventricular outflow tract obstruction. Periodic bedrest in the left lateral decubitus position is recommended for all patients with hypertrophic cardiomyopathy and even mild symptoms.

In patients who have severe symptoms and severe outflow tract obstruction, septal reduction therapy is recommended before proceeding with pregnancy. Septal myectomy is considered the 'gold standard' for symptomatic patients who have persistent symptoms despite optimal medical therapy.[35] In young healthy women, the risk of the operation *in experienced centers* is less than 1%.[36] Septal myectomy relieves the gradient and produces an excellent reduction in symptoms. Surgical myectomy has been performed during pregnancy in the rare patient with a large outflow gradient who develops severe intractable symptoms during pregnancy.

Table 13.1 General recommendations for management of patients with hypertrophic cardiomyopathy during pregnancy

Document degree of left ventricular outflow tract (LVOT) obstruction and risk stratification
Risk stratification for sudden death
Beta blockade for symptoms
Avoid decrease in preload (dehydration, over diuresis)
Avoid inotropes (dopamine or dobutamine) and vasodilators (nifedipine)
In the hypotensive patient balance fluids and vasoconstrictor

Septal ablation has been considered an alternative to septal myectomy in patients with hypertrophic cardiomyopathy and left ventricular outflow tract obstruction.[37] However, the long-term effect of this procedure is unknown. It is not known whether or not creating a large infarct in patients already at risk of ventricular arrhythmias may enhance the propensity to develop dangerous arrhythmias or cause adverse ventricular remodeling with time.[38] Therefore, in women of child-bearing age, septal myectomy has been considered the procedure of choice in our institution (Mayo Clinic)to which such rare patients are referred.

Arrhythmias are uncommon in patients with hypertrophic cardiomyopathy undergoing pregnancy.[25,26] Should atrial fibrillation or flutter occur, cardioversion should be considered if there is hemodynamic compromise as a result of the loss of atrial contraction and fast ventricular response. Beta blockers are usually the drug of choice in preventing further episodes, although low-dose amiodarone can be used if recurrent episodes are present. Amiodarone has been used safely in pregnancy. Fetal hypothyroidism may occur so that a neonatal assessment after delivery is warranted but no congenital abnormalities have been noted.

Aggressive risk stratification to determine those at risk for sudden death should be performed on all patients with hypertrophic cardiomyopathy. The major risk factors that predict sudden death include previous out-of-hospital arrest or documented sustained ventricular tachycardia, and a strong family history of hypertrophic cardiomyopathy with sudden death. Other 'minor' risk factors for the occurrence of sudden death include severe hypertrophy (thickness >3 cm), non-sustained ventricular tachycardia on Holter monitoring, a drop in blood pressure with exercise and perfusion defects on MRI. If multiple risk factors are present, implantation of an automatic defibrillator has been recommended.[6] Successful shocks with automated defibrillators have been reported in pregnant patients with hypertrophic cardiomyopathy.[39] Amiodarone may be a useful suppressive antiarrhythmic agent in the rare event of recurrent intractable ventricular tachycardia during pregnancy.

Labour and delivery

Delivery should take place in high-risk centers experienced in the management of this condition and where continuous ECG and blood pressure monitoring are possible. Continued beta blockade and fluid replacement are necessary in the presence of dynamic outflow tract obstruction. Normal vaginal delivery is safe and cesarean section is indicated only for obstetric purposes. The use of prostaglandins for induction of labour is inadvisable because of their vasodilator effect, but oxytocic agents are well tolerated. Epidural anesthesia should be avoided because of the production of hypotension, and blood loss should be replaced promptly. After completion of the third stage, the patient should sit up to avoid pulmonary congestion and may require intravenous frusemide. (Table 13.2)

Table 13.2 Management of delivery in patients with hypertrophic cardiomyopathy

Delivery in hospital with continuous ECG and blood pressure monitoring
Normal vaginal delivery
Do not use prostaglandins
Prompt blood loss replacement
Sit the patient up after completion of the third stage to avoid pulmonary edema
Antibiotic prophylaxis

Table 13.3 Outcomes in pregnant patients with hypertrophic cardiomyopathy

Reference	No. of patients	No. of pregnancies	Cardiac symptoms during pregnancy[a]	Worsening of symptoms during pregnancy	Intrauterine deaths	Observed deaths
Thaman et al.[26]	127	271	36 (28%)	10 (<10%)	3 (2%)	0
Autore et al.[25]	100	199	Not reported	6 of 40 patients (15%)	Not reported	2
Probst et al.[28]	41	150	27%	0%	0	0

[a]Numbers in parentheses are percentages.

If there is evidence of left ventricular outflow tract obstruction with hemodynamic deterioration after delivery, fluids and vasoconstriction with phenylephrine to increase afterload are recommended. Beta-adrenergic agents such as dopamine or dobutamine should be avoided as a result of the increase in contractility, outflow tract gradient and worsening hypotension that they cause. Continuous monitoring by right heart catheterization may be needed in selected cases and transesophageal echocardiography has been used to assess the hemodynamics. Antibiotic prophylaxis is needed for dental procedures during pregnancy and to cover surgical delivery.

Conclusion

With care in high risk patients the outcome of pregnancy in women with hypertophic cardioimyopathy is usually good (Table 13.3).

References

1 Maron BJ, Gottdiener JS, Epstein SE. Patterns and significance of distribution of left ventricular hypertrophy in hypertrophic cardiomyopathy. A wide angle, two dimensional echocardiographic study of 125 patients. *Am J Cardiol* 1981;**48**:418–28.
2 Davies MJ. The current status of myocardial disarray in hypertrophic cardiomyopathy. *Br Heart J* 1984;**51**:361–3.

3 Nishimura RA, Holmes DR, Jr. Hypertrophic obstructive cardiomyopathy. *N Engl J Med* 2004;**350**:1320–7.

4 Teare D. Asymmetrical hypertrophy of the heart in young adults. *Br Heart J* 1958;**20**:1–8.

5 Brock R. Functional obstruction of the left ventricle; acquired aortic subvalvar stenosis. *Guy's Hospital Rep* 1957;**106**:221–38.

6 Maron BJ, McKenna WJ, Danielson GK et al. American College of Cardiology/ European Society of Cardiology Clinical Expert Consensus Document on Hypertrophic Cardiomyopathy: a report of the ACC Foundation Task Force on Clinical Expert Consensus Documents and the European Society of Cardiology Committee for Practice Guidelines. *J Am Coll Cardiol* 2003;**42**:1687–713.

7 Maron BJ. Hypertrophic cardiomyopathy: a systematic review. *JAMA* 2002;**287**: 1308–20.

8 Richardson P, McKenna RW, Bristow M et al. Report of the 1995 World Health Organization/International Society and Federation of Cardiology Task Force on the definition and classification of cardiomyopathies. *Circulation* 1996;**93**:841–2.

9 Maron BJ, Casey SA, Poliac LC, Gohman TE, Almquist AK, Aeppli DM. Clinical course of hypertrophic cardiomyopathy in a regional United States cohort. *JAMA* 1999;**281**:650–5.

10 Niimura H, Bachinski LL, Sangwatanaroj S et al. Mutations in the gene for cardiac myosin-binding protein C and late-onset familial hypertrophic cardiomyopathy. *N Engl J Med* 1998;**338**:1248–57.

11 Nagueh SF, McFalls J, Meyer D et al. Tissue Doppler imaging predicts the development of hypertrophic cardiomyopathy in subjects with subclinical disease. *Circulation* 2003;**108**:395–8.

12 Nagueh SF, Bachinski LL, Meyer D et al. Tissue Doppler imaging consistently detects myocardial abnormalities in patients with hypertrophic cardiomyopathy and provides a novel means for an early diagnosis before and independently of hypertrophy. *Circulation* 2001;**104**:128–30.

13 Ho CY, Sweitzer NK, McDonough B et al. Assessment of diastolic function with Doppler tissue imaging to predict genotype in preclinical hypertrophic cardiomyopathy. *Circulation* 2002;**105**:2992–7.

14 Maron MS, Olivotto I, Betocchi S et al. Effect of left ventricular outflow tract obstruction on clinical outcome in hypertrophic cardiomyopathy. *N Engl J Med* 2003;**348**:295–303.

15 Sherrid MV, Gunsburg DZ, Moldenhauer S, Pearle G. Systolic anterior motion begins at low left ventricular outflow tract velocity in obstructive hypertrophic cardiomyopathy. *J Am Coll Cardiol* 2000;**36**:1344–54.

16 Klues HG, Maron BJ, Dollar AL, Roberts WC. Diversity of structural mitral valve alterations in hypertrophic cardiomyopathy. *Circulation* 1992;**85**:1651–60.

17 Frank S, Braunwald E. Idiopathic hypertrophic subaortic stenosis. Clinical analysis of 126 patients with emphasis on the natural history. *Circulation* 1968;**37**:759–88.

18 Ryan MP, Cleland JGF, French JA et al. The standard electrocardiogram as a screening test for hypertrophic cardiomyopathy. *Am J Cardiol* 1995;**76**:689–94.

19 Van Driest SL, Ommen SR, Tajik AJ, Gersh BJ, Ackerman MJ. Sarcomeric genotyping in hypertrophic cardiomyopathy. *Mayo Clin Proc* 2005;**80**:463–9.

20 Watkins H, Rosenzweig A, Hwang D et al. Characteristics and prognostic implications of myosin missense mutations in familial hypertrophic cardiomyopathy. *N Engl J Med* 1992;**326**:1108–14.

21 Van Driest SL, Ackerman MJ, Ommen SR et al. Prevalence and severity of 'benign' mutations in the beta-myosin heavy chain, cardiac troponin T, and alpha-tropomyosin genes in hypertrophic cardiomyopathy. *Circulation* 2002;**106**:3085–90.

22 Ackerman MJ, VanDriest SL, Ommen SR, et al. Prevalence and age-dependence of malignant mutations in the beta-myosin heavy chain and troponin t genes in hypertrophic cardiomyopathy: a comprehensive outpatient perspective. *J Am Coll Cardiol* 2002;**39**:2042–8.

23 Spirito P, Bellone P, Harris KM, Bernabo P, Bruzzi P, Maron BJ. Magnitude of left ventricular hypertrophy and risk of sudden death in hypertrophic cardiomyopathy. *N Engl J Med* 2000;**342**:1778–85.

24 Charron P, Heron D, Gargiulo M et al. Prenatal molecular diagnosis in hypertrophic cardiomyopathy: report of the first case. *Prenat Diagn* 2004;**24**:701–3.

25 Autore C, Conte MR, Piccininno M et al. Risk associated with pregnancy in hypertrophic cardiomyopathy. *J Am Coll Cardiol* 2002;**40**:1864–9.

26 Thaman R, Varnava A, Hamid MS et al. Pregnancy related complications in women with hypertrophic cardiomyopathy. *Heart* 2003;**89**:752–6.

27 Oakley GD, McGarry K, Limb DG, Oakley CM. Management of pregnancy in patients with hypertrophic cardiomyopathy. *BMJ* 1979;**i**:1749–50.

28 Probst V, Langlard JM, Desnos M, Komajda M, Bouhour JB. [Familial hypertrophic cardiomyopathy. French study of the duration and outcome of pregnancy.] *Arch Mal Coeur Vaiss* 2002;**95**:81–6.

29 Turner GM, Oakley CM, Dixon HG. Management of pregnancy complicated by hypertrophic obstructive cardiomyopathy. *BMJ* 1968;**4**:281–4.

30 Pelliccia F, Cianfrocca C, Gaudio C, Reale A. Sudden death during pregnancy in hypertrophic cardiomyopathy. *Eur Heart J* 1992;**13**:421–3.

31 Shah DM, Sunderji SG. Hypertrophic cardiomyopathy and pregnancy: report of a maternal mortality and review of literature. *Obstet Gynecol Surv* 1985;**40**:444–8.

32 Benitez RM. Hypertrophic cardiomyopathy and pregnancy: maternal and fetal outcomes. *J Maternal-Fetal Invest* 1996;**6**:51–5.

33 Minnich ME, Quirk JG, Clark RB. Epidural anesthesia for vaginal delivery in a patient with idiopathic hypertrophic subaortic stenosis. *Anesthesiology* 1987;**67**:590–2.

34 Oakley GD, McGarry K, Limb DG, Oakley CM. Management of pregnancy in patients with hypertrophic cardiomyopathy. *BMJ* 1979;**i**:1749–50.

35 Maron BJ, Dearani JA, Ommen SR et al. The case for surgery in obstructive hypertrophic cardiomyopathy. *J Am Coll Cardiol* 2004;**44**:2044–53.

36 McCully RB, Nishimura RA, Tajik AJ, Schaff HV, Danielson GK. Extent of clinical improvement after surgical treatment of hypertrophic obstructive cardiomyopathy. *Circulation* 1996;**94**:467–71.

37 Sigwart U. Non-surgical myocardial reduction for hypertrophic obstructive cardiomyopathy. *Lancet* 1995;**346**:211–14.

38 Maron BJ. Surgery for hypertrophic obstructive cardiomyopathy: alive and quite well. *Circulation* 2005;**111**:2016–18.

39 Piacenza JM, Kirkorian G, Audra PH, Mellier G. Hypertrophic cardiomyopathy and pregnancy. *Eur J Obstet Gynecol Reprod Biol* 1998;**80**:17–23.

CHAPTER 14

Peripartum cardiomyopathy, other heart muscle disorders and pericardial diseases

Celia Oakley

Peripartum cardiomyopathy

Peripartum cardiomyopathy is a dilated cardiomyopathy that occurs in the peripartum period. Heart failure had been known of since the eighteenth century but was first described in 1937 as 'Idiopathic myocardial degeneration associated with pregnancy and especially the puerperium'.[1] With the emergence and classification of the different forms of cardiomyopathy in the 1960s it became known as a dilated cardiomyopathy with a temporal relationship to pregnancy.[2] Biopsy shows myocarditis in a high proportion of cases[3,4] and further work has pointed to a probable autoimmune mechanism, although this is still not fully understood.[5]

The sudden onset of heart failure in a previously healthy young woman who had been looking forward to the birth brings bleak fear to the patient and her family, and something similar to her doctors as the future is unknown to each. Some patients rapidly deteriorate and will die without a device or transplantation whereas others make an astonishing almost complete recovery and it is impossible to know which way 'the cat will jump'. More often the onset is less dramatic and the failure less severe but improvement slow or absent. There is no doubt that many mild cases are missed altogether. As the condition is rare (although less rare than generally believed), personal experience is limited and the literature tends to reflect a limited personal experience that may be likened to a blind person describing an elephant, having felt only one part of it.

Definition

Peripartum cardiomyopathy (PPCM) is a dilated cardiomyopathy with a temporal relationship to pregnancy. It was defined arbitrarily by Demakis et al.[6] in 1971 as unexplained left ventricular systolic dysfunction developing in the last month of pregnancy or within 5 months of delivery. The definition required that there be no other identifiable cause for the heart failure and excluded pa-

Table 14.1 Diagnostic criteria

- Cardiac failure developing in the last month of pregnancy or within 5 months of delivery
- Absence of other detectable cause
- Apparent absence of myocardial disease before the last month of pregnancy
- Left ventricular systolic dysfunction demonstrated by echocardiography:
  - ejection fraction <45%
  - fractional shortening <30% and/or
  - end-diastolic dimension >2.7 cm/m^2

---

tients with a previous history of possible myocardial disease.[6] At a workshop in 1997 the addition was made that the left ventricular dysfunction should be demonstrated echocardiographically[7] (Table 14.1).

Although the definition aims to separate patients out with previously unsuspected dilated cardiomyopathy exacerbated by the pregnancy, it is not practicable for all seemingly healthy women to have echocardiography studies on first booking and, in practice, the differentiation is difficult and will largely depend on when heart disease is first recognized. Any patient with a family history of cardiomyopathy should have echocardiography performed even if she is apparently fully fit.

Patients with pre-existing heart disease are not immune from developing a PPCM and may be more likely to develop symptoms because of their reduced cardiovascular reserve.[8,9]

Epidemiology and prevalence

The prevalence of PPCM is not known because recognition and accurate diagnosis depend on the availability and application of echocardiography. This would require its routine use in every parturient woman within sizeable defined populations for insight to be gained about the true prevalence. M-mode echocardiography was only just becoming available in the cardiology departments of major hospitals in the 1960s and so had not contributed to the diagnosis of the retrospective series of patients described in the key papers from New Orleans in 1965[2] or from Chicago in 1971.[6] Even now cases go undiagnosed and this is true of major centers as well as less highly developed ones.

The condition has been described from all around the world in both small personal series and reviews of accumulated cases from many sources, and over different observation periods, so providing little idea of true prevalence.[10–16] It is no wonder that estimates are in truth just wild guesses. They vary widely from 1 in 1485 to 1 in 15 000 live births even within the USA.[10–14] Much higher figures come from South Africa (1 in 1000) and from Haiti (1 in 350–400) live births.[15] The high prevalence reported from Nigeria was caused by heart failure induced by a local custom that decrees that parturient women eat excessive local salt (*kanwa*) and lie on heated mud beds for 40 days post partum.[17–18]

A consensus opinion from the workshop in 1997 was of an incidence in between 1 in 3000 and 1 in 4000 in the USA[7,19] which suggests that there may be 750–1000 cases a year in the UK.

Etiology

Traditional predisposing causes of PPCM include multiple pregnancy, multiparity, African race, older maternal age, pre-eclampsia and a history of previous peripartum cardiomyopathy. Selenium deficiency,[20] infection, tocolytic therapy and surgical delivery have also been suggested.[21,22]

The hemodynamic burden is greater during pregnancy than in the puerperium. Multiple pregnancy magnifies this. If twin pregnancy is a cause of PPCM such patients should develop symptoms during the second trimester, as do patients with structural heart disease or a pre-existing dilated cardiomyopathy when they exhaust a reduced cardiac reserve. With delivery and uterine contraction maternal blood volume is expanded by return of uteroplacental blood and at the same time afterload increases resulting from loss of the low-resistance placental bed. These volume shifts are exaggerated in multiple pregnancy. Postpartum blood loss is needed to alleviate the hypervolemia but iatrogenic overhydration may contribute to pulmonary edema after surgical delivery.

Over 90% of cases of PPCM present in the puerperium when the increased hemodynamic load of pregnancy has diminished. This is inconsistent with the condition being simply an exacerbation of a pre-existing dilated cardiomyopathy, but would conform with an autoimmune origin developing as the dormant immune system is reactivated after delivery.[24–26]

The reported incidence of myocarditis ranges from 8.8% to 78%. The frequent finding of myocarditis when endomyocardial biopsies are taken within a month of onset of symptoms is in conformity with the autoimmune theory, as is the marked capacity for hemodynamic recovery that is also shown by some patients with acute myocarditis seen outside pregnancy. The true prevalence of myocarditis in PPCM may have been underestimated because many biopsies may be taken after the changes have regressed and, even in fulminant cases, myocarditis tends to be focal, bringing the possibility of sampling errors. The diagnosis may also be missed if immunohistochemical staining is not performed. Failure to include these in the so-called 'Dallas criteria' may have contributed to the difficulty in recruiting patients to the trial of immunosuppression in acute myocarditis.[27,28] It is probable that the most good would be done by immunosuppressive treatment if it is started as early as possible after onset. The difficulty in recognizing heart failure in late pregnancy, when many women complain of shortness of breath and develop swollen legs, means that insidious onset at that time would be very likely to remain undiagnosed.

Viruses have long been suspected of playing a part in initiating both the inflammatory process in dilated cardiomyopathy and an autoimmune process against exposed or damaged myocardial proteins, although no infective agent has been found in cases of PPCM and the causative agent is probably not an infective one. Fetal cells are known to enter the maternal circulation during pregnancy and to remain there without rejection. If such foreign cells enter cardiac tissue during the immunosuppressed state of pregnancy, they might well be responsible for triggering a vigorous reaction after restoration of immune competence and would explain cases of PPCM with a new partner after previous healthy pregnancies. Persuasive support for abnormal immunological activation comes from the finding of high titers of autoantibodies both peripartum and in dilated cardiomyopathy. In addition, several autoantibodies have been found that were unique to PPCM and not present in patients with dilated cardiomyopathy.[24–26]

Some patients with PPCM give a family history of dilated cardiomyopathy and autoantibodies are found in both conditions.[29–31] Dilated cardiomyopathy is familial in about a quarter of cases but the heredity is far from straightforward. Genetic studies may shed some light on PPCM in which a family history of either dilated cardiomopathy or PPCM seems too frequent for chance. Both facilitative and protective factors would account for the fewer than expected numbers in cardiomyopathy families in which 'latent cases' with only mild echocardiographic abnormality are a feature. As well as these and possible lurking infective agents are the unique hormonal environment and possible maladaptive responses to the hemodynamic changes of pregnancy, all of which have been suggested as possible contributory causes.[32–34]

Although the time of clinical onset does not necessarily mark the time of onset of the cardiac dysfunction, fulminant cases usually present in the first few days post partum but give no hint of a preceding cardiac problem. Milder cases tend to present later in the puerperium with a much more insidious onset that the women are unable to date. Only 9% of patients present in the last month of pregnancy and it is likely that the problem almost universally starts early after delivery, as would be in keeping with the immunological explanations for the condition.

Pre-eclampsia has been cited as a possible contributory cause and is sometimes associated but pre-eclampsia does not cause systolic heart failure in healthy young women, and cardiomyopathy is not found even in patients who have been under close observation in hospital. Moreover PPCM usually develops post partum whereas delivery cures pre-eclampsia.

PPCM is no doubt polygenic with links to idiopathic dilated cardiomyopathy, its expression determined by the interplay of many other endogenous and environmental factors yet to be determined.

Diagnosis

Diagnosis rests on the recognition of left ventricular dysfunction around the time of parturition that is believed to be new and for which other possible causes have been excluded.

Heart failure

The recognition of heart failure or even that the patient is ill is not easy before delivery when dyspnea, fatigue and edema are normally common in late pregnancy. Cough, orthopnea, paroxysmal nocturnal dyspnea, palpitation, chest pain and abdominal pain may develop.

Most women are kept in hospital for only a few hours before being discharged back into the care of their midwives, on whom much of the responsibility of noticing something wrong will fall. Diagnosis should become obvious if symptoms worsen at a time when they should have improved, but the heart failure may be missed until the new mother tries to resume her normal activities, together with the added work and loss of sleep involved in looking after a new baby.

The condition does not differ clinically from dilated cardiomyopathy. Examination will reveal a resting tachycardia, low blood pressure and pulse pressure, raised cervical venous pressure, gallop rhythm, lung crackles and enlarged liver. A mitral regurgitant murmur is sometimes heard. Fluid overload is a prominent feature, particularly in patients who have just had a surgical delivery, and there may be ascites.

Chest pain

As in myocarditis outside pregnancy, chest pain is frequently the herald symptom that leads to diagnosis. It may suggest myocardial infarction and demand urgent investigation.[35] Myocardial infarction is also a rare complication of pregnancy that usually occurs in the peripartum period. The differential diagnosis may remain in doubt until coronary angiography, because cardiac markers may be raised and echocardiography does not always show uniformly global hypokinesia. Cocaine abuse can cause vasospasm with ischemic chest pain and even cardiac infarction, which is often caused by a spontaneous coronary artery dissection; if it involves the left anterior descending artery it may lead to extensive anteroapical dysfunction and severe left ventricular failure. A few infarcts being seen now are occurring in older women, smokers with the metabolic syndrome and atheroma. Either way urgent coronary angiography is needed for diagnosis and prompt appropriate treatment.

Embolism

Endocardial thrombosis is frequent and either pulmonary or systemic embolism may be the first clinical event that brings the cardiac problem to light.[36–39] Echocardiography, a routine first investigation for a possible embolic source, may show ventricular thrombus and severe biventricular dysfunction that had previously escaped notice because of lack of formal cardiovascular examination or pulmonary auscultation. This is because there may have been little in the way of cardiac symptoms before the embolus despite the marked compromise. Most peripartum women are healthy and pass from home to hospital and back with little time for anything apart from the actual birth. Even after such patients have been re-admitted to hospital on account of embolism, the signs of cardiac dysfunction are sometimes missed. Although this emphasizes the huge cardiovascular reserve that exists, it also indicates the subtlety of the clinical signs or their elusiveness unless clinicians' thoughts turn to the heart. Even florid failure with edema may be attributed to other causes.

The higher prevalence of intracardiac thrombosis and embolism in peripartum cardiomyopathy than in dilated cardiomyopathy outside pregnancy is attributable to the hypercoagulable state existing in pregnancy, which increases the risk of intracavitary thrombus caused by stasis in poorly contracting chambers or endocardial inflammation.

Echocardiography reveals the problem but only if it is performed. This is more likely if the patient has an embolus or is short of breath after delivery, but much less likely if she complains only of fatigue or chest pain and is not examined. This could mean an unknown but possibly large number of milder non-fatal cases remaining unrecognized and either improving spontaneously or presenting later with a dilated cardiomyopathy.

Arrhythmias

The increased tendency to cardiac arrhythmias seen in pregnancy is attributed to an increased sympathetic drive that is intensified by the neuroendocrine activation of cardiac failure.

Arrhythmias are frequent and palpitation is often the presenting feature of a PPCM. Frequent ectopic beats, supraventricular and ventricular tachycardias (Figure 14.1b, c), atrial flutter and fibrillation may all be seen in the same patient and contribute to hemodynamic instability.[40,41] A new mother, tired and therefore harassed, may ignore the rapid heart beat attributing it to her fatigue. Her ventricular dysfunction may then be worsened and it may be uncertain whether the arrhythmia caused the ventricular dysfunction, 'tachycardia failure,' or whether it was caused by an underlying PPCM.

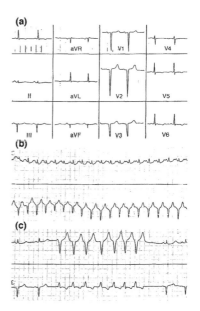

Figure 14.1 (a) ECG from a patient with a fulminant peripartum cardiomyopathy showing low voltage and QS waves in leads V1–V3, poor R-wave progression and T-wave inversion in left ventricular leads, suggesting (old rather than evolving) anteroapical infarction. (b,c) Rhythm strips from the same patient showing supraventricular tachycardia (b) and a burst of ventricular tachycardia (c).

Table 14.2 Differential diagnosis

- Pre-existing dilated cardiomyopathy
- Peripartum myocardial infarction (coronary artery dissection, thrombosis or embolism, cocaine-induced spasm)
- Pulmonary embolism – thrombus or amniotic fluid
- Fluid overload

Differential diagnosis

The clinical differential diagnosis is from other causes of heart failure, other cardiomyopathies, pre-existing dilated cardiomyopathy, acute myocardial infarction, ritodrine-induced pulmonary edema in patients given the drug by infusion in saline, fluid overload after surgical delivery, tachycardia-induced failure, massive pulmonary embolism, amniotic fluid embolism, and infective, metabolic and toxic causes of heart failure (Table 14.2).

Investigations

Laboratory blood tests

Hematology and biochemical findings are usually normal, but atrial and brain natriuretic peptides are elevated and the D-dimer will be raised above the usually raised upper limits for pregnancy and the puerperium in patients with intracardiac thrombi or those who have had emboli. Cardiac markers, especially troponin, may be above normal or enzymes may be within normal with a raised troponin.

The laboratory work-up will include renal and liver function tests, thyroid function, serological tests for viral and rickettsial infections, syphilis and HIV, and tests for alcohol and cocaine, plus autoimmune studies to exclude collagen vascular disease, sarcoidosis and pheochromocytoma as clinically indicated.

Electrocardiogram

Sinus tachycardia is often interrupted by multiple supraventricular and ventricular ectopic beats, bursts of tachycardia, atrial flutter or fibrillation. Low voltage is usual particularly in the standard leads. The QRS may be widened, reflecting left ventricular dilatation. Left or right bundle-branch block may come and go or a QS pattern in the chest leads may suggest myocardial infarction (see Figure 14.1). Occasionally the ECG is within normal limits or just shows non-specific ST- and T-wave abnormalities or T-wave inversion.

The chest radiograph

Portable anteroposterior films are not very helpful and if possible a departmental posteroanterior film should be obtained. The cardiac diameter is usually increased and the lungs show pulmonary congestion or frank pulmonary edema. Small pleural effusions are commonly present.

Echocardiography

All four cardiac chambers are usually dilated and there is marked left ventricular hypokinesia. This is typically global but may be more focal, suggesting possible infarction. Wall thicknesses are normal. All valves except the aortic may show regurgitation. All the indices of contractility are reduced. Spontaneous echo contrast reflects slowed flow (Figure 14.2) and thrombus may be seen in either or both ventricles or in the atria if they are fibrillating. A small pericardial effusion is commonly present.

Cardiac catheterization and angiocardiography

Hemodynamic measurement is not needed if the diagnosis is clear. When performed, pulmonary artery wedge pressure and ventricular diastolic pressures will be elevated, but pulmonary artery pressure is usually normal or barely raised. If significant pulmonary hypertension is recorded this suggests a pre-existing condition and is not seen in acute PPCM.

Coronary angiography shows normal coronary arteries and left ventricular angiography is contraindicated if echocardiography has shown ventricular thrombus and the added contrast load is better avoided because all the information is available from echocardiography.

Endomyocardial biopsy

The indications for biopsy in dilated cardiomyopathy are controversial but biopsy is needed when a specific cause is suspected. This should include PPCM in which the prevalence of myocarditis remains uncertain. Biopsy should be performed only if the operator is experienced in the technique and has access to an experienced pathologist for interpretation. Biopsies should be taken from the right ventricle if echocardiography has shown this to be free from thrombus. If biopsy is to be performed it should be done as soon as practicable after onset and after prior consultation with the cardiac histopathologist, who should be fully informed of the clinical details. Biopsies should be obtained from as many different sites in the ventricle as possible.

Treatment

Patients with PPCM should be made known to and discussed with cardiologists in a specialist cardiac intensive care unit. If they do poorly and need transfer they can then be moved without delay so that a ventricular assist device can be installed as a bridge to recovery or transplantation performed. The condition of these patients often changes quickly (for both better and worse) and decisions must be made (and if necessary changed) equally rapidly.

The patient with acute-onset heart failure needs to be managed in a cardiac unit so that her vital signs, heart rate and blood pressure, cardiac rhythm, oxygen saturation and urinary output can be monitored, treatment adjusted and appropriate action taken in case of sudden arrhythmia or cardiac arrest. This can be difficult in severely ill patients with prenatal presentation, in whom invasive monitoring during delivery will be advisable and when continuous

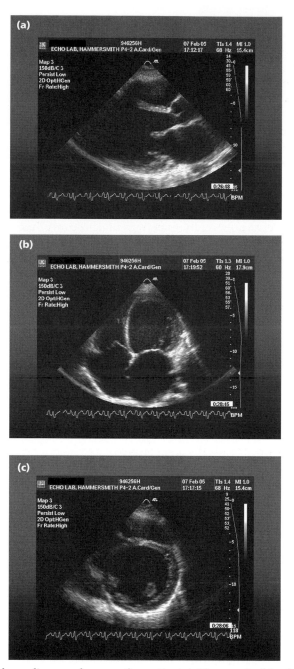

Figure 14.2 Echocardiograms from another patient. (a) Long-axis, (b) apical four-chamber and (c) short-axis views at the level of the papillary muscles, showing a moderately dilated and globally poorly contracting left ventricle (end-diastolic dimension 66 mm, ejection fraction 25%). The left atrium is also dilated and the apical four-chamber view shows spontaneous echo contrast in the left ventricle.

assessment of the fetus is also essential. Fortunately such cases are exceptionally rare.

The timing and mode of delivery need to be discussed among cardiologists, obstetricians and anesthetists. In most cases this will be vaginal delivery waiting for spontaneous labour if the cardiac condition has been stabilized and the fetus is well. Labour should be induced if she fails to respond. If there is concern about the baby surgical delivery may be necessary, but otherwise vaginal delivery with good pain relief and accelerated second stage are to be preferred. Epidural anesthesia is contraindicated if the patient is still heparinized. The patient and her partner should be kept fully informed by the consultant throughout and concerns, doubts and options discussed.

Heart failure is treated conventionally except that angiotensin-converting enzyme (ACE) inhibitors and angiotensin receptor blockers (ARBs) are contraindicated if the patient is still undelivered. Reliance has to be placed on hydralazine and nitrates. Carvedilol and amlodipine may also be used before delivery when needed. Diuretics are needed for volume overload, but remember the risk of uteroplacental hypoperfusion in undelivered patients. Spironolactone is helpful in severe failure. Low blood pressure need not be a deterrent to pressing ahead cautiously with vasodilators, provided that urine output and cerebration are unaffected. If the cardiac output is rising in response to unloading, the low blood pressure will not fall further and a systolic pressure of 80 mmHg is well tolerated by a young patient. Beta blockers should be introduced slowly because they cause transient deterioration before improvement, but are particularly useful for deterring arrhythmias. Digoxin is indicated only if needed for control of atrial fibrillation. The addition of pentoxifylline has been claimed to improve the outcome.[42]

Intravenous dobutamine should be used when inotropic support is needed. A Swan–Ganz catheter is not needed if peripheral perfusion and oxygen saturations are satisfactory, the lung bases clear and urine output is good. It is only in the sickest patients on a balloon pump, and needing frequent adjustment of drug infusion rates, that a Swan–Ganz catheter adds the information on which fine adjustments are made. Continuous hemofiltration may be needed to remove excess fluid pending hemodynamic improvement.

Transplantation[43] is always a last resort in this condition, with the capacity for such dramatic improvement. A left ventricular assist device may be needed as a bridge to recovery or to transplantation, and buys time. Priority is given to such young patients but assessment and preparation take time and organs are not always available, all of which underline the need for cardiologists in hospitals without these facilities not to keep hold of these patients.

Anticoagulant treatment

Anticoagulant treatment is important in these patients with their high thrombotic risk and should be started immediately whether or not ventricular thrombi have been shown or whether embolism has occurred or spontaneous echo contrast is seen. They should be continued until all thrombi have disappeared,

D-dimer has returned to normal and while ventricular function remains impaired.

Unfractionated heparin should be used in undelivered patients because the level of anticoagulation can be assessed from the activated partial thromboplastin time and low-molecular-weight heparin cannot be as quickly reversed with protamine. Warfarin is used after delivery. All the drugs mentioned are compatible with breast-feeding.

Immunosuppressive treatment
Immunosuppressive treatment should probably be given to all patients in whom biopsy has shown myocarditis, although benefit is not yet evidence based. Many patients improve rapidly without it and others deteriorate despite it. The myocarditis trial was unsatisfactory for many reasons—biopsy criteria, delayed onset of treatment and protocol violations—as well as being unrelated to the condition in pregnancy.[28]

Immunoglobulins
A small study of intravenous immunoglobulin in women with PPCM suggested that improvement in ejection fraction was greater in patients given this treatment than in those who did not receive it.[44]

Follow-up
It may be wise to continue left ventricular support with an ACE inhibitor and a beta blocker for a year after recovery of ventricular function. Patients whose left ventricular ejection fraction is still depressed should remain on treatment, probably also including warfarin, and all patients should be followed up long term with at least annual echocardiography irrespective of whether or not they have apparently recovered fully.

Prognosis
Prognosis depends on recovery of left ventricular function.[45–50] As with the figures for prevalence the reported mortality rate from small series around the world varies widely (from 7% to 56%). A realistic figure for the short-term mortality rate is between 20 and 25%, and almost half of deaths occur in the first 3 months. The mortality rate was 28% in a series of black women from South Africa. Cytokine levels were highest in the women who died.[45] About a third of patients show a return to normal left ventricular function within 6 months and more than half show significant improvement. The long-term prognosis depends on whether left ventricular function eventually returns to normal or the patient develops a dilated cardiomyopathy.

There is still very little information about the response to any subsequent pregnancies. Women who have recovered from PPCM may have reduced contractile reserve on dobutamine stress testing, and it has been suggested that such women might not tolerate a subsequent pregnancy although there are as yet no follow-up data for this suggestion.[51]

In a retrospective series from Brazil, 11 of 18 patients had persistent left ventricular function. Deterioration was not seen in subsequent pregnancies in any of those who had recovered.[46] Information on 44 patients was recovered by questionnaire from members of the American College of Cardiology by Elkayam.[47] The recurrence rate was 21%, but with no deaths among 28 patients who had recovered completely, and 44% with 3 deaths among 16 patients who had shown persistent left ventricular dysfunction. Improvement of ejection fraction after the first subsequent pregnancy was to much the same level as before it, in both those who had and those who had not recovered completely. These data suffer from both the inclusion of patients with left ventricular dysfunction diagnosed within 6 months of delivery and possible observer bias.

Patients who have recovered normal left ventricular function seem to have a good prognosis. If such patients wish to have a further pregnancy they should have a dobutamine echo stress test of contractile reserve. If this is normal they can be told that a further pregnancy should be safe but that information is still sparse. If contractile reserve is shown to be reduced the advice should be more guarded. Women with persistently depressed left ventricular function should be advised against embarking on another pregnancy.

Dilated cardiomyopathy

Patients with idiopathic dilated cardiomyopathy are discouraged from getting pregnant and there are few reports in the literature in which left ventricular function has been well documented before the pregnancy. The few patients described had not tolerated the increased blood volume and cardiac output and developed heart failure or pulmonary edema in midtrimester. More often patients have developed unexpected dyspnea and dry cough, which were at first attributed to a chest infection. The left ventricle is usually already >6 cm with an ejection fraction of 30% or less. Some improvement is expected after delivery but others behave like patients with PPCM and deteriorate further although considerable recovery may follow in survivors.[52–55]

A teenager with cardiomyopathy known from infancy deteriorated at 20 weeks, requiring ventilation and inotropic support, but recovered after termination of the pregnancy[53] and a 40 year old with an ejection fraction of 30% and left ventricular end-diastolic dimension of 7 cm, who had been stable for 8 years, went into failure at 26 weeks, deteriorated further after cesarean delivery and died.[54]

The small published and personal experience suggests that patients with pre-existing dilated cardiomyopathy have a poorer clinical outcome than patients with PPCM but hint at a link. A family history of dilated cardiomyopathy may be a clue to pre-existing but occult dysfunction in a patient who first develops symptoms within the time envelope assigned to 'peripartum' cardiomyopathy. It is recommended that echocardiography should be performed, if possible before conception, in all patients desiring pregnancy who have a family history of either dilated cardiomyopathy or PPCM.

Advice has to be on an individual basis. The history is important. Some patients who are stable and asymptomatic will tolerate pregnancy but the high chance of deterioration both during pregnancy and post partum suggests that pregnancy should be avoided or termination advised if the end-diastolic volume is already above normal or if the ejection fraction is <50%.[55] Patients who embark on pregnancy should have their left ventricular function regularly monitored throughout by echocardiography so that need for adjustment in therapy or hospital admission can be anticipated and clinical deterioration prevented if possible.

ACE inhibitors should be withdrawn and hydralazine substituted with a long-acting nitrate added later if needed. Diuretic dosage should be as low as possible. A beta blocker such as metoprolol should be introduced gradually if there are frequent ectopic beats, or especially if there is a resting sinus tachycardia that reflects failure to increase stroke volume. The approach to delivery will involve the whole team. Usually patients should be delivered vaginally with full pain relief and an expeditious second stage with relief from the need to push.

Sudden onset of pulmonary edema is a risk after delivery. Blood loss should be minimal and the patient should be sat up promptly and given 20 mg intravenous frusemide. Oxytocic agents are not contraindicated.

Patients with a secondary dilated cardiomyopathy caused by a known toxin or other cause are more predictable and differ from patients with idiopathic or familial dilated cardiomyopathy. Depression of left ventricular function after previous chemotherapy may not be known to have caused damage until years afterwards. Deterioration may occur in midtrimester or even earlier, with a risk of pulmonary edema in the third stage but with improvement in the puerperium. Two patients had been asymptomatic after surgery and doxorubicin for bone cancer years before. (Both also had a kyphoscoliosis.) The first patient developed dyspnea at 28 weeks and pulmonary edema at 36 weeks, with an ejection fraction of 10% requiring infusion of dopamine; after delivery she again became asymptomatic. The second patient developed pulmonary edema on day 5 post partum in her first pregnancy, and at 35 weeks in her second and third pregnancies, recovering to become asymptomatic again but with a reduced ejection fraction on each occasion.[56]

Restrictive cardiomyopathies

Patients with a restrictive cardiomyopathy and diastolic ventricular dysfunction with preserved systolic function usually have rapid left ventricular filling and, although fluid retention may be disabling and sudden pulmonary edema life threatening, cardiac output is often well maintained by a compensatory tachycardia with normal fetal growth and a favorable outcome. They are, however, a heterogeneous collection. Some families show a dominant inheritance.

Although a few cases have a superficial similarity to patients with constrictive pericarditis, they do not show the marked interdependence seen in constriction; left-sided diastolic pressures are higher than those on the right, often causing pulmonary hypertension and tricuspid regurgitation with a large right atrium. A normal pericardial space is visible on echocardiograms.

Most women with familial cardiomyopathies tend to tolerate pregnancy well, either because they are mildly affected or because significant cardiac dysfunction does not develop until later in life. If this were not the case their disorders would die out except for spontaneous mutations but their children are sometimes affected earlier and more severely (anticipation) (see Chapter 22).

Arrhythmogenic right ventricular cardiomyopathy

This diagnosis is more frequently made in men than women and there is little published experience about pregnancy. The propensity of arrhythmias to get worse during pregnancy, uncertain prognosis and lack of published experience to draw upon are probably a deterrent to cardiologists called on for advice. All but a few patients have good hemodynamic function and a stable patient with an implanted cardioverter–defibrillator should be fit to undertake pregnancy. The dominant inheritance and individual family history will weigh in the decision-making. A published case with atrial flutter, atrioventricular block and embolic stroke was mistaken for PPCM.[57]

X-linked cardiomyopathies

In most of the X-linked disorders associated with cardiomyopathy female carriers are either totally spared or affected to only a mild extent and pregnancy is safe.

The ECG and echocardiographic abnormalities in female carriers of Duchenne and Becker muscular dystrophies are similar to those in affected males, although usually less marked. They usually show tall right-sided R waves and deep Q waves in left ventricular leads associated with diminished posterior left ventricular wall movement seen on echocardiography. Female carriers of Emery–Dreifuss muscular dystrophy may develop conduction abnormalities and need pacemaker implantation.

Female carriers of Fabry's disease develop a milder form of the disease, with later onset and mainly cardiac involvement with thickening of the ventricular walls, simulating hypertrophic cardiomyopathy. This is caused by storage of a glycosphingolipid resulting from lack of the enzyme alpha galactosidase. The condition can be diagnosed by immuno-quantification of this enzyme. Significant cardiac abnormality is not usually seen until after affected women have passed their child-bearing years.

The advice of a clinical geneticist should be sought and the possibility of potential embryo selection considered in patients contemplating pregnancy.

Pericardial diseases

A small increase in the amount of pericardial fluid is seen in the third trimester in about 40% of pregnant women. Sometimes the effusion is more sizeable but still clinically silent, associated with excessive water retention and weight gain.[58,59]

There is no reason to believe that pregnancy affects the incidence or spectrum of the various pericardial diseases in women. It is therefore uncommon in association with pregnancy and the literature reflects this with numerous accounts of a wide variety of single cases. Acute idiopathic pericarditis and pericardial involvement in autoimmune diseases are most often seen and are the most frequent cause of large effusions.[58]

Tamponade is rare in acute idiopathic pericarditis which usually presents with chest pain and typical ECG changes. Systemic lupus erythematosus and other autoimmune diseases are the leading causes of pericarditis and cardiac tamponade in pregnancy.[60] An autoimmune screen should be performed in any patient presenting with tamponade, pericarditis or constriction of unknown origin (see Chapter 11). Dissection of the aortic root may lead to cardiac tamponade and sudden death in pregnancy, most often in older multiparous women with hypertension, Marfan syndrome, bicuspid aortic valve or coarctation of the aorta (including those whose coarctations have been surgically corrected) This is associated with thinning of the aortic wall in pregnancy.[61]

Constrictive pericarditis causes increased systemic congestion and fluid retention in pregnancy but pulmonary congestion is rarely a problem. Output may be maintained by tachycardia and the diagnosis is often overlooked. Mild cases can be managed with support stockings and frugal use of diuretics. Pericardiectomy, when essential, can be performed during pregnancy without the need for cardiac bypass in patients not responding to medical therapy.

Most pericardial diseases can be managed as in non-pregnant patients but indometacin and high-dose aspirin can cause premature closure of the ductus and colchicine is contraindicated in pregnancy.

References

1 Gouley BA, McMillan TM, Bellet S. Idiopathic myocardial degeneration associated with pregnancy and especially the puerperium. *Am J Med Sci* 1937;**19**:185–99.
2 Walsh JJ, Burch GE, Black WC, Ferrans VJ, Hibbs RG. Idiopathic myocardiopathy of the puerperium (postpartal heart disease). *Circulation* 1965;**32**:19–31.
3 Melvin KR, Richardson PJ, Olsen EG, Daly K, Jackson G. Peripartum cardiomyopathy due to myocarditis. *N Engl J Med* 1982;**307**:731–4.
4 Midvei MG, DeMent SH, Feldman AM, Hutchins GM, Baughman KL. Peripartum myocarditis and cardiomyopathy. *Circulation* 1990;**81**:922–8.
5 Ansari AA, Fett JD, Carraway RE, Mayne AE, Onlamoon N, Sundstrom JB. *Clin Rev Allergy Immunol* 2002;**23**:301–24.
6 Demakis JG, Rahimtoola SH, Sutton GC et al. Natural course of peripartum cardiomyopathy. *Circulation* 1971;**44**:1053–61.
7 Pearson GD, Veille J-C, Rahimtoola SH et al. Peripartum cardiomyopathy: National Heart, Lung and Blood Institute and Office of Rare Diseases (National Institutes of Health) workshop recommendations and review. *JAMA* 2000;**283**:1183–8.

8 Oakley CM, Nihoyannopoulos P. Peripartum cardiomyopathy with recovery in a patient with coincidental Eisenmenger ventricular septal defect. *Br Heart J* 1992;**67**:190–2.

9 Purcell IF, Williams DO. Peripartum cardiomyopathy complicating severe aortic stenosis. *Int J Cardiol* 1995;**52**:163–6.

10 Costanzo-Nordin MR, O'Connell JB. Peripartum cardiomyopathy in the 1980s: etiologic and prognostic consideration and review of the literature. *Prog Cardiol* 1989;**2**:225–39.

11 Brown CS, Bertolet BD. Peripartum cardiomyopathy: a comprehensive review. *Am J Obstet Gynecol* 1998;**178**:409–14

12 Veille JC, Zaccaro D. Peripartum cardiomyopathy: summary of an international survey on peripartum cardiomyopathy. *Am J Obstet Gynecol* 1999;**181**:315–39.

13 Heider AL, Kuller JA, Strauss RA, Wells SR. Peripartum cardiomyopathy: a review of the literature. *Obstet Gynecol Surv* 1999;54:26–31.

14 Avila WS, de Carvalho ME, Tschaen CK et al. Pregnancy and peripartum cardiomyopathy. A comparative and prospective study. *Arq Bras Cardiol* 2002;**79**:484–93.

15 Fett JD, Carraway RD, Dowell DL, King ME, Pierre R. Peripartum cardiomyopathy in the Hospital Albert Schweitzer District of Haiti. *Am J Obstet Gynecol* 2002;**186**: 1005–10.

16 Ferrero S, Colombo BM, Fenini F, Abbamonte LH, Arena E. Peripartum cardiomyopathy. A review. *Minerva Ginecol* 2003;**55**:139–51.

17 Brockington IF. Postpartum hypertensive heart failure. *Am J Cardiol* 1971;**27**:650–8.

18 Davidson NM, Parry EHO. Peripartum cardiac failure. *Q J Med* 1978;**47**:431–61.

19 Ventura SJ, Peters KD, Martin JA, Maurer JD. Births and deaths: United States, 1996. *Mon Vital Stat Rep* 1997;**46**(1 suppl 2):1–40.

20 Fett JD, Ansari AA, Sundstrom JB, Coombs GF. Peripartum cardiomyopathy; a selenium disconnection and an autoimmune connection. *Int J Cardiol* 2002;**86**:311–16.

21 Dijibo A. A low plasma selenium is a risk factor for peripartum cardiomyopathy. A comparative study in Sahelian Africa. *Int J Cardiol* 1991;**36**:57–9.

22 Beus E, Mook NKA, Ramsay G, Stappers JLM, Putten HWHM. Peripartum cardiomyopathy: a condition intensivists should be aware of. *Intensive Care Med* 2003;**29**: 167–74.

23 Billieux PS, Petignat P, Fior A et al. Pre-eclampsia and peripartum cardiomyopathy in molar pregnancy: clinical implication for maternally imprinted genes. *Ultrasound Obstet Gynecol* 2004;**23**:398–401.

24 Ansari AA, Fett JD, Carraway RE et al. Autoimmune mechanisms as the basis for human peripartum cardiomyopathy. *Clin Rev Allergy Immunol* 1998;**23**:301–24.

25 Artlett CM, Jimenez SA, Smith JB. Identification of fetal DNA and cells in skin lesions from women with systemic sclerosis. *N Eng J Med* 1998;**338**:1186–91.

26 Nelson JL. Pregnancy, persistent microchimerism and auto-immune disease. *J Am Med Women's Assoc* 1998;**53**:31–2.

27 Chow LH, Radio LH, Sears TD, McManus BM. Insensitivity of right ventricular endomyocardial biopsy in the diagnosis of myocarditis. *J Am Coll Cardiol* 1989;**14**: 915–20.

28 Mason JW, O'Connell JB, Herskowitz A et al. A clinical trial of immunosuppressive therapy for myocarditis. *N Engl J Med* 1995;**333**:269–75

29 Fett JD, Sundstrom JB, Etta King M, Ansari AA. Mother–daughter peripartum cardiomyopathy. *Int J Cardiol* 2002;**86**:331–2.

30 Massad LS, Reiss CK, Mutch DG, Hasket EJ. Family peripartum cardiomyopathy after molar pregnancy. *Obstet Gynecol* 1993;**81**:886–8.

31 Pearl W. Familial occurrence of peripartum cardiomyopathy. *Am Heart J* 1995;**129**: 421–2.

32 Julian DG, Szekely P. Peripartum cardiomyopathy. *Prog Cardiovasc Dis* 1985;**27**: 223–6.

33 Mone SM, Sanders SP, Colan SD. Control mechanisms for physiological hypertrophy of pregnancy. *Circulation* 1996;**94**:667–72.

34 Geva T, Mauer MB, Striker L, Kirshon B, Pivarnik JM. Effects of physiological load of pregnancy on left ventricular contractility and remodeling. *Am Heart J* 1997;**133**: 53–9.

35 Dickfeld T, Gagliardi JP, Marcos J, Russell SD. Peripartum cardiomyopathy presenting as an acute myocardial infarction. *Mayo Clin Proc* 2002;**77**:500–1.

36 Carlson KM, Browning JE, Eggleston MK, Ghjerman RB. Peripartum cardiomyopathy presenting as lower extremity arterial thromboembolism. A case report. *J Reprod Med* 2000;**45**:351–3.

37 Lasinska-Kowara M, Dudziak M, Suchorzewska J. Two cases of peripartum cardiomypathy initially misdiagnosed for pulmonary embolism. *Am J Anaesth* 2001; **48**:773–7.

38 Nishi I, Ishimitsu T, Isiizu T et al. Peripartum cardiomyopathy and biventricular thrombi. *Circ J* 2002;**66**:863–5.

39 Kaufman I, Bondy R, Benjamin A. Peripartum cardiomyopathy and thromboembolism; anaesthetic management and clinical course of an obese, diabetic patient. *Can J Anaesth* 2003;**50**:161–5.

40 Tan HL, Lie KL. Treatment of tachyarrhythmias during pregnancy and lactation. *Eur Heart J* 2001;**22**:458–64.

41 Colombo J, Lawal AH, Bhandari A, Hawkins JL, Atlee JL. Case 1: a patient with severe peripartum cardiomyopathy and persistent ventricular fibrillation supported by a biventricular assist device. *J Cardiothorac Vasc Anesth* 2002;**16**:107–13.

42 Sliwa K, Skudicky D, Candy G. The addition of pentoxifylline to conventional therapy improves outcome in patients with peripartum cardiomyopathy. *Eur J Heart Fail* 2002;**3**:701–5.

43 Aziz TM, Burgess MI, Acladious NN et al. Heart transplantation for peripartum cardiomyopathy: a report of three cases and a literature review. *Cardiovasc Surg* 1999;**7**:565–7.

44 Bozkurt B, Villaneuva FS, Holubkov R et al. Intravenous immune globulin in the therapy of peripartum cardiomyopathy. *J Am Coll Cardiol* 1999;**34**:177–80.

45 Sliwa K, Skudicky D, Bergemann A. Peripartum cardiomyopathy: analysis of clinical outcome, left ventricular function, plasma levels of cytokines and Fas/APO-1. *J Am Coll Cardiol* 2000;**35**:701–5.

46 Albanesi Filho FM, da Silva TT. Natural course of subsequent pregnancy after peripartum cardiomyopathy. *Arq Bras Cardiol* 1999;**73**:47–57.

47 Elkayam U, Tummala PP, Rao K et al. Maternal and fetal outcomes of subsequent pregnancies in women with peripartum cardiomyopathy. *N Engl J Med* 2001;**344**:1567–71.

48 de Souza JL, Jr, de Carvalho Frimm C, Nastari L, Mady C. Left ventricular function after a new pregnancy in patients with peripartum cardiomyopathy. *J Card Fail* 2001;**7**:30–5.

49 Baughman KL. Risks of repeat pregnancy after peripartum cardiomyopathy: double jeopardy. *J Card Fail* 2001;**7**:36–7.

50 Elkayam U. Pregnant again after peripartum cardiomyopathy: to be or not to be? *Eur Heart J* 2002;**23**:753–6.
51 Lampert MB, Lang RM. Peripartum cardiomyopathy. *Am Heart J* 1995;**130**:860–70.
52 Chan F, Ngan Kee WD. Idiopathic dilated cardiomyopathy presenting in pregnancy. *Can J Anaesth* 1999;**46**:1146–9.
53 Yacoub A, Martel MJ. Pregnancy in a patient with primary dilated cardiomyopathy. *Am Coll Obstet Gynecol* 2002;**99**:928–30.
54 Kozelj M, Novak-Antolic Z, Noc M, Antolic G. Idiopathic dilated cardiomyopathy in pregnancy. *Acta Obstet Gynaecol Scand* 2003;**82**:389–90.
55 Expert Consensus Document on management of cardiovascular diseases during pregnancy. The task force on the management of cardiovascular diseases during pregnancy. *Eur Heart J* 2003;**24**:761–81.
56 Pan P, Moore CH. Doxorubicin-induced cardiomyopathy during pregnancy: three case reports of anesthetic management for cesarean and vaginal delivery in two kyphoscoliotic patients. *Anesthesiology* 2002;**97**:513–15.
57 Lui CY, Marcus FI, Sobonya RE. Arrhythmogenic right ventricular dysplasia masquerading as peripartum cardiomyopathy with atrial flutter, advanced atrioventricular block and embolic stroke. *Cardiology* 2002;**97**:49–50.
58 Spodick DH. Pericardial disorders during pregnancy. In: Spodick DH (ed.), *The Pericardium: a comprehensive text book*. New York: Dekker, 1997: pp 89–92.
59 Ristic AD, Seferovic PM, Ljubic A et al. Pericardial disease during pregnancy. *Hertz* 2003;**28**:209–15.
60 Averbuch M, Bojko A, Levo Y. Cardiac tamponade in the early post partum period as the presenting and predominant manifestation of systemic lupus erythematosus. *J Rheumatol* 1986;**13**:444–5.
61 Anderson, Fineron FW. Aortic dissection in pregnancy-induced changes in the vessel wall and bicuspid valve in pathogenesis. *Br J Obstet Gynaecol* 1994;**101**:1085–8.

CHAPTER 15
Coronary artery disease

Celia Oakley

Symptomatic coronary artery disease is still infrequent in women of child-bearing age but an increase in its prevalence in pregnancy has been attributed to modern changes in women's lifestyles. Even so most coronary events complicating pregnancy are still not the result of atheroma and are not preceded by angina.

Coronary atheroma

More angina is being seen in women of child-bearing age because young women with jobs and careers are postponing having children. Their coronary disease may first show itself in pregnancy when poor diet, relative physical inactivity, obesity, hypertension, raised cholesterol, diabetes and smoking are beginning to take their toll.

Many young working women are still smoking, when many of the rest of the population have stopped, travel by car to their sedentary jobs and have no time for exercise. This contrasts with the much more active lives of 'non-working' housewives and mothers.

They may still be unaware that coronary disease is the most common cause of death in women or think that it is confined to postmenopausal women, and this belief still seems to be held by some healthcare workers. These misconceptions lead women to think that they can safely postpone measures to reduce their risk.

The prevalence of various risk factors differs between men and women with diabetes and high blood pressure more prominent in women. Women with diabetes have 2.6 times the risk of dying from coronary heart disease compared with a 1.8-fold risk in men with diabetes. Hypertension increases women's risk two or three times. Clustering of risk factors in the metabolic syndrome multiplies this particularly in women who have diabetes and smoke.[1,2]

Genetic and environmental factors are both important. Familial hypercholesterolemia causes premature coronary atheroma, with the time of onset of symptoms, angina and myocardial infarction determined by the cholesterol level particularly low-density lipoprotein (LDL).

Previous radiotherapy to the mediastinum may be followed by coronary artery narrowing and secondary atheroma years later.[3] Coronary arteritis in polyarteritis nodosa,[4] anti-phospholipid syndrome,[5] Still's disease[6] and previous Kawasaki's disease[7] may cause acute coronary thrombosis in otherwise normal-looking coronary arteries, or they may heal with fibrosis and narrowing or occlusion with an angiographic appearance identical to that of atheromatous disease.

Myocardial infarction

Myocardial infarction is rare and estimated to complicate fewer than 1 in 10 000 pregnancies.[8] It usually develops unannounced by preceding angina because, even though the prevalence of coronary heart disease has increased among pregnant women, the underlying cause is still not usually atheroma. It accounted for just 9 out of 70 cases of myocardial infarction reviewed by Hankins et al.,[8] although premature atherosclerotic coronary disease is probably under-reported.

The use of crack cocaine has increased and is suspected when myocardial infarction occurs in thin young women without apparent risk factors. The mechanism may be intense spasm, sometimes followed by dissection and thrombosis.[9–11]

The most common pathology underlying pregnancy-related myocardial infarction is probably spontaneous dissection although numerous other pathogenic factors may contribute, all of them rare. These may be peculiar to or aggravated by pregnancy or coincidental (Tables 15.1 and 15.2). They include coronary embolism, hypercoagulable states, drug-induced spasm and congenital coronary anomalies. About 80% of cases occur in the peripartum period.

Table 15.1 Causes of myocardial infarction during pregnancy or the puerperium predisposed to by pregnancy or peculiar to it

Spontaneous coronary artery dissection
Hypercoagulable states
  Coronary thrombosis
  Inherited thrombophilias
  Coronary embolism:
    from prosthetic mitral or aortic valves
    from the left atrium in mitral stenosis
    from the left atrium or ventricle in peripartum or other cardiomyopathy
    paradoxical in atrial septal defect or patent foramen ovale or in cyanotic congenital heart disease
    from the placenta in molar pregnancy or chorion carcinoma
Oxytocic drugs
  Ergot derivatives
  Bromocriptine
Maternal pre-eclampsia

Table 15.2 Causes of myocardial infarction during pregnancy that are probably coincidental

---

Coronary atheroma
Coronary arteritis
  Polyarteritis nodosa
  Anti-phospholipid syndrome
  Still's disease
  Takayasu's arteritis
  Old Kawasaki's disease
  Behçet's disease
Coronary embolism
  Infective endocarditis
  Left atrial myxoma
Cocaine abuse
In pheochromocytoma

Coronary artery dissection

Dissection of the aorta in pregnancy has been long recognized and is not confined just to patients with hypertension, Marfan syndrome or a previous coarctation, although these causes should always be suspected. It has been attributed to thinning and weakening of the aortic wall associated with reduced collagen synthesis in pregnancy.[12,13] The same mechanism may account for dissection of a coronary artery. This is usually in the peripartum period and in older multiparous women.[13,14] When not associated with pregnancy it has been linked to the use of oral contraceptives[15] and women before the menopause.[16]

Myocardial infarction has been reported in association with multiple pregnancy and the subsequent development of pre-eclampsia.[17] Hemodynamic stress, changes in collagen and hypercoagulability are probably all maximal late in pregnancy.

The hormonal influences on vessel wall collagen synthesis may lead to weakening of the integument and predispose to dissection. The occurrence of multivessel coronary artery dissection is consistent with this,[18–23] with it happening at times of hemodynamic stress during heavy physical exercise[23] and especially in relation to labour and delivery, particularly in women with hypertension[22] or connective tissue defects.[24,25]

Cystic medial necrosis at the dissection site has been suggested but not consistently found.[26,27] Reduced collagen synthesis was shown *in vitro* in cultured skin fibroblasts of one patient.[12] Eosinophilic infiltration in the adventitia was described in eight fatal cases,[28] but was not found in two cases treated by heart transplantation.[29,30]

The site is usually the left anterior descending coronary artery, typically originating within 2 cm of the coronary ostium.[31] As the diagnosis has hitherto

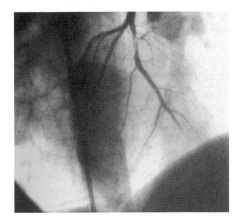

Figure 15.1 A left coronary angiogram (right anterior oblique view) of a 37 year old woman with a spontaneous dissection in the proximal anterior descending coronary artery which caused acute anterior myocardial infarction (reproduced with permission from the British Journal of Cardiology).[24]

usually been made *post mortem*, a preponderance of anterior descending artery dissections may reflect the higher mortality of anterior infarction rather than a true difference in vulnerability between the coronary arteries.

The mortality rate was 60% in medically treated cases and 0% in surgically treated cases in a review of 31 pregnancy-associated cases of coronary artery dissection from the literature who were admitted alive.[32] In a later literature review of 42 cases, in which 21 of 43 presented with sudden death (20.8%), deaths in women who survived more than 24 h after infarction were usually the result of a second coronary artery dissection.[33]

Successful cardiac transplantation was reported in two cases of dissection associated infarction in pregnancy[29,30] and in a case of dissection and infarction outside pregnancy after unsuccessful revascularization and some days on a cardiac assist device.[34]

Spontaneous coronary artery dissections can be recognized at angiography, (Figure 15.1) sometimes at the site of coronary spasm and occasionally in patients with coronary atheroma. The association of dissection with coronary artery spasm probably explains infarction precipitated by crack cocaine[9–11] or ergot derivatives, the latter used for prevention of postpartum hemorrhage or termination of pregnancy.[35–37] These drugs may cause acute chest pain sometimes followed by myocardial infarction, as happened in one of our patients, previously apparently perfectly healthy, who developed a fatal infarct after routine ergometrine. Bromocriptine is a dopaminergic drug that has been reported to cause spasm and infarction after its use to suppress lactation.[38] These vasoconstrictor agents can cause constriction of coronary arteries, thought to result in endothelial breaches that lead to hemorrhagic dissection of the media but also attract platelets and subsequent thrombus formation.

Patients with myocardial infarction complicating pregnancy should always be fully investigated by coronary angiography although earlier reported cases had not been so studied and suggestions about causation have been speculative except in fatal cases.

Coronary embolism

Myocardial infarction caused by embolism from prosthetic valves, the left atrium in mitral stenosis or vegetations in infective endocarditis may occur in pregnancy.[39,40] Coronary embolism has also been reported from intracavitary thrombus in peripartum cardiomyopathy.[41] Anterior infarction occurred in one of our patients with prosthetic mitral and aortic valves who had stopped warfarin on her own volition when she found that she was pregnant. The hypercoagulable state associated with pregnancy may be responsible for thrombus formation in the left atrial appendage, even in patients who are in persistent sinus rhythm. One of our patients, a recent immigrant, was referred with abdominal pain and a suspected ectopic pregnancy, but was found to have a large inferoposterior infarct, tight mitral stenosis and an 8 weeks' gestation *in utero*. Echocardiography failed to reveal any further thrombus. The pregnancy proceeded to a successful outcome after relief of the mitral stenosis and she remained in sinus rhythm throughout the ensuing 10 years during which she has had several further successful pregnancies.

Inherited thrombophilias may first declare themselves through primary coronary thrombosis.

Angina

When angina first develops in pregnancy full investigation is needed because ischemia is likely to get worse and the risk of plaque disruption and thrombosis probably increases. This should ideally be performed before conception but such patients may not have been known to be at risk.

Exercise testing is notoriously less reliable in women than men. This is because of the frequency of atypical chest pain in a population with a low prevalence of coronary disease. Equivocal results, false positives and failed tests are common, but this is especially so in older women who do not undertake enough exercise on the treadmill to stress their hearts. The test is still worth doing because younger pregnant women are likely to be more active and a strongly positive test is unequivocal. Otherwise stress echocardiography is not subject to false positives and avoids radiation, but it requires skill and is more expensive. Coronary angiography should be performed if the stress test is positive. Percutaneous intervention with deployment of drug-eluting stents should be planned for the same session to reduce radiation and be performed after the first trimester with careful uterine shielding, followed by clopidogrel and aspirin. It is more effective as well as safer than rising anti-anginal drug dosage. If a beta blocker is needed it is usual to change atenolol to metoprolol because of a trial that showed lower birthweights among the children of mothers treated with atenolol for high blood pressure (although the cause may well have been the hypertension rather than the drug).[42]

Coronary angiography can spring surprises. Old Kawasaki's disease may re-emerge in pregnancy with angina or infarction caused by thrombosis in an aneurysm, and it is likely to need surgery rather than angioplasty.

Pregnancy may be undertaken after successful coronary bypass surgery. This may have been performed for severe familial hypercholesterolemia. These patients and the rare homozygotes or combined heterozygotes may also develop left ventricular outflow obstruction, caused by narrowing of the aortic root both proximal and distal to the valve.[43] Surgery involves widening of the root with aortic valve replacement and reimplantation of the coronary arteries, which needs to be performed before undertaking pregnancy. Advice from a clinical geneticist is needed, because with autosomal dominant inheritance the children of homozygotes will be obligate heterozygotes and severe heterozygotes have a 50% chance that they will pass the disease on, possibly in a more severe form. Even so these women are not easily deterred. There is no information about the possible adverse effects of statins on the fetus, so it is usual to advise a change to cholestyramine. Pregnancy is likely to be associated with progression of the disease.

Diagnosis of myocardial infarction

Apart from the fact that it usually comes as a bolt from the blue and that the context is all wrong, myocardial infarction presents in the same ways as it does outside pregnancy and the puerperium. It carries a high mortality. If cardiac arrest occurs outside hospital the outcome is almost always fatal. Other presentations may be with cardiogenic shock, severe chest pain or pulmonary edema. Diagnosis and treatment in patients with sudden chest pain may be slow because a heart attack is thought to be unlikely, there is hesitation over management and coronary angiography is delayed or not done.

The diagnosis will be confirmed by ECG changes, echocardiography, coronary angiography and release of cardiac troponin. As creatine kinase CK MB concentration rises post partum because of release from the myometrium;[44] reliance needs to be on serial troponin estimations but this will be retrospective because of the need for urgent action.

Differential diagnosis of myocardial infarction

Most cardiovascular disasters in pregnancy can be recognized by echocardiography, which should be performed without delay because confirmation will bring a need for rapid action to save life.

Peripartum cardiomyopathy

This may closely mimic myocardial infarction (Table 15.3), may have an acute onset and present with chest pain, pulmonary edema or arrhythmia with ECG changes, suggestive of infarction as well as elevation of cardiac troponin.

Table 15.3 Differential diagnosis of myocardial infarction in pregnancy

Peripartum cardiomyopathy ± coronary embolism
Pulmonary embolism
  Venous thrombus
  Amniotic fluid
Aortic root dissection
Pericarditis
Fluid overload
  After surgical delivery
  Ritodrine infusion

Even echocardiography may show seemingly focal rather than global left ventricular dysfunction, in peripartum cardiomyopathy although the whole ventricle will be hypokinetic as well as the right ventricle. Coronary angiography provides final differentiation.

Dissection of the aortic root

This usually has a cataclysmically sudden onset whereas the pain of myocardial infarction tends to build up. The pain typically goes through to the back and may travel down. The dissection may extend to involve a coronary artery (usually the right) causing infarction and frequently leads to aortic regurgitation.

Pulmonary embolism

This is a cause of collapse but, even with clinical cardiac arrest, the ECG usually shows maintained sinus rhythm (electromechanical dissociation). It can cause ischemic chest pain and ST depression on ECG, with release of troponin, but echocardiography rapidly differentiates.

Acute pericarditis

This tends to cause pain with a pleuritic component and is eased by leaning forward. The ECG changes resemble extensive anterior infarction but the patient has no sign of circulatory embarrassment and echocardiography shows a well-contracting left ventricle. Cardiac markers rise only slightly and the evolution is benign.

Overhydration after cesarean delivery or a ritodrine infusion to delay premature delivery, given in saline rather than 5% glucose, may lead to sudden pulmonary edema but echocardiography shows vigorous contraction and a high output.

Management of myocardial infarction

Treatment needs to be swift and urgent as it is outside pregnancy, because of the very high mortality. This is because most dissections, the probable underlying cause, usually involve the whole territory of a major coronary artery and sometimes more than one. Moreover, the patients had previously healthy coronary arteries and have not developed a collateral circulation.

As a result of the variety of possible mechanisms and the urgency of need for revascularization, immediate coronary angiography should be performed with all possible speed and echocardiography performed in the catheter laboratory, or before, to look at left ventricular function, and exclude peripartum cardiomyopathy, pulmonary embolism and intracardiac thrombus. Left ventricular angiography can then be omitted.

Patients with pregnancy associated ST-elevation myocardial infarction should be treated aggressively with no concessions apart from abdominal shielding if the patient is still pregnant. There is no time to deliver the baby first and in any case the risk would be high. Primary angioplasty and stenting should be performed whenever possible, but in the absence of interventional facilities on site or nearby there should be no hesitation in employing thrombolysis. Stenting may seal off a dissection and promote healing with the lumen intact, but urgent coronary bypass may be needed if this fails or for anterior descending artery dissections that are too extensive. Pain relief, anti-platelet agents, beta blockers and angiotensin-converting enzyme (ACE) inhibitors will be needed (but ACE inhibitors should be omitted until after delivery and carvedilol considered as the beta blocker of choice in antepartum patients).

Every effort should be made to maintain the pregnancy until the infarct has healed and to deliver at term. The mode of delivery should be designed to reduce physical stress as much as possible with epidural analgesia, and assisted second stage for vaginal delivery in a multigravida, epidural or general anesthesia for cesarean delivery if this is chosen.

In the event of cardiac arrest before delivery, resuscitation should be carried out with the uterus displaced laterally to avoid aortocaval compression. If resuscitation fails and the fetus is viable cesarean section within 15 min may save the baby.

If no dissection is present a source for embolism may be revealed by echocardiography. If none is found the explanation may have been paradoxical embolism through a patent foramen ovale, which can be shown by injection of echo contrast during a Valsalva maneuver. Evidence of leg vein thrombosis may be found and a perfusion lung scan may reveal defects caused by unsuspected pulmonary embolism. Consideration needs to be given to device closure of a foramen if found.

Postinfarct support is very important because the patient has been through the harrowing experience of a life-threatening heart attack at a young age and at a most vulnerable time. The new mother is going to be emotionally as well as physically exhausted and will need reassurance, encouragement and practical help. Drug treatment will need to be the same as for non-pregnancy-associated postinfarct patients with a beta blocker, ACE inhibitor, statin, clopidogrel and aspirin. This is because maximum protection from possible future atheroma-associated events is sensible in a young woman with an already smitten left ventricle. None of the drugs contraindicates breast-feeding, which should be encouraged and measures set in place to maintain a lifelong healthy lifestyle.

Congenital coronary anomalies

Congenital coronary anomalies are occasionally encountered in pregnancy and patients with repaired tetralogies and other defects have now lived long enough to be seen with acquired atheromatous coronary disease. Occasional patients with previously unrecognized corrected transposition are referred with angina and 'mitral' regurgitation thought to be ischemic in origin. They often have poor function of the systemic right ventricle and atrial fibrillation or atrioventricular conduction defects.

A continuous murmur caused by a coronary cameral fistula may first be detected during antenatal examination. It is usually distinguishable from a patent duct by an unusual location. Echocardiography will usually display the anomaly but small ones may be hard to spot (Figure 15.2). Even large fistulae may be symptom free and cause no trouble in pregnancy but should be closed after the pregnancy. Small fistulae should be left alone. Connections can be multiple and are best tackled percutaneously.

Anomalous origin of a coronary artery (usually the left) from the pulmonary artery, with poor left ventricular function as a result of neonatal infarction or progressive ischaemia caused by increasing fistulous flow from right to left coronary artery, may present with angina,[45] mitral regurgitation or left ventricular failure. The patient illustrated in Figure 15.3 had undergone two uneventful pregnancies before she was referred with angina, mitral regurgitation and failure. She did well after ligation of the left coronary artery at its ostium and

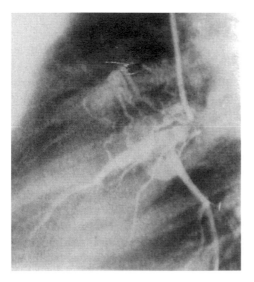

Figure 15.2 One frame from a left coronary angiogram of a young girl who was found to have a murmur at a routine examination. This was continuous and placed maximally at the third left interspace too low for a patent ductus. Echocardiography showed flow into the main pulmonary artery just distal to the valve. Coronary angiography showed a coronary artery fistula with abnormal branches from the anterior descending coronary artery draining into the main pulmonary artery which is opacified from the left coronary injection. This rare abnormality carries no adverse prognostic significance.

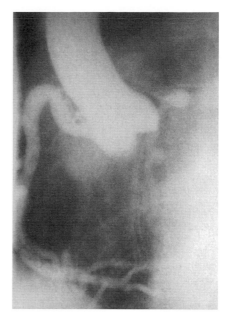

Figure 15.3 Aortogram showing the dilated right coronary artery in a patient with anomalous origin of the left coronary artery from the pulmonary artery (described in the text). The left coronary artery is faintly opacified by fistulous flow from the right coronary artery but has no connection with the aorta.

internal mammary artery bypass into the left anterior descending artery and mitral valve replacement.

Pregnancy after myocardial infarction

The occurrence of a heart attack in pregnancy is deeply distressing and likely to be followed by considerable depression and insecurity even if recovery is good. Little is known about the risk of further pregnancies, which depends on the mechanism and the residual left ventricular function. Subsequent successful pregnancies have been reported but both patients and their doctors will usually be fearful because the risk of repetition of dissection is unknown.

Conclusion

Myocardial infarction is a rare complication of pregnancy with a high mortality. Rapid intervention with coronary stenting or bypass is usually indicated. The most common cause is probably spontaneous dissection but the prevalence of atheroma has increased in association with the older age of many pregnant women.

References

1 Wenger NK. Coronary heart disease: the female heart is vulnerable. *Prog Cardiovasc Dis* 2003;**46**:199–229.
2 Von der Lohe E. *Coronary Heart Disease in Women*. Berlin: Springer, 2003.

3 Brosius FC, Waller BF, Roberts WC. Radiation heart disease: analysis of 16 young (aged 15–33 years) necropsy patients who received over 3500 rads to the heart. *Am J Med* 1981;**70**:519–30.

4 Mallilos-Perez M, Orteger-Carnicer O, Gutierrez-Millet V, Pazmino-Narvaez L. Post partum acute myocardial infarction associated with polyarteritis nodosa. *Med Clin* 1982;**78**:32–4.

5 Rallings P, Exner T, Abraham R. Coronary artery vasculitis and myocardial infarction associated with antiphospholipid antibodies in a pregnant woman. *Aust NZ J Med* 1989;**19**:347–50.

6 Parry G, Goudevenos J, Williams DO. Coronary thrombosis postpartum in a young woman with Still's disease. *Clin Cardiol* 1992;**15**:305–7.

7 Nolan TE, Savage RW. Peripartum myocardial infarction from presumed Kawasaki's disease. *Southern Med J* 1990;**83**:1360–1.

8 Hankins GDV, Wendel GD, Leveno KL, Stoeham J. Myocardial infarction during pregnancy: a review. *Obstet Gynecol* 1985;**65**:139–46.

9 Jaffe BD, Broderick TM, Leier CV. Cocaine induced coronary artery dissection. *N Eng J Med* 1994;**330**:510–11.

10 Liu SS, Forrester RM, Murphy GS, Chen K, Glassenberg R. Anaesthetic management of a parturient with myocardial infarction related to cocaine use. *Can J Anaesth* 1992;**39**:858–61.

11 Livingston JC, Mabie BC, Ramanathan J. Crack cocaine, myocardial infarction and troponin I levels at the time of caesarean delivery. *Anesth Analg* 2000;**91**:913–15.

12 Bonnet J, Aumailley M, Thomnas D, Grosgogeat Y, Broustet JP, Bricaud H. Spontaneous coronary artery dissection; case report and evidence for a defect in collagen metabolism. *Eur Heart J* 1986;**7**:904–9.

13 Anderson RA, Fineron FW: Aortic dissection in pregnancy: importance of pregnancy induced changes in the vessel wall and bicuspid aortic valve in pathogenesis. *Br J Obstet Gynaecol* 1994;**101**:1085–18.

14 Basso C, Morgagni GL, Thiene G. Spontaneous coronary artery dissection: a neglected cause of acute myocardial ischaemia and sudden death. *Heart* 1996;**75**:451–4.

15 Dhawan R, Singh G, Fesniack H. Spontaneous coronary artery dissection: the clinical spectrum. *Angiology* 2002;**53**:5383–93.

16 Maeder M, Ammann P, Angehrn W, Rickli H. Idiopathic spontaneous coronary artery dissection: incidence, diagnosis and treatment. *Int J Cardiol* 2005;**101**:363–9.

17 Sheikh AU, Harper MA. Myocardial infarction during pregnancy: management and outcome of two pregnancies. *Am J Obstet Gynecol* 1993;**163**:279–83.

18 Antoniucci D, Magdidilgenti I. Spontaneous dissection of the three major coronary arteries. *Eur Heart J* 1990;**11**:1130–4.

19 Black MD, Catzavelos C, Boyd D, Walley VM. Simultaneous spontaneous dissections in three coronary arteries. *Can J Cardiol* 1991;**7**:34–6.

20 Emori T, Goto, Y, Maeda T, Chiba Y, Haze K. Multiple coronary artery dissections diagnosed in vivo in a pregnant woman. *Chest* 1993;**104**:289–90.

21 Togni M, Ammann FW, Follath F. Spontaneous multivessel coronary artery dissection in a pregnant woman treated successfully with stent implantation. *Am J Med* 1999;**107**:407–8.

22 Greenblatt JM, Kochar GS, Albornoz MA. Multivessel spontaneous coronary artery dissection in a patient with severe systolic hypertension: a possible association. A case report. *Angiology* 1999;**50**:509–13.

23 Choi JW, Davidson CJ. Spontaneous multivessel coronary artery dissection in a long distance runner successfully treated with oral antiplatelet therapy. *J Invasive Cardiol* 2002;**14**:675–8.

24 De Maio JJ Jr, Kinsella SH, Silverman ME. Clinical course and long term prognosis of spontaneous coronary artery dissection. *Am J Cardiol* 1989;**64**:471–4.

25 Jorgensen MB, Aharonian V, Mansukhani V, Mahrer PR. Spontaneous coronary dissection; a cluster of cases with this rare finding. *Am Heart J* 1994;**127**:1382–7.

26 Dowling GP, Buja LM. Spontaneous coronary artery dissection occurs with and without periadventitial inflammation. *Arch Pathol Lab Med* 1987;**111**:470–2.

27 Chanler Smith J. Dissecting aneurysms of coronary arteries. *Arch Pathol* 1975;**99**:1127–31.

28 Robinowitz M, Virmani R, McAllister H. Spontaneous coronary dissection and eosinophilic inflammation: a cause and effect relationship? *Am J Med* 1982;**72**:923–8.

29 Curiel P, Petrella A et al. Postpartum coronary artery dissection followed by heart transplantation. *Am J Obstet Gynecol* 1990;**163**:538–9.

30 Movsesiam MA, Wray RB. Postpartum myocardial infarction. *Br Heart J* 1989;**62**:154–6.

31 Thayer JO, Healy RW, Maggs PR. Spontaneous coronary artery dissection. *Ann Thorac Surg* 1987;**44**:97–102.

32 Engelman DT, Thayer J, Derossi J, Scheinerman J, Brown N. Pregnancy related coronary artery dissection: a case report and collective review. *Conn Med* 1993;**57**:135–9.

33 Koller PT, Cliffe CM, Ridley DJ. Immunosuppressive therapy for peripartum-type spontaneous coronary artery dissection: case report and review. *Clin Cardiol* 1998;**21**:40–6.

34 Ferrari E, Tozzi P, von Segesser LK. Spontaneous coronary artery dissection in a young woman: from emergency coronary artery bypass grafting to heart transplantation. *Eur J Cardiothorac Surg* 2005;**28**:349–51.

35 Liao JK, Cockrill BA, Yurchak PM. Acute myocardial infarction after ergonovine administration. *Am J Cardiol* 1991;**68**:623–4.

36 Fujiwara Y, Yamanaka O, Nakamura T, Yokoi H, Yamaguchi H. Acute myocardial infarction induced by ergonovine administration for artificially induced abortion. *Jpn Heart J* 1993;**34**:803–8.

37 Hayashi Y, Ibe T, Kawato H, Futamura N et al. Post partum acute myocardial infarction induced by ergonovine administration. *Intern Med* 2003;**42**:983–6.

38 Ruch A, Duhring JL. Postpartum myocardial infarction in a patient receiving bromocriptine. *Obstet Gynecol* 1989;**74**:448–9.

39 Ottman EH, Gall SA. Myocardial infarction in the third trimester of pregnancy secondary to an aortic valve thrombus. *Obstet Gynecol* 1993;**81**:804–5.

40 Janion M, Kurzawski J, Konstantinowicz H et al. Myocardial infarction in pregnancy. *Kardiologia Polska* 1993;**38**:351–3.

41 Box LC, Hanak V, Arciniegas JG. Dual coronary emboli in peripartum cardiomyopathy. *Tex Heart Inst J* 2004;**31**:442–4.

42 Butters L, Kennedy S, Rubin PC. Atenolol in essential hypertension during pregnancy. *BMJ* 1990;**301**:587–9.

43 Hameed AB, Tummala PP, Goodwin TM et al. Unstable angina during pregnancy in two patients with premature atherosclerosis and aortic stenosis in association with familial hypercholesterolaemia. *Am J Obstet Gynecol* 2000;**182**:1152–5.

44 Leiserowitz GS, Evans AT, Samuels SJ, Omand K, Kost GJ. *J Reprod Med* 1992;**37**:910–16.
45 Zavalloni D, Belli G, Caratti A, Presbitero P. Anomalous origin of the left coronary artery from the pulmonary artery in an adult pregnant patient: surgical and percutaneous myocardial revascularisation. *Ital Heart J* 2005;**6**:348–52.

CHAPTER 16
Heart rhythm disorders

David Lefroy, Dawn Adamson

Cardiac arrhythmias occur commonly during pregnancy and are a frequent cause for concern for the well-being of both the mother and the fetus. For some mothers the arrhythmias may simply be a recurrence of a previously diagnosed arrhythmia or a manifestation of known heart disease. However, in most cases, there is no previous history of heart disease, and the new occurrence of a cardiac problem generates considerable alarm. Fortunately, most arrhythmias that occur during pregnancy are benign, and simply troublesome, rather than incapacitating or life threatening. Advice about appropriate actions during symptomatic episodes, together with reassurance, is usually all that is needed. In the remaining minority of cases, judicious use of anti-arrhythmic drugs will lead to a safe and successful outcome for both mother and baby. Maternal death from arrhythmia is extremely rare.

The aims of investigating a suspected cardiac arrhythmia apply irrespective of whether or not the patient is pregnant. The first aim is accurate diagnosis of the arrhythmia by clinical assessment and appropriate ECG investigation. This enables the clinician to give a reliable opinion about the prognosis and appropriate treatment. The temptation to treat symptoms empirically should be resisted because it will frequently lead to the use of ineffective, inappropriate and possibly harmful therapy.[1,2]

The second aim is to determine whether or not there is additional heart disease associated with the arrhythmia. For this the echocardiogram is an invaluable adjunct to the clinical examination, e.g. a patient with atrial fibrillation may be found to have previously undiagnosed mitral stenosis, and this in turn will have an important implication for the use of anticoagulation during pregnancy.

The third aim is that systemic disorders may present with arrhythmias and should be actively sought and excluded by appropriate clinical investigation, e.g. abnormalities of thyroid function should always be excluded, and hemorrhage, pulmonary embolism, infections and inflammatory states must be considered in cases of unexplained sinus tachycardia.

Practice points
Essential investigations for suspected arrhythmia during pregnancy include:
- Resting 12-lead ECG
- ECG recorded during tachycardia, 12-lead if at all possible
- Echocardiogram
- Thyroid function tests.

It is in the realm of treatment that the management of arrhythmias during pregnancy varies significantly from the approach used in the non-pregnant patient. There are a number of reasons for this. First, the potential for harm to the fetus mandates against the use of procedures that require X-ray fluoroscopy, including radiofrequency catheter ablation or pacemaker implantation, which are standard treatments for arrhythmias in non-pregnant patients. Second, concern about adverse effects on the fetus may preclude the use of several anti-arrhythmic drugs. Third, the altered physiological state of pregnancy may have profound effects on the pharmacokinetics of anti-arrhythmic drugs, leading to unpredictable plasma levels that may limit the safety and efficacy of drug treatment. Finally, compared with a non-pregnant patient, a pregnant woman may better accept arrhythmia symptoms without recourse to drug treatment simply because her symptoms are likely to improve spontaneously after delivery.[3–5]

This chapter is intended to serve as a guide to understanding and managing arrhythmias in pregnant women by covering the underlying principles and discussing individual arrhythmias that may be encountered.

Incidence and prevalence of arrhythmia during pregnancy

The sinus rate increases by about 10 beats/minute during pregnancy, and sinus tachycardia greater than 100 beats/min is common.[1,2] Ectopic beats, intermittent sinus tachycardia and non-sustained arrhythmia are very commonly encountered in more than 50% of pregnant women who are investigated for symptoms of arrhythmia.[6,7] Sustained tachycardias are less common, and the prevalence in women of child-bearing age has been estimated at around 2–3/1000.[1,5] Some arrhythmias that occur during pregnancy represent a recurrence of a pre-existing problem, but a substantial number of cases present for the first time in pregnancy.[8,9] Bradyarrhythmias presenting during pregnancy are rare with a prevalence of about 1–20 000, and are usually caused by sinoatrial disease or congenital complete heart block. Death as a result of maternal tachyarrhythmia is extremely rare, with none recorded in the UK during a 12-year period in women with no evidence of underlying structural heart disease.[1]

Tachycardia mechanisms and arrhythmogenic effects of pregnancy

The cardiovascular adaptations to pregnancy include increased resting heart rate, raised intravascular volume, increased cardiac output, reduced systemic vascular resistance, dilatation of the cardiac chambers, augmented stroke volume and enhanced catecholaminergic tone. Atrial and ventricular myocardial wall stress is probably increased, and stretch-dependent ionic currents in cardiac myocytes may be activated. In addition to these changes, a state of heightened visceral awareness in pregnancy may lead a patient to pay attention to symptoms of sinus tachycardia or occasional ectopic activity which are within normal limits and which otherwise would have been ignored.[3,4]

Tachycardias are initiated and perpetuated by one or more of three mechanisms—focal, re-entrant or ion channelopathy—all of which may be initiated or modified by the physiological changes of pregnancy.

Focal tachycardia

A focal tachycardia can arise from a small cluster of abnormal cells called an 'ectopic focus'. An ectopic focus may occur anywhere within atrial or ventricular myocardium, but some locations are more common, such as right ventricular outflow tract and the regions adjacent to the atrial connections of the pulmonary and caval veins. An ectopic focus is able to generate depolarizations that pre-empt the next sinus beat, thus generating atrial or ventricular ectopic beats. These may occur singly or in runs of tachycardia. An individual ectopic focus has a unique ECG signature in the form of an abnormal P wave (in the case of an atrial focus) or abnormal QRS complex (in the case of a ventricular focus).

The cardiovascular adaptations to pregnancy promote the activity of ectopic foci, and ectopic beats are particularly common during pregnancy. Sustained focal atrial or ventricular tachycardia may present for the first time during pregnancy. A focal mechanism for tachycardia is suspected clinically when there are frequent ectopic beats and recurrent self-terminating episodes of tachycardia.

Focal tachycardias may be triggered by physical exertion and terminate spontaneously when exercise ceases. They often respond to anti-arrhythmic drugs that act on nodal tissue such as beta blockers, verapamil or digoxin.

Re-entrant tachycardia

An abnormal electrical circuit ('re-entry circuit') may be present within the heart and consists of one or more of the following components: atrial myocardium, ventricular myocardium, atrioventicular (AV) node, accessory AV pathway (Figure 16.1). The common feature of re-entrant arrhythmias is that a depolarizing impulse can travel repeatedly around the re-entry circuit, generating one heart beat for each cycle. The greater the distance that the impulse has to travel around the re-entry circuit, the more likely it is that each part of the circuit will have recovered electrical excitability by the time the impulse returns for the next cycle. This condition for sustained re-entry can be expressed as follows:

Length of re-entry circuit (mm) > Impulse propagation speed (mm/ms) × Refractory period (ms)

The physiological changes of pregnancy make it more likely that this condition will be fulfilled. Dilatation of the cardiac chambers increases the length of a re-entrant circuit, and the increased catecholaminergic tone reduces the refractory period.

Re-entrant tachycardias are more common than focal tachycardias and tend to have a more stable heart rate. Class I and III anti-arrhythmic drugs, which act

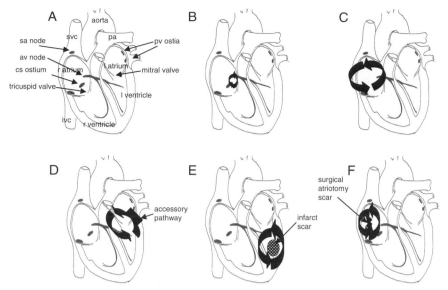

Figure 16.1 Diagram of re-entrant circuits. Panel A: anatomy of diagram. av, atrioventricular; cs, coronary sinus; ivc, inferior vena cava; l, left; pa, pulmonary artery; pv, pulmonary vein; r, right; svc, superior vena cava. Panel B: AVNRT re-entrant circuit in the region of the AV node. Panel C: Reentrant circuit for the common form of atrial flutter which is anticlockwise around the tricuspid annulus in the right atrium. Panel D: Atrioventricular re-entrant circuit using an accessory pathway to complete the retrograde limb of the circuit in a patient with Wolff–Parkinson–White syndrome. Panel E: Reentrant ventricular tachycardia around a region of infarct scar in the left ventricle. Panel F: Reentrant tachycardia around an old healed surgical incision in the right atrium.

on atrial and/or ventricular myocardium, tend to be more effective. They work by prolonging the myocardial refractory period and thus preventing the condition for sustained re-entry described above.

Ion channelopathy

Mutations of the genes coding for cardiac K$^+$ and Na$^+$ channel proteins result in impaired and delayed cardiac repolarization and cause various forms of congenital long QT syndrome. Genetic polymorphisms may also underlie the susceptibility of individuals to drug-induced and other forms of the acquired long QT syndrome. Other ion channel mutations have been implicated as the cause of some cases of familial atrial fibrillation and Brugada syndrome, in which affected individuals have a characteristic ECG with partial right bundle-branch block and ST segment elevation in leads V1–3, and are prone to syncope and sudden death as a result of ventricular tachycardia.

The effect of pregnancy on cardiac ion channels, long QT syndrome and poly-morphic ventricular tachycardia has not been studied in detail. The preponder-ance of long QT syndrome in women, despite most cases being autosomal dominant, strongly suggests that expression of the condition is dependent on sex hormones, which in turn suggests that expression of the relevant cardiac ion channels may be affected by the changing hormonal milieu of pregnancy.

Tachycardia mechanisms: practice points

Focal tachycardias
- Frequent ectopic beats of same QRS morphology as tachycardia
- Tendency for frequent 'stop–starts'
- May be exacerbated by exercise and increased catecholaminergic tone
- Usually the heart is structurally normal
- Typically respond to beta blockers and verapamil
- Cardioversion is often unhelpful; early re-initiations are common.

Re-entrant tachycardias
- Re-entry is the most common tachycardia mechanism
- The echocardiogram and resting ECG may be normal or show evidence of underlying disease
- Ectopic beats occur occasionally, may initiate and terminate tachycardias, and are usually different from the morphology of tachycardia
- Class I and III anti-arrhythmic drugs are useful, particularly when the AV node is not part of the re-entrant circuit
- Cardioversion is an option.

Ion channelopathies and long QT syndrome
- There are abnormalities of the ST segment and/or T wave on the resting ECG
- Syncope and cardiac arrest may occur
- Polymorphic ventricular tachycardia and pause-dependent initiation
- Acquired forms are related to certain drug classes or electrolyte depletion
- Familial tendency
- Beta blockers are effective, but other anti-arrhythmic drugs should be avoided because they make the problem worse.

Clinical presentation and investigation

History

Palpitations are the most common presenting symptom, are usually intermit-tent and only rarely indicate a serious problem. From the history, the inter-mittent thumping and missed beats caused by ectopic beats can be readily distinguished from the rapid palpitation of tachycardia. Ectopic beats that are most noticeable at rest but disappear during physical exertion are benign.

The irregularity of atrial fibrillation distinguishes it from regular tachycardia. An abrupt onset of symptoms at the start of an episode is common to many tachycardias, but an abrupt cessation of symptoms, either spontaneously or with a self-administered vagotonic maneuver such as breath-holding, straining or taking a cold drink, is fairly typical for supraventricular tachycardia (SVT), and may help distinguish this from a sinus tachycardia, which typically slows down over a few minutes.

Presyncope or syncope at the start of a first episode of SVT, with rapid recovery of consciousness, is quite common, but occurs rarely with recurrent SVT because the patient learns to recognize the warning symptoms and take action to avoid syncope by sitting or lying down. Presyncope or syncope at the end of an episode of palpitations may suggest an 'offset' pause resulting from delay in resumption of sinus rhythm; this is a marker of intrinsic sinus node disease which may be exacerbated by beta blockers.

Recurrent syncope with or without palpitation is a worrying symptom because the fetus may be endangered by the reduction in placental blood flow, and, in some cases, it may be a harbinger of sudden maternal death. Syncope caused by cardiac arrhythmia involves complete and abrupt loss of consciousness, and frequently results in injury. Syncope that occurs during or immediately after exertion is worrying and indicates a catecholaminergic-dependent arrhythmia mechanism. In contrast, syncope caused by vasovagal mechanisms is typically more gradual in onset, and the patient is able to avoid injury. When the loss of cerebral blood flow is prolonged, the patient may suffer a secondary convulsion, leading to a misdiagnosis of epilepsy. If there is no head injury or convulsion, recovery of consciousness and full orientation are rapid and occur within a few minutes. The presence of residual focal neurological deficit raises the possibility of a neurological cause of syncope and warrants urgent investigation.

Patients with arrhythmia may also present with fatigue, breathlessness, peripheral edema and chest discomfort resulting from cardiac insufficiency. Symptoms of thromboembolism may be the presenting feature of atrial fibrillation or atrial flutter.

A history of previous heart disease increases the likelihood that an arrhythmia is threatening. Inquiry should be made about the family history, particularly with reference to cases of premature sudden death. Patients with congenital heart disease that has been surgically treated in childhood are now frequently surviving to adulthood. They are particularly vulnerable to arrhythmias, which may be hemodynamically compromising and warrant special consideration. Patients who have received atrial surgery, such as a Mustard procedure for transposition, or a Fontan procedure, are particularly vulnerable to atrial flutter, as are those with any cause of right ventricular impairment. Patients who have undergone correction of Fallot's tetralogy may experience atrial flutter or ventricular tachycardia arising from the right ventricular outflow tract, particularly if the correction was incomplete and there is a residual hemodynamic abnormality.

Examination

The pulse may be abnormal during symptoms, variation in the intensity of the first heart sound, and intermittent cannon waves in the jugular venous pulse during symptoms, suggest AV dissociation, and are features of third-degree AV block or ventricular tachycardia. The clinician should focus on looking for signs of heart disease that may be associated with arrhythmia, including scars from previous surgery, murmurs of structural heart disease and signs of cardiac failure. It is also important to look for systemic problems such as thyrotoxicosis that may manifest as an arrhythmia.

Resting 12-lead ECG

A patient without previous heart disease will usually have a normal ECG between episodes of arrhythmia. Infrequently, a patient may have 12-lead ECG abnormalities indicative of primary 'electrical' disease, such as frequent ectopic beats or Wolff–Parkinson–White syndrome (Figure 16.2).

In patients with suspected bradycardia, abnormalities that should be sought include evidence of sinus node disease such as resting sinus bradycardia or intermittent pauses, and conduction system disease causing prolongation of the P–R interval, QRS-axis deviation or bundle-branch block.

A patient with previous heart disease may have an abnormal resting ECG that reflects their condition and any surgical intervention that they may have received in the past. There may be Q waves from previous myocardial infarction, increased QRS voltage and QRS axis shift, with repolarization changes caused by ventricular hypertrophy, P wave abnormalities associated with atrial enlargement and right bundle-branch block in patients with repaired Fallot's tetralogy.

The 12-lead ECG during arrhythmia

The 12-lead ECG recorded during symptoms is most helpful for arrhythmia diagnosis, but is not always available. A tachycardia with chaotically irregular QRS complexes is usually the result of atrial fibrillation. Less frequently, it is caused by atrial tachycardia or flutter with variable AV conduction. A regular narrow QRS complex (<120 ms) tachycardia (rate > 100/min) is either the result of sinus tachycardia if normal P waves precede each QRS complex, or of SVT if there are no visible P waves or the P waves are abnormal (Figure 16.3). Vagotonic maneuvers such as carotid sinus massage or adenosine injection may help differentiate sinus tachycardia from SVT. A regular broad QRS complex (>12 ms) tachycardia is usually the result of SVT with bundle–branch aberrant conduction or ventricular tachycardia, or SVT with pre-excitation caused by an accessory pathway (Table 16.1). In a patient with a pacemaker, broad QRS tachycardia may be the result of a pacemaker-mediated tachycardia. A careful search should be made for pacing spikes on the ECG, which may be very low amplitude if the pacing system is bipolar and the ECG is highly filtered.

Bradycardia is the result of either reduced sinus node automaticity (P–P intervals >1 s on ECG), or second- or third-degree AV block (fewer QRS complexes than P waves on surface ECG with P wave rate < 100/min).

(a)

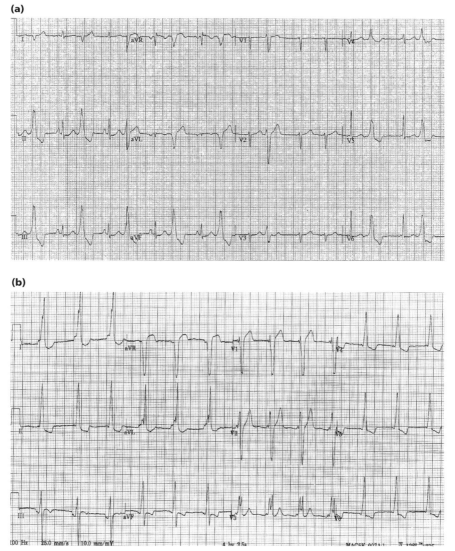

(b)

Figure 16.2 (a) 12-lead ECG from a 34-year-old pregnant woman with syncope and
a structurally normal heart. There are frequent ventricular ectopic beats with a left
bundle-branch block (LBBB) morphology and a QRS axis of around +100°, indicating
a right ventricular outflow tract origin. The patient was successfully treated with beta
blockers during pregnancy and had a successful ablation after delivery. (b) 12-lead ECG
from a 31-year-old pregnant women with frequent tachycardias and Wolff–Parkinson–
White syndrome. Delta waves (slurring of the upstroke to the QRS complex) together
with a short P–R interval are seen in this ECG during sinus rhythm. The tachycardias
were controlled with flecainide plus atenolol, and the pathway was successfully ablated
after delivery.

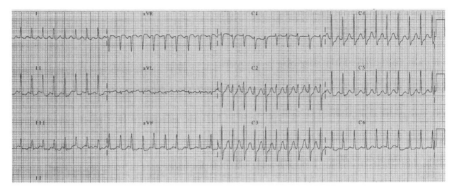

Figure 16.3 Supraventricular tachycardia in a 36-year-old pregnant woman. There is a narrow QRS tachycardia, at 230 beats/min with no clearly discernible P waves. The acute episode was treated with adenosine, and her subsequent ECGs were normal. She had no further episodes and did not require additional anti-arrhythmic drug treatment. She was offered ablation after delivery, but declined.

Prolonged ECG recording

Arrhythmia symptoms are typically intermittent and a 12-lead ECG recording during symptoms may not be available. Prolonged ECG monitoring with either inpatient bedside monitoring or a portable Holter monitor may pick up an episode in a patient with frequent symptoms (Figure 16.4). Where symptoms are less frequent, it is appropriate for the patient to wear a cardiac rhythm event monitor for 7 days or longer, with a patient-activation function for use during episodes of symptoms. It is helpful for the patient to keep a diary of symptoms, which can then be related to the recorded rhythm. Most types of recorder will also record asymptomatic episodes when the heart rate falls outside certain pre-programmed limits. The patient should be encouraged to pursue all her normal activities during the recording, in particular those activities that have previously triggered her symptoms.

Implantable loop recorders are increasingly being used to diagnose unexplained syncope. There is no published experience of the use of these devices in pregnancy but there is no contraindication to their use. The battery life is typically around 18 months and the diagnostic yield is more than 50% in most published series in non-pregnant patients.

Echocardiography

Echocardiography is of undisputed value in the diagnosis and follow-up of structural and functional heart disease, and should be considered an integral part of the investigation of any pregnant patient with arrhythmia. It is non-invasive and poses no risk to the fetus. It is the best way to exclude puerperal cardiomyopathy.

Exercise ECG

Exercise ECG testing can reasonably be used during pregnancy except in cases where bedrest is indicated for obstetric reasons, and is particularly useful in

Table 16.1 Criteria that distinguish ventricular tachycardia from SVT with bundle-branch block aberrant conduction in cases of broad QRS complex tachycardia

---

Ventricular tachycardia likely
Past history of:
Myocardial infarction
Cardiomyopathy
Ventricular surgery (e.g. Fallot repair)
Other ventricular damage or scarring

Examination shows:
Variable intensity of the first heart sound
Intermittent cannon waves in the JVP

Tachycardia ECG shows:
Dissociated P waves
Fusion and capture beats
QRS concordance in the pre-cordial leads
QRS morphology atypical for bundle-branch block

Sinus rhythm ECG shows:
Broad QRS complex with a substantially different pattern to tachycardia QRS complexes

No response to carotid sinus massage of high doses of adenosine
SVT will bundle-branch aberrant conduction likely
Past history of:
Recurrent similar episodes over many years with no evidence of disease progression
Previous known SVT
Rapid throbbing in neck in time with pulse

Tachycardia ECG shows:
Typical RBBB or LBBB pattern
Sharp upstroke/downstroke to QRS complexes

Sinus rhythm ECG shows:
No abnormality
Wolff–Parkinson–White syndrome

Tachycardia slows transiently or terminates with carotid sinus massage or adenosine

---

JVP, jugular venous pulse; LBBB, left bundle-branch block; RBBB, right bundle-branch block; SVT, supraventricular tachycardia.

cases where symptoms are repeatedly provoked by exercise, but the arrhythmia has not been documented by other means. Care should be taken during the test not to exceed greatly the patient's accustomed maximal level of physical exertion during her daily routine. Hypotension during exercise poses a risk to the fetus and should result in immediate cessation of the test.

Tilt-table testing

Tilt-table testing is useful to confirm the presence of vasovagal mechanisms as the cause for recurrent syncope when this is suspected from the history. As the test may induce quite profound and long-lasting hypotension, there are some concerns that it may endanger the fetus. However, there are reports that it can be safely carried out.[10] Vasovagal syncope rarely presents for the first time during pregnancy because women are relatively protected by the increased circulating blood volume and catecholaminergic tone. It is more commonly seen in the postpartum period, when rapid fluid losses, relative intravascular volume depletion and readjustment to non-pregnant physiology may increase vulnerability.

Invasive cardiac electrophysiological testing and catheter ablation

Electrophysiological testing is nowadays usually undertaken as a prelude to catheter ablation of tachycardia, but both procedures confer risk to the fetus as a result of exposure to ionizing radiation. In nearly all cases, the arrhythmia can successfully be managed till delivery by drugs, and ablation can be undertaken subsequently. In patients with uncontrollable and life-threatening arrhythmias, ablation can be undertaken. Exposure of the fetus to radiation can be minimized by lead shielding of the mother's abdomen, and the use of

(a)

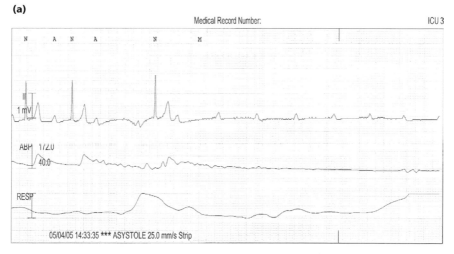

Figure 16.4 (a) Recording from a bedside monitor in a 33-year-old pregnant woman who had recurrent syncopal episodes at 32 weeks of pregnancy. A dual chamber pacemaker was implanted while the abdomen was shielded, and X-ray exposure kept to a minimum.

(b)

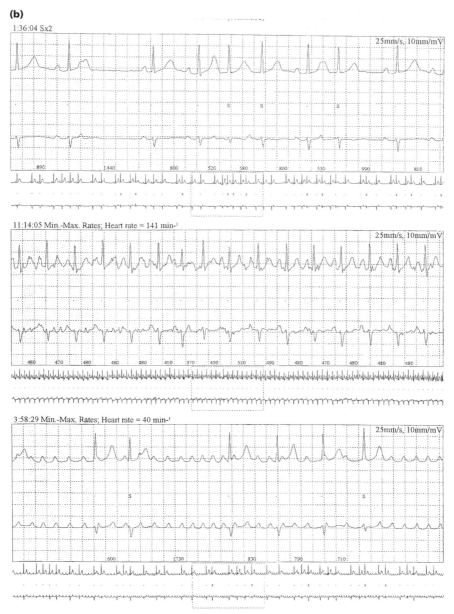

Figure 16.4 *Continued* (b) Ambulatory Holter monitor recording from a patient with paroxysmal atrial fibrillation, probably caused by a pulmonary vein focus and a structurally normal heart. The top ECG strip shows sinus rhythm with frequent atrial ectopic beats. The P waves of the ectopic beat fall on the T waves of the preceding beats, and so are not clearly seen. The middle strip shows atrial fibrillation. The bottom strip shows a rapid atrial flutter. The patient's symptoms were controlled with beta blockers and she received thromboprophylaxis with aspirin. The arrhythmias subsided spontaneously after delivery.

echocardiography or non-fluoroscopic catheter locator systems (such as CARTO or EnSite NavX) to guide catheter placement.

Pharmacological challenge

In certain circumstances, a pharmacological challenge may provide important diagnostic information. The use of adenosine during narrow QRS-complex tachycardia will either terminate the tachycardia (AV nodal re-entrant tachycardia or AVNRT, AV re-entrant tachycardia or AVRT, some cases of atrial tachycardia) or transiently slow the tachycardia before it resumes at its former rate (atrial flutter, atrial tachycardia, sinus tachycardia) (Figure 16.5). In cases where the SVT does not terminate, slowing of tachycardia is usually sufficient to reveal the characteristics of the underlying P waves or flutter waves to allow the correct diagnosis. In broad QRS-complex tachycardia, adenosine can usefully be used to differentiate between SVT (slowing or termination) and VT (no effect). Adenosine selectively slows AV nodal conduction, while not affecting accessory pathway conduction. It may therefore reveal latent pre-excitation in patients with Wolff–Parkinson–White syndrome, where pre-excitation is not apparent on the resting 12-lead ECG.

In some patients, Brugada syndrome may be considered, because of either a family history of sudden death or typical or suggestive ECG changes. A flecainide provocation test may be helpful in elucidating the characteristic ECG changes where the diagnosis is in doubt (Figure 16.6).

Genetic testing

Several cardiac conditions increase the vulnerability to arrhythmias and have a defined genetic basis. The list is growing and includes long QT syndrome, Brugada syndrome, hypertrophic cardiomyopathy, familial dilated cardiomyopathy and arrhythmogenic right ventricular dysplasia. Although routine genetic testing for these conditions is not currently available for the evaluation of arrhythmia risk in pregnancy, a detailed family history should always be taken,

Adenosine 12 mg

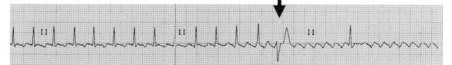

Figure 16.5 Rhythm strip from a pregnant women with a previous mitral valve replacement who had an abrupt onset of a narrow QRS complex tachycardia. The diagnosis of atrial flutter became clear when the ventricular rate was transiently slowed by intravenous adenosine.

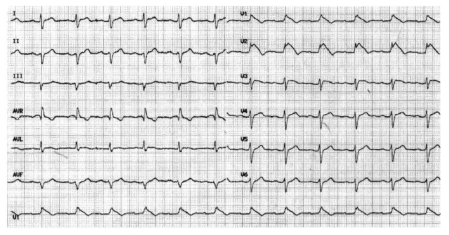

Figure 16.6 A patient with recurrent syncope and a normal echocardiogram. Subtle non-specific change on the baseline ECG became markedly abnormal after the administration of flecainide 80 mg intravenously. The ST-segment elevation in leads V1–3 is diagnostic of Brugada syndrome. This is associated with the risk of sudden death and this patient received an implantable cardioverter defibrillator.

and include specific questioning about premature sudden death. Counseling about the risk of transmission of these conditions to offspring is essential, and it is likely that there will be an increasing role for pre-implantation diagnosis of these conditions in affected families.

Anti-arrhythmic drugs

The physiological changes of pregnancy affect drug absorption, action and metabolism in several ways. It may therefore be difficult to achieve adequate therapeutic drug levels while avoiding toxicity. This may explain why some women experience recurrence of symptoms of arrhythmia during pregnancy despite continuing therapy that had previously been effective.[4]

The greatest risk of drug-induced congenital malformation occurs during fetal organogenesis, which occurs during weeks 3–11, and is therefore complete by the end of the first trimester. Thereafter, the risk is mainly of impaired growth and functional development, or direct toxicity to fetal tissues. Drugs given shortly before term or during labour may have adverse effects on labour or the neonate after delivery. Most antiarrhythmic drugs are categorized by the US Food and Drug Administration (FDA) as category C during pregnancy which signifies that:

'. . . risk (to the foetus) cannot be ruled out. Adequate well-controlled human studies are lacking, and animal studies have shown a risk to the foetus or are lacking as well. There is a chance of foetal harm if the drug is administered during pregnancy; but the potential benefits may outweigh the risks.'[4,5]

Drug treatment should be used if there is either hemodynamic compromise, or a risk of tachycardia cardiomyopathy, or there are other disabling symptoms. Drug treatment is not required for a benign tachycardia that is well tolerated. A low dose should be used initially with titration according to response, and this must be accompanied by regular monitoring. The selection of an appropriate drug depends on knowledge of the arrhythmia mechanisms, and only those drugs that have a safe track record in pregnancy should be used.

Adenosine

Adenosine is useful for the emergency management of SVT and broad QRS-complex tachycardias, and has been used safely in pregnant women.[4,5,11] It is administered as a bolus dose and it has a very short duration of action of no more than 5–10 s. It depresses sinus and AV nodal function causing transient brady-cardia and AV block in the mother, but it has no detectable effect on the fetal cardiac rhythm. Adenosine is contraindicated in patients with brittle asthma, in whom it may cause bronchospasm, and in those taking dipyridamole because of the risk of prolonged asystole.

Digoxin

There is a long history of digoxin use during pregnancy and it is considered to be safe.[5] It crosses the placenta, but is not teratogenic. It is renally cleared, although renal excretion is inhibited by concomitant use of amiodarone. It is mainly used for the control of ventricular rate in patients with persistent atrial fibrillation, but may also be effective in some cases of focal atrial tachycardia.

Beta blockers

Propranolol is the beta blocker with the longest track record and is considered safe in pregnancy.[5] Beta blockers are not teratogenic, but beta$_1$-selective blockers such as atenolol or metoprolol may be preferred because they may interfere less with beta$_2$-receptor-mediated uterine relaxation. However, beta$_1$-selective agents achieve less complete cardiac beta blockade because there are functional beta$_2$-receptors on cardiac myocytes, and these may therefore be less effective anti-arrhythmic agents. There have been reports linking beta blockers to fetal bradycardia, hypotonia, hypoglycemia and intrauterine growth retardation.

Sotalol

Sotalol is a combined beta blocker and class III anti-arrhythmic drug. It does cross the placenta and is renally excreted. It has achieved class B classification with the FDA and its use in pregnant patients has been reported with no adverse outcome.[4,5]

Flecainide

Flecainide has been used frequently during pregnancy and is a reasonable choice for patients with a structurally normal heart.[4,5] It should probably be avoided in those with myocardial disease, and in particular patients with ventricular tachycardia or vulnerability to myocardial ischaemia.

Amiodarone

The conflict between the interests of the mother and the well-being of the fetus is thrown into sharp relief with amiodarone. Amiodarone is a very effective anti-arrhythmic drug to treat and prevent life-threatening ventricular arrhythmias in patients with ventricular disease. However, there is a real concern about fetal hypothyroidism and brain damage.[12,13] Amiodarone crosses the placenta and achieves fetal concentrations of around 10% of maternal serum values.[14] Maternal amiodarone use may cause a goiter, which in turn compromises the upper airway in the neonate. For these reasons, amiodarone should be used only when the mother's life is significantly threatened and no other agent will do.[4,5]

Verapamil

There are no reports of teratogenicity, but verapamil does cross the placenta and may have cardiovascular effects in the fetus.[15] Intravenous verapamil is a useful alternative to adenosine for emergency termination of SVT, and oral verapamil may be used in patients to prevent SVT recurrence when beta blockers are contraindicated or not tolerated.[4]

DC cardioversion

DC cardioversion may be used to terminate sustained tachycardias. It should be carried out with general anesthesia, or deep sedation with midazolam or diazepam. Traditionally, the cardioversion electrodes are placed at the right sternal edge and cardiac apex, but for atrial fibrillation, it may be more effective to use an anterior–posterior configuration. Firm downward pressure on the sternal paddle reduces the electrode separation and increases the intensity of the electrical field, thus maximizing the chance of success. A waveform that reverses polarity during delivery (biphasic waveform) achieves cardioversion at energy thresholds that are half those required when a monophasic waveform is used. For all tachyarrhythmias except ventricular fibrillation, the shock should be synchronized to the R wave to minimize the risk of inducing ventricular fibrillation.

Patients with atrial flutter or fibrillation are particularly vulnerable to systemic thromboembolism after restoration of sinus rhythm. DC cardioversion should not be carried out on patients who have been in atrial fibrillation for longer than 24 hours unless the arrhythmia results in serious cardiovascular compromise, or the patient has been fully anticoagulated since the onset of arrhythmia or the absence of thrombus in the left atrium has been verified by transesophageal echocardiography. Anticoagulation should be continued for a minimum of 4 weeks after DC cardioversion.

DC cardioversion seems to be quite safe in all stages of pregnancy because the intensity of the electrical field to which the fetus is exposed is low. Nevertheless, the fetus should be carefully monitored throughout the procedure. In the latter stages of pregnancy, some anesthetists prefer to carry out the procedure using full general anesthesia and intubation in view of the more difficult airway and increased risk of gastric aspiration.

Practice points
Tips for DC cardioversion during pregnancy
- Anticoagulation is needed in patients with atrial flutter or fibrillation
- DC cardioversion when should be performed under a general anesthetic
- Fetal monitoring is necessary
- Anterior and posterior paddle positions work best for atrial arrhythmia
- Apply firm pressure on the anterior paddle
- Use a defibrillator with a biphasic waveform if available
- Start with 50 J for regular tachycardias
- Start with maximal output (e.g. 360 J) for atrial fibrillation.

Implantable cardioverter defibrillators

Women with an implanted cardioverter defibrillator (ICD) may undergo pregnancy successfully with a good reported outcome. Potentially threatening arrhythmias are promptly detected and automatically terminated by an ICD by either a series of rapid pacing impulses delivered via an endocardial right ventricular pacing lead or delivery of a synchronized shock between a coil electrode in the right ventricular cavity and a second electrode formed by the ICD box, which is located in the pre-pectoral position on the left. Prompt detection and termination of an arrhythmia by an ICD minimize the hemodynamic disturbance and thereby limit the risk of harm to the fetus. ICDs are configured to concentrate the maximal electrical field strength to the mother's ventricular myocardium, and the electrical energy to which the fetus is exposed is minimal. Delivered energies (2–40 J) are about a tenth of those used for external DC cardioversion. One study of 44 women with ICDs who became pregnant showed an 82% rate of successful completion of pregnancy without complication. There were no maternal deaths, and only one stillborn child, despite eight women receiving one or more ICD shocks.[16]

Management of specific arrhythmias

Bradycardia

Bradycardia results from either dysfunction of the sinus node characterized by a P-wave rate of <60/min on the ECG, or high-grade (second- or third-degree) AV block where some or all P waves are not conducted.

The presence of new-onset sinus bradycardia with a resting heart rate of <60 beats/min may indicate hypothyroidism or hypothermia. Heart rate-slowing drugs such as beta blockers, calcium channel blockers or digoxin may cause moderate sinus bradycardia of 45–60 beats/min at therapeutic concentrations. Extreme bradycardia of <45 beats/min is often associated with symptoms

Table 16.2 Causes of AV nodal block

Idiopathic
Congenital complete heart block, maternal lupus with anti-Ro anti-La antibodies
Vagal overactivity
Myocardial ischemia or infarction
Electrolyte imbalance
Drug toxicity
Iatrogenic post-cardiac surgery or post-catheter ablation
Infective endocarditis
Lyme disease
Sarcoidosis
Amyloidosis

of excessive fatigue, effort intolerance, pre-syncope or syncope, and may result from high doses of rate-slowing drugs, or even from moderate doses in patients with underlying sinus node disease. Intermittent sinus bradycardia may be seen in cases of sinoatrial disease, or occur with heightened vagal tone in patients susceptible to vasovagal syncope. Sinus bradycardia and sinus pauses may occur in patients with obstructive sleep apnea.

Congenital complete heart block is usually detected in childhood, and asymptomatic patients with a mean heart rate of >50 beats/min probably do not require a pacemaker. Acquired second- or third-degree AV nodal block is usually the result of idiopathic conduction system disease but may occasionally have an identifiable cause. Patients with symptomatic bradycardia that cannot be alleviated by addressing an underlying cause require implantation of a permanent pacemaker (Table 16.2).

Ectopic beats

An increase in the frequency of atrial and ventricular ectopic beats occurs very commonly during pregnancy. When these are symptomatic, a 12-lead ECG during symptoms is helpful to define the origin. A Holter monitor may show runs of ectopic beats and tachycardia. An echocardiogram is helpful for reassurance when symptoms are persistent and troublesome, and is usually normal. Reassurance is usually sufficient, but propranolol or another beta blocker can be used if necessary.

Sinus tachycardia

Sinus tachycardia >100 beats/min is not uncommon during pregnancy and a rate that is persistently in excess of 110/min should prompt consideration of underlying causes of secondary tachycardia, including infection, inflammatory disease, thyrotoxicosis and cardiomyopathy. A Holter monitor may be helpful to differentiate the normal circadian variation in heart rate of a sinus tachycardia from the virtually fixed heart rate of incessant atrial tachycardia. This distinction is important because a ventricular rate that remains high throughout

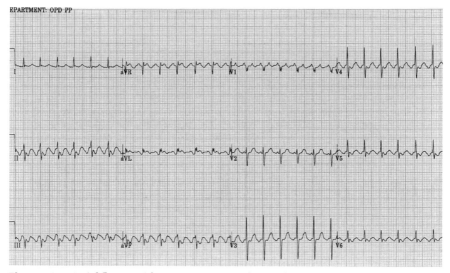

EPARTMENT: OPD PP

Figure 16.7 Atrial flutter with 2 : 1 atrioventricular conduction. The typical sawtooth pattern flutter waves are seen in leads II, III and aVF. The flutter waves occur at 300/min, and in this case every alternate wave is conducted to the ventricle, giving a ventricular rate of 150/min.

the night may result in tachycardia cardiomyopathy, and therefore requires treatment. Debilitating sinus tachycardia associated with pregnancy may be treated with propranolol and typically resolves within days of delivery.

Supraventricular tachycardia

Supraventricular tachycardia is readily diagnosed when the QRS complexes are narrow, regular and rapid, and the P waves abnormal or absent (see Figure 16.3). Broad QRS-complex tachycardia may be caused by SVT with aberrant conduction in a left or right bundle-branch block pattern, or by VT. Discrimination between SVT and VT in a case of broad QRS-complex tachycardia is guided by the characteristics indicated in Table 16.1.

Atrial flutter is usually distinguishable from other forms of SVT by the typical saw-tooth pattern of the baseline, best seen in ECG leads II, III and aVF (Figure 16.7). AVNRT, AVRT and atrial tachycardia typically present with regular narrow QRS-complex tachycardia in a patient with an otherwise normal heart. Analysis of the onset and termination of the arrhythmia, the P-wave morphology and relationship of the P wave to the QRS complex, and the response to adenosine, will often allow differentiation between different SVT mechanisms, but this is not always the case. Whatever the precise mechanism, vagotonic maneuvers such as carotid sinus massage may terminate the episode, and can be self-administered by the patient to deal with recurrences. When vagotonic maneuvers fail, intravenous bolus adenosine can be used, with escalating boluses up to a maximum of 18–24 mg until the desired response is achieved.

Wolff–Parkinson–White syndrome

Wolff–Parkinson–White (WPW) syndrome is diagnosed on the basis of the 12–lead ECG in sinus rhythm where delta waves are seen (see Figure 16.2). These are inscribed at the beginning of the QRS complex and cause a slurring of the initial up- or downstroke of the QRS complex, together with an increase in the width of the QRS complex and shortening of the P–R interval. The delta wave represents 'pre-excitation' of a portion of the ventricular myocardium via an accessory AV pathway. Accessory pathways are located around the annuli of the mitral or tricuspid valves. In up to 10% of cases, there is more than one accessory pathway.

In most cases, the heart is otherwise normal, but WPW syndrome may be associated with hypertrophic cardiomyopathy or Ebstein's anomaly. Patients with WPW syndrome are prone to AVRT (see Figure 16.1), which may become more frequent during pregnancy. WPW syndrome patients are also vulnerable to atrial fibrillation, which may be conducted with high rates to the ventricles via the accessory pathway, resulting in ventricular rates that may exceed 300 beats/min in some cases. This is a life-threatening situation with a significant risk of degeneration to ventricular fibrillation and cardiac arrest. Drugs that modulate AV nodal function, such as beta blockers, verapamil and digoxin, are useless in this situation, and may even enhance conduction via the accessory pathway. A class I drug such as flecainide will suppress or block conduction via the accessory pathway and also have an anti-fibrillatory action on the atria, and this is therefore the drug of choice for the emergency treatment of this condition and prevention of recurrence. Patients should be referred for catheter ablation of the pathway after delivery.

A patient with a WPW syndrome pattern on the ECG who has never had symptoms of arrhythmia does not require treatment. If the patient has had self-limiting palpitations but no documented tachycardia, assessment with Holter monitoring is appropriate. Sometimes, delta waves are present only intermittently, and this is a reassuring finding that indicates that the risk is very low.

Atrial flutter and fibrillation

Atrial flutter and fibrillation are uncommon in pregnant women who do not have structural heart disease. Heart conditions that increase hemodynamic stress to the left atrium (e.g. mitral stenosis) tend to cause fibrillation, whereas those affecting the right atrium (e.g. a Fontan circulation) tend to cause atrial flutter. When the atria fibrillate or flutter, blood within the left atrial appendage stagnates and may thrombose. The thrombus thus formed is often only loosely adherent to the atrial endocardium, and may fragment and embolize to the systemic arterial tree. The risk of thromboembolism and stroke is compounded by the presence of mitral stenosis, left atrial dilatation or impaired ventricular function, or a previous history of thromboembolism. The risk of embolization is particularly high in the first few days after cardioversion to sinus rhythm, as coordinated atrial contractile function gradually returns to normal, and may

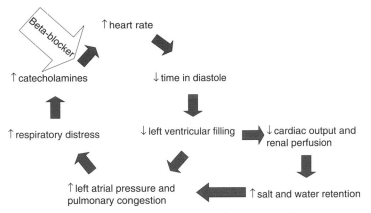

Figure 16.8 The downward cycle of hemodynamic deterioration that may occur in patients with restricted filling of the left ventricle caused by either mitral stenosis or cardiomyopathy. Beta blockers interrupt the cycle and can be life saving.

result in pre-formed thrombus being squeezed out of the left atrial appendage like toothpaste from a tube.

If there is an associated impediment to ventricular filling such as mitral stenosis or diastolic ventricular dysfunction, the high ventricular rates associated with atrial fibrillation or flutter will curtail ventricular filling because the proportion of the cardiac cycle spent in diastole decreases as the heart rate increases. This results in an increase in filling pressures and reduced forward flows, together with peripheral vasoconstriction and reflex salt and water retention (Figure 16.8). Unless checked, this process may progress to acute pulmonary edema with frightening rapidity. The intense catecholaminergic drive that occurs in pulmonary edema further increases the heart rate and filling pressures, resulting in a rapidly escalating crisis. As well as the usual treatment for pulmonary edema of diuretics, morphine and nitrates, a beta blocker, given intravenously if necessary, is essential and may be life saving in this situation.

If the atrial fibrillation or flutter has been present for several weeks or longer and is well tolerated by the patient, it is usually pragmatic to aim to control the ventricular rate with AV node-blocking drugs, together with using long-term anticoagulation, rather than to attempt to regain sinus rhythm. In cases of poorly tolerated atrial flutter or fibrillation, cardioversion will be required and can often be achieved either pharmacologically with sotalol or flecainide, or using DC cardioversion. Amiodarone is also effective and is known to be safe in patients with impaired ventricular function. If the patient is not already established on long-term anticoagulation, she should be anticoagulated as soon as the arrhythmia is diagnosed.

Atrial flutter can be effectively eliminated by radiofrequency catheter ablation, and this is the treatment of choice to prevent subsequent recurrences, although it should be delayed until after delivery. Significant progress has been made in recent years towards achieving a curative ablation approach to atrial

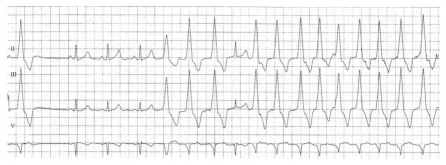

Figure 16.9 Monomorphic ventricular tachycardia recorded from the same patient as in Figure 16.2a.

fibrillation. However, reported success rates vary, long-term follow-up information is absent and there is a worrying incidence of major or catastrophic procedural complications, so this technique is currently best reserved for only the most problematic cases.

Idiopathic ventricular tachycardia

There are two types of VT that can occur in an otherwise structurally and functionally normal heart, and these are termed 'idiopathic VT'. Unlike all other types of VT, idiopathic VT (IVT) almost never accelerates to an unstable rhythm and cardiac arrest, and the prognosis is considered to be benign.

The most common type of IVT to occur in pregnancy arises from a focus in the right ventricular outflow tract just below the pulmonary valve. Typically, patients experience frequent ventricular ectopy, bigemini and bursts of repetitive non-sustained VT (Figure 16.9). Ectopic beats may comprise 1–50% or more of the total beats during Holter monitoring. The QRS morphology of the ectopic and tachycardia beats is usually of a left bundle-branch block (LBBB) pattern, and the QRS axis is between +90° and +110° with very positive QRS complexes in leads II, III and aVF. Occasionally, the QRS complex in V1 is biphasic or positive rather than a typical LBBB, and this may indicate a focal origin in the left ventricular outflow tract, or even in the aortic root in the left coronary sinus of Valsalva. This tachycardia responds well to beta blockers in most cases, and is best treated with curative radiofrequency. Catheter ablation after delivery is advised, because future recurrences are common.

Idiopathic left ventricular VT is much less commonly encountered during pregnancy. It is recognized by the typical RBBB pattern of the QRS in lead V1 during tachycardia, with a QRS axis of around −60°. It is a re-entrant arrhythmia arising from a circuit within the terminal portion of the left posterior fascicle of the LBB and, unusually for VT, it responds to verapamil.

Monomorphic VT secondary to structural heart disease

Any disease process that affects the ventricular myocardium to cause scarring, hypertrophy or infiltration may disrupt the electrical integrity of the myocardium. Examples include myocardial infarction, dilated cardiomyopathy such as puerperal cardiomyopathy, hypertrophic cardiomyopathy, arrhythmogenic right ventricular cardiomyopathy, sarcoidosis, tumors and amyloid. Diseased regions of myocardium may form barriers to the normal propagation of cardiac depolarization. Such barriers may contribute the necessary components to form a re-entrant circuit (see Figure 16.1) that will sustain VT. Under these conditions, multiple re-entry circuits may be present, some with a short pathlength that can sustain very rapid VT. Rapid VT causes hypotension, reduced myocardial coronary perfusion and subendocardial ischemia, an unstable situation that degenerates into ventricular fibrillation. VT in the presence of structural heart disease is associated with a significant risk of sudden death and requires emergency treatment.

The emergency treatment of VT associated with structural heart disease may include intravenous lidocaine, intravenous amiodarone and DC cardioversion. Amiodarone may be used to prevent recurrence and is the only anti-arrhythmic drug known to reduce the risk of sudden death in patients with ventricular disease. Such patients should also be referred for consideration for an ICD, which is known to confer survival benefit over and above optimal drug therapy in patients with a left ventricular ejection fraction of 35% or less.

A normal resting 12-lead ECG and a normal, carefully performed echocardiographic study effectively exclude the presence of underlying structural heart disease in patients with suspected VT, and these investigations are essential for the risk stratification of such patients.

Polymorphic VT
Polymorphic VT is distinguished from monomorphic VT by the continuously changing shape of the QRS complex from one beat to the next, associated with significant irregularity of the heart rate. Unless polymorphic VT spontaneously terminates within a few seconds, it invariably causes collapse. If it is sustained, it degenerates into ventricular fibrillation. Polymorphic VT may be the result of either acute myocardial ischaemia or disorders of cardiac repolarization, including the long QT syndrome and Brugada syndrome.

Torsade de pointes ('twisting of the points [of the QRS axis]') is a particular type of polymorphic VT associated with acquired long QT syndrome (Figure 16.10). Drugs that are implicated in causing this problem are class I and III anti-arrhythmic drugs, macrolide antibiotics, non-sedating antihistamines, antidepressants and some antipsychotics. Women are more susceptible than men and electrolyte imbalances heighten the risk. Typically, the arrhythmia occurs in rapid bursts, causing pre-syncope or syncope, each burst being initiated by a 'short–long–short' sequence of R–R intervals. There is a very high risk of progression to ventricular fibrillation. The emergency treatment includes correction of electrolyte deficiencies, including magnesium and removing any potential culprit drugs from the drug chart. Temporary overdrive ventricular pacing at a rate of 100–120 beats/min will immediately abolish the arrhythmia by preventing the relative pause on which the initiation of each episode depends.

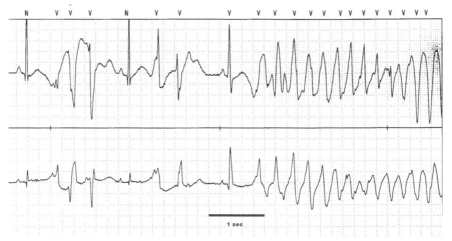

Figure 16.10 *Torsade de pointes* tachycardia in a patient with acquired long QT syndrome caused by erythromycin given for a chest infection.

Congenital long QT syndrome is the result of a genetically determined abnormality of cardiac ion channels, and most frequently affects K⁺ or Na⁺ channels. Women with long QT syndrome do not increase their risk of arrhythmia during pregnancy, but the risk of arrhythmia is increased by up to fivefold in the post-partum period, when prophylactic beta blockade is advisable.[17] Beta blockers are highly effective at preventing arrhythmias in most cases of long QT syndrome. In some individuals it may be necessary to implant a pacemaker to allow a sufficient dose of beta blocker. In cases where tachycardias persist despite beta-blocker treatment, defibrillator implantation is required. Beta blockers are ineffective for Brugada syndrome, and defibrillator implantation is mandatory in symptomatic cases.

Cardiac arrest

Fortunately cardiac arrest is uncommon in pregnant women, occurring in about 1 in 30 000 deliveries,[18] but it is important to be aware of differences in cardiopulmonary resuscitation techniques in pregnant women. An obstetrician and pediatrician should be involved at the earliest possible stage, and cesarean section should be seriously contemplated both to save the fetus and to facilitate resuscitation in cases of more than 25 weeks' gestational age. Amniotic fluid embolism, pulmonary embolism, puerperal cardiomyopathy, and acute coronary or aortic dissection are important causes of cardiac arrest in the pregnant or recently delivered woman. In the later stages of pregnancy, the uterus can reduce venous return because of aortocaval compression, particularly in the supine position.[19] This obstruction can be relieved by using sandbags or a foam wedge under the right side of the patient to tilt the patient onto the left side, thus displacing the uterus to the left. Chest compression is best accomplished higher up the chest than usual because of the cranial displacement of the diaphragm and heart by the enlarged uterus. Gastric emptying is delayed in pregnancy and so early intubation is recommended to prevent aspiration.

Postpartum management

Many arrhythmias that are troublesome during pregnancy are amenable to curative radiofrequency catheter ablation. Patients may be referred for this procedure after delivery, by which time it is common for the arrhythmia to have resolved and the patient to be asymptomatic. At this point, many new mothers are understandably reluctant to undergo an invasive cardiac procedure despite the very small (but non-zero) risk of serious or catastrophic complication. They should be advised to consider ablation even if currently asymptomatic, particularly if they are contemplating further pregnancy in the future. The risk of recurrence of a previously troublesome arrhythmia in subsequent pregnancies is high.

Conclusions

Arrhythmias during pregnancy are common and can almost always be managed successfully with a conservative approach, and the relatively infrequent and judicious use of anti-arrhythmic drugs. Arrhythmias associated with structural cardiac abnormality or an abnormal ECG in sinus rhythm are a cause for concern. Close collaboration of the obstetric, fetal medicine and cardiology services is required to guarantee optimal management and achieve the best possible outcome for the mother and baby.

References

1 Anderson MH. Rhythm disorders. In: Oakley C (ed.), *Heart Disease in Pregnancy*. London: BMJ Publishing, 1997: pp 248–81.
2 Conti JB, Curtis AB. Arrhythmias during pregnancy. In: Saksena S, Camm AJ (eds), *Electrophysiological Disorders of the Heart*. Philadelphia: Elsevier, 2005: pp 517–32.
3 Ferrero S, Colombo BM, Ragni N. Maternal arrhythmias during pregnancy. *Arch Gynecol Obstet* 2004;**269**:244–53.
4 Tan HL, Lie KI. Treatment of tachyarrhythmias during pregnancy and lactation. *Eur Heart J* 2001;**22**:458–64.
5 Blomstrom-Lundqvist C, Scheinman MM, Aliot EM et al. ACC/AHA/ESC guidelines for the management of patients with supraventricular arrhythmias. *Circulation* 2003;**108**:1871–909.
6 Shotan A, Ostrzega E, Mehra A, Johnson JV, Elkayam U. Incidence of arrhythmias in normal pregnancy and relation to palpitations, dizziness, and syncope. *Am J Cardiol* 1997;**79**:1061–4.
7 Gowda RM, Khan IA, Mehta NJ, Vasavada BC, Sacchi TJ. Cardiac arrhythmias in pregnancy: clinical and therapeutic considerations. *Int J Cardiol* 2003;**88**:129–33.
8 Tawam M, Levine J, Mendelson M, Goldberger J, Dyer A, Kadish A. Effect of pregnancy on paroxysmal supraventricular tachycardia. *Am J Cardiol* 1993;**72**:838–40.

9 Lee SH, Chen SA, Wu TJ et al. Effects of pregnancy on first onset and symptoms of paroxysmal supraventricular tachycardia. *Am J Cardiol* 1995;**76**:675–8.

10 Grubb BP. Neurocardiogenic syncope. In Grub BP, Olshansky B (eds), *Syncope: Mechanisms and Management*. Armonk, NY: Futura Publishing Co., 1998: p 73.

11 Mason BA, Ricci-Goodman J, Koos BJ. Adenosine in the treatment of maternal paroxysmal supraventricular tachycardia. *Obstet Gynecol* 1992;**80**:478–80.

12 Ovadia M, Brito M, Hoyer GL, Marcus FI. Human experience with amiodarone in the embryonic period. *Am J Cardiol* 1994;**73**:316–17.

13 Magee LA, Downar E, Sermer M, Boulton BC, Allen LC, Koren G. Pregnancy outcome after gestational exposure to amiodarone in Canada. *Am J Obstet Gynecol* 1995;**172**:1307–11.

14 Chow T, Galvin J, McGovern B. Antiarrhythmic drug therapy in pregnancy and lactation. *Am J Cardiol* 1998;**82**:58I–62I.

15 Klein V, Repke JT. Supraventricular tachycardia in pregnancy: cardioversion with verapamil. *Obstet Gynecol* 1984;**63**:16S–18S.

16 Natale A, Davidson T, Geiger MJ, Newby K. Implantable cardioverter-defibrillators and pregnancy: a safe combination? *Circulation* 1997;**96**:2808–12.

17 Rashba EJ, Zareba W, Moss AJ et al. Influence of pregnancy on the risk for cardiac events in patients with hereditary long QT syndrome. LQTS Investigators. *Circulation* 1998;**97**:451–6.

18 Kloeck W, Cummins RO, Chamberlain D et al. Special resuscitation situations: an advisory statement from the International Liaison Committee on Resuscitation. *Circulation* 1997;**95**:2196–210.

19 Lee RV, Rodgers BD, White LM, Harvey RC. Cardiopulmonary resuscitation of pregnant women. *Am J Med* 1986;**81**:311–18.

CHAPTER 17
Pulmonary embolism

Celia Oakley

Venous thromboembolism is one of the most serious threats to the life of the pregnant woman. The risk rises in women with heart disease or obstetric problems and the problem lies in the management of a rare condition that is hard to diagnose even though it is the leading non-obstetric cause of maternal mortality.

Diagnosis and the necessarily rapid choice of management strategy present special difficulty in pregnancy or the parturient woman. Accurate diagnosis is mandatory because, if confirmed, pulmonary embolism requires prolonged anticoagulant treatment but a missed diagnosis may well herald a fatal outcome. Although all diagnostic tests for pulmonary embolism can be used without known risk to the fetus and the indications for anticoagulant treatment are the same as they are outside pregnancy, physicians feel unsure about diagnostic and management strategies during pregnancy and, thankfully, most obstetricians have little experience of it.

Both pulmonary embolism and the preceding deep vein thrombosis (DVT) have often been silent or not diagnosed, which is why many patients with pulmonary embolism (PE) die without warning or before diagnosis has been made and treatment instituted. Rarely, recurrent PE leads to long-term disability from pulmonary hypertension with shortness of breath and lifespan. Other women suffer from post-thrombotic syndrome with edema, skin discoloration, varicose veins and ulceration.

Pulmonary embolism used to be regarded as a complication of the puerperium. Early mobilization and other measures have led to a fall in the number of postpartum deaths during the past few decades. More recently, the proportion of antepartum deaths has risen with up to half of all the deaths occurring during pregnancy, the numbers distributed throughout, but the most dangerous period still being the first 24 hours after delivery (vaginal or surgical), and the heightened risk continuing although diminishing over the next 6 weeks. Absolute numbers have not notably fallen further in recent years nor will they do so until substantial advances have been made in the prevention and accurate detection of venous thrombosis because its early treatment greatly reduces the risk of fatal PE.

Epidemiology
The incidence of PE in pregnancy and the puerperium is said to lie between 1 in 1000 and 1 in 3000 deliveries[1,2] and the mortality at about 1 per 100 000

Table 17.1 Predisposing factors to venous thromboembolism

Normal pregnancy	Additional factors	Obstetric factors
Increased blood coagulability	Family history of thrombosis	Placental insufficiency
Slow blood flow in the legs	Bedrest	Placenta praevia
Endothelial damage	Obesity	
Smoking	Hypertension	
	Diabetes	
	Older age	
	Surgery	
	Infection	
	Polycythemia	

pregnancies.[3] In contrast to the numbers of fatal cases that are documented through the Confidential Enquiries into Maternal Deaths (now the Confidential Enquiries into Maternal and Child Health [CEMACH]), it is more difficult to obtain accurate figures for non-fatal DVT and PE because these are not reported. Newer data on the incidence of 'near-miss' PE in the UK, its management and sequelae will become available[4] although it is likely that many 'near misses' are not recognized.

Pathogenesis

There is increased risk of venous thromboembolism in pregnancy (Table 17.1).

Virchow's three postulates remain valid. Pregnancy induces both a hyper-coagulable state and alterations in blood flow. Endothelial factors are released with delivery, especially when it is surgical.

The plasma concentration of clotting factors (fibrinogen and factors VII, VIII and X) increases and fibrinolytic activity diminishes in pregnancy as a result of an increased level of plasminogen activator inhibitor, increased adhesion and activation of platelets, and decreased levels of protein C and the activated protein C (APC) ratio.[5–8]

Hormonally driven vascular dilatation slows venous return from the legs. During the third trimester, blood flow is further reduced in the supine or sitting position by compression of both the inferior vena cava and the aorta by the uterus, particularly after engagement of the fetal head.

Additional predisposing factors

The normal balance between coagulation and anticoagulation is further adversely tilted in pregnancy by obesity, smoking, older age, dehydration, surgery, immobilization, infection, hypertension, diabetes, polycythemia and a family history of thrombosis.[7–15] Contributory obstetric causes are placenta praevia and placental insufficiency.

Blood viscosity is increased by polycythemia in patients with cyanotic congenital heart disease who frequently need bedrest in pregnancy.

Thrombophilias

Thrombophilias may be inherited or acquired. Afflicted individuals may declare themselves with a first-ever thrombotic episode in pregnancy or the puerperium.

Inherited abnormalities in the coagulation syndrome include deficiency of protein C, protein S or antithrombin III. Congenital or acquired deficiency of these natural anticoagulants is responsible for 10% of thromboses in apparently healthy people. The factor V Leiden mutation, which causes resistance to degradation by activated protein C is the most common cause of familial venous thromboembolism and is found in about 5% of the population but in at least 20% of unexpected thromboses. These familial defects may have caused no trouble until the development of another predisposing factor such as oral contraceptive use or pregnancy. Raised levels of homocysteine have been identified recently as a risk factor for venous thrombosis as well as for premature atherosclerosis.[5–15]

Among acquired coagulopathies antibodies against phospholipids particularly the lupus anticoagulant and, to a lesser extent, antibodies against cardiolipin, bring increased risk of thrombosis and sometimes lie behind repeated fetal loss particularly in mid trimester.[14]

Natural history of venous thromboembolism

The risk of first DVT is increased 2-fold in pregnancy and 14-fold in the puerperium but, as more than half of patients with an acutely swollen calf do not have thrombosis, a rapid, safe and effective method of ruling it out is needed. Diagnosis is based on clinical probability, blood tests and imaging.[16–18] Thrombosis starts in the venous valves where fibrin and red cells plus sparse platelets form red thrombus. This may be lysed or organized, break up, break off or progress to occlude the vein. In pregnancy most venous thrombi are found in the left femoral veins, but some start in the pelvic veins or, in heart disease, sometimes in the right heart chambers.

Most pulmonary emboli are multiple and most of them travel to the lower lobes. Small thrombi are likely to reach the peripheral pulmonary artery branches where, if they block the artery, they may cause subsegmental infarction and hemoptysis or pleuritic pain if they set up an inflammatory reaction.

Large thrombi may lodge at the bifurcation of the main pulmonary artery, causing instant death or cardiogenic shock if more than half to two-thirds of the cross-sectional area of the pulmonary arteries is obstructed. Sudden blocking of at least a third of the capacity of the pulmonary bed in either central branches or multiple smaller emboli leads to failure of the overloaded right ventricle. This is followed by acute or subacute low-output congestive failure or unexplained syncope. Spontaneous hemodynamic recovery may follow through remodeling of the emboli or their onward movement with re-embolization down the pulmonary arterial tree to where the cross-sectional area is greater and natural lysins are active. Less critical emboli with a better-tolerated response to the suddenly increased afterload cause right ventricular dysfunction, which may be cryptic despite dilatation and a drop in stroke output and blood pressure. If more emboli follow before resolution of the first, the output of the enfeebled right ventricle may be insufficient to continue to support life.

Endogenous lysis of pulmonary emboli normally occurs rapidly with break-up and shrinkage, re-embolization down the lungs and almost complete resolution within 2 weeks of onset of anticoagulant treatment. Exogenous lysins accelerate this process during the vital early period. In fatal cases several generations of emboli are not infrequently found even in patients with a history of only a single embolic episode. Rarely, multiple emboli arriving over a longer period and failing to resolve cause chronic pulmonary hypertension although pulmonary hypertension from such non-resolution is uncommon.[18]

Pathophysiology of pulmonary embolism
Pulmonary embolism causes an increase in physiological dead space and consequent hyperpnea but the vagally induced increased drive to breathe often also leads to alveolar hyperventilation with a fall in arterial Pco_2. Ventilation–perfusion mismatch may develop as a result of intrapulmonary shunts, low cardiac output or reversed shunting through a patent foramen ovale, and also of regional loss of surfactant, which is responsible for patchy atelectasis in embolized segments after a few days. Hypoxemia may develop for any of these reasons but is not invariable and a quarter of patients with proven pulmonary embolism in the PIOPED study had a normal Po_2.[19,20]

The unprepared thin-walled right ventricle dilates and its systolic pressure rarely reaches more than 50 or 60 mmHg, with the high diastolic pressure leading to bulging of the septum into the left ventricle. This may reduce left ventricular filling (ventricular interdependence) and is the reason why right ventricular fluid loading may be detrimental. Low blood pressure, tachycardia with shortened diastole and high ventricular diastolic pressures (Figure 17.1), and sometimes also hypoxemia, combine to reduce coronary oxygen delivery and cause myocardial ischemia. This not only exacerbates right ventricular failure but can also affect the left ventricle, causing patchy posterobasal infarction. In the clinical context of major PE, raised cardiac markers including troponins do not indicate a concomitant coronary artery event.[21]

Diagnosis

Clinical presentation
Pulmonary embolism presents in diverse ways, which vary from non-specific to catastrophic (Table 17.2). Early surgical studies showed that two-thirds of fatal cases die within an hour of the onset of symptoms.[22] Action must be swift if lives are to be saved (Figure 17.2).

About half of all patients with PE do not have detectable DVT and many patients with venous thrombosis have asymptomatic pulmonary emboli. The

Figure 17.1 Simultaneous brachial artery (BA) and pulmonary artery (PA) pressures from a patient with massive pulmonary embolism showing tachycardia, 120/min, with pulsus paradoxus. Blood pressure has been well maintained in the supine position but is spiky with a narrow base, indicating a low stroke volume. The PA pressure is 55/30 mmHg and the end-diastolic pressure in the right ventricle (RV) is even higher; the pulmonary valve remains open throughout the cycle and a closure sound is absent.

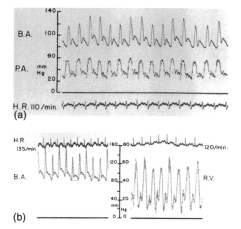

Table 17.2 Symptoms and signs of pulmonary embolism

Symptoms of pulmonary embolism	Signs of pulmonary embolism
Acute onset of shortness of breath	Tachypnea
Collapse, syncope, faintness	Tachycardia
Pleuritic chest pain	Chest tenderness
Non-pleuritic chest pain	Raised jugular venous pressure
Hemoptysis	Right ventricular heave and gallop
Leg swelling or pain	Deep vein thrombosis

problem is that a complaint of shortness of breath is common in pregnancy. A high index of suspicion is needed and PE should be excluded in any pregnant or parturient patient with unexplained respiratory symptoms, especially if of sudden onset. Dyspnea is the most frequent symptom and tachypnea the most frequent sign.[23]

Clinical syndromes (Table 17.3)

Minor PE

No PE is minor in import because it may herald major and fatal embolism. Symptoms may be absent with presentation resulting from DVT. The most frequent symptoms are shortness of breath, substernal discomfort or pleuritic pain and dry cough. In the absence of infarction, physical symptoms and signs may be entirely absent or limited to anxiety or tachpnea and tachycardia.

Pulmonary infarction

Acute onset of pleuritic chest pain, with consequent shortness of breath and sometimes hemoptysis, indicates PE until it has been excluded. Examination

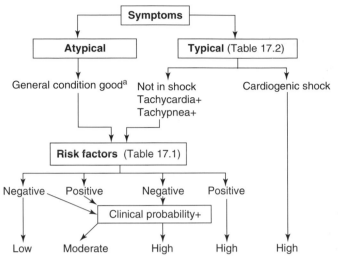

Figure 17.2 Clinical probability of pulmonary embolism according to symptoms and risk factors. ªGeneral condition good; no tachycardia or dyspnea.

Table 17.3 Clinical syndromes

Acute minor pulmonary embolism
Pulmonary infarction
Subacute massive pulmonary embolism
Massive pulmonary embolism
Recurrent pulmonary embolism
Paradoxical embolism
Non-thrombotic embolism

may show limitation of movement of the involved hemithorax. A surprising number have chest wall tenderness, probably caused by inflammation of the parietal pleura. Pleuritic pain should not be attributed to infection without fever and purulent sputum. The emboli are usually small, distal and basal. Infarction is delayed some days after the embolism. Fever, leukocytosis and changes on the chest radiograph then develop.

Subacute massive PE
Faintness on effort or actual syncope, with shortness of breath and apprehension, may mark subacute massive PE and be accompanied by pleuritic pain, dry cough, hemoptysis or fever, or any combination of these. Fleeting syncope may be the only symptom if it was caused by transient blockage of the right ventricular exit, which was then cleared by onward passage of the emboli, or it may be followed by continuing faintness on effort if the partially obstructed right ventricle fails to maintain sufficient output and blood pressure falls on exercise.

Physical signs are often deceptively few. Clinical signs of acute right ventricular failure can be subtle. Tachypnea is the most frequent followed by tachycardia. The jugular venous pressure may be raised and there may be increased left parasternal pulsation, a third heart sound gallop and widely split second sound. The lungs are usually clear but there may be focal crackles as surfactant is lost from non-perfused segments of lung. At this stage the arrival of further emboli will very probably be fatal, but otherwise the evidence of acute cor pulmonale has usually resolved in just a day or two.

Massive PE

The patient, who may have seemed quite fit up to then, has suddenly collapsed and is in shock, pale, cold, clammy and shut down or in actual circulatory arrest. In patients with maintained consciousness, tachypnea and hyperpnea are striking with poor peripheral perfusion. Substernal chest pain may be confusing. The lungs are usually clear with good air entry. Rarely, PE may trigger bronchospasm in people with asthma. The pulse is rapid and ill-sustained and blood pressure maintained only with the patient supine. There may be pulsus paradoxus as filling of the left ventricle and stroke volume fall on inspiration (see Figure 17.1). The venous pressure will be raised but this cannot be observed clinically because the patient is lying flat and also because of her heightened respiratory efforts. A third heart sound gallop is prominent but pulmonary valve closure is soft (not accentuated as generally stated) and may be absent if the right ventricular diastolic pressure has risen to equal the diastolic pressure in the pulmonary artery. In less severe cases the second heart sound is widely split. A systolic murmur of tricuspid regurgitation may be audible but it is often silent because right ventricular pressure and flow may be insufficient to produce audible turbulence, and indeed all the heart sounds become soft as the circulation fails. When circulatory arrest occurs sinus rhythm is commonly maintained (persistent electrical activity).

A low P_{CO_2} may be coupled with a low P_{O_2} sometimes contributed to by central right-to-left shunting if the foramen ovale is patent. This can lead to concomitant stroke, which may dominate the clinical scene. The association of hypoxemia with hypocapnia and a respiratory alkalosis is always highly suggestive of pulmonary embolism but hypoxemia is not invariable.[24,25]

Recurrent PE

Patients with shortness of breath and features of pulmonary hypertension may have had recurrent episodes of PE or give no such history but show widespread perfusion defects on scanning.

An underlying thrombophilia is likely but sometimes tests reveal autoimmune disease with lupus or Behçet syndrome, and the pulmonary hypertension has resulted from pulmonary arteritis with thrombosis *in situ* rather than embolism. In rare cases pulmonary angiography or cardiac magnetic resonance imaging (CMRI) may show multiple pulmonary artery branch stenoses.

Paradoxical embolism

Elevation of right atrial pressure favors paradoxical passage of emboli if the foramen ovale is patent. A devastating stroke or unexplained systemic embolism should lead to a search for a cardiac source and suspicion of paradoxical embolism, so concomitant PE and occult DVT should also be sought.[26,27]

Echocardiography with injection of a sonicated indicator while the patient performs a Valsalva maneuver will force a right-to-left shunt, with passage of bubbles through the defect and their appearance in the left atrium. The technique is more sensitive if imaging is performed from the transesophageal approach. If patency of the foramen ovale is revealed after systemic embolism, device closure should be performed.

Non-thrombotic PE

Amniotic fluid, fat, tumor or air may embolize to the lungs.[28,29] Fat embolism may occur after major fractures. Progressive pulmonary hypertension may result from multiple microtumor embolism in chorioncarcinoma. This sometimes develops years after a normal pregnancy or abortion. A pregnancy test should be performed if there is clinical suspicion. Air embolism is a complication of central venous lines and special care is necessary when the right atrial pressure is raised, in case of patency of the foramen ovale. A much smaller amount of air than is tolerated on the right side can have devastating consequences when released into the systemic circulation.

Embolism of amniotic fluid is usually asymptomatic and is common peripartum but, rarely, it causes sudden collapse during or after delivery, particularly after surgical delivery in multiparous patients but is distinguished by the disseminated vascular coagulopathy that usually follows.

Diagnostic strategy

The diagnostic strategy depends on the initial hemodynamic presentation.[30–32] Suspected PE always requires urgent confirmation or exclusion.

In patients whose general condition is good and who are hemodynamically stable there is time for diagnostic imaging. Suspicion rests on clinical probability (see Figure 17.2) and diagnosis will follow the results of the baseline tests and scans (Figure 17.3).

Diagnostic delay must be minimized in patients needing urgent reperfusion (Figure 17.4). There is no time for imaging tests apart from immediate on-site echocardiography. Patients who are in cardiogenic shock need reperfusion treatment right away. Echocardiography also plays a central role in identifying those patients without shock but whose hemodynamic instability and poorer outlook are shown by right ventricular dilatation.

Baseline tests

Blood gases, ECG and chest radiograph are basic. They may be uninformative diagnostically if they are all normal but they say much about the general condition of the patient and are useful in exclusion of other conditions.

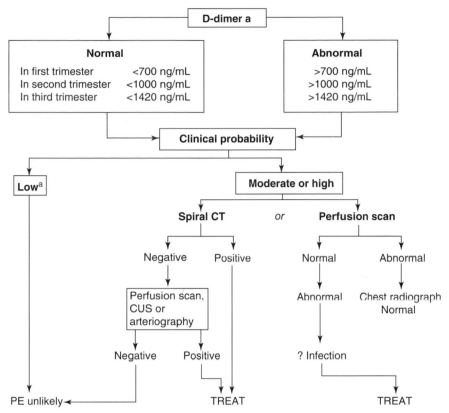

Figure 17.3 Diagnostic strategy for pulmonary embolism (PE) in stable patients. CT, computed tomography; CUS, compression ultrasonography. [a]Reliability in pregnancy needs further confirmation.

Arterial blood gases

These are helpful but not specific and may be normal. A normal alveolar–arterial oxygen gradient does not exclude PE but a reduced Po_2 in an apparently fit patient is highly significant, especially when combined with a low Pco_2. Arterial samples should be taken with the patient sitting up if possible.[25,33]

The electrocardiogram

The ECG (Table 17.4) may reveal evidence of right ventricular overload with clockwise rotation and right-sided T-wave inversion, low voltage, right axis and rSr in V1 or occasionally right bundle-branch block.[24]

The chest radiograph

This is usually normal but a near-normal film in the setting of severe respiratory and circulatory compromise is highly suggestive of massive PE. The chest radiograph is useful in ruling out other lung pathology such as pneumonia or pneumothorax. It may show non-specific abnormality such as patchy basal atelectasis or pleural effusion or, rarely, one of the classic signs, a wedge-shaped

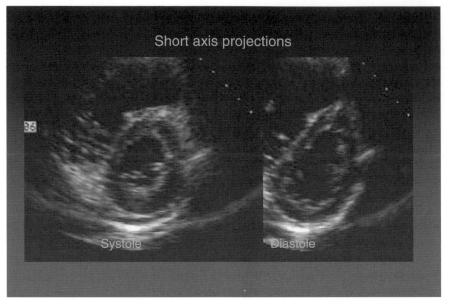

Figure 17.4 Transthoracic echocardiogram, short-axis projection, systole on the left, diastole on the right, showing diastolic bowing of the ventricular septum toward the left ventricle and reduced left ventricular volume in acute pulmonary embolism.

Table 17.4 The ECG in pulmonary embolism

T-wave inversion in leads III, aVF and right-sided chest leads
Right axis and clockwise rotation, dominant S–V5
rSr in V1; complete right bundle-branch block (rare)
Low voltage in limb leads
Qs in leads III and aVF

opacity caused by segmental infarction or focal oligemia (Westermark's sign), indicating massive central embolic occlusion.[24]

D-dimers
These are breakdown products of fibrin clot. They indicate on-going fibrinolysis. A normal level is a rapid test, currently much used to rule out thromboembolism but pregnancy itself increases the plasma D-dimer concentration above the normal upper limit of 500 ng/mL.

Normal ranges at different stages of pregnancy were recently established from quantitative assays in 50 normal pregnant women using a US Food and Drug Agency (FDA)-approved ELISA (enzyme-linked immunosorbent assay) method. D-dimer levels increased through pregnancy and exceeded 500 ng/mL in 50%, 75% and 100% of women in the three trimesters. The study indicated that levels above 700, 1000 and 1420 have >50% likelihood of being abnormal

Table 17.5 Diagnostic imaging in suspected pulmonary embolism

No lung scan needed if leg scan positive	
Chest radiograph	Usually normal or non-specific
Echocardiography	Immediate availability Shows RV (TTE), main PA branches (TOE)
Perfusion scan	Positive scan with normal chest radiograph; start heparin Useful if SCT negative and clinical probability high
Ventilation scan	Useful if both radiograph and perfusion scan are abnormal If abnormal consider antibiotics If normal start heparin or both
Spiral CT scan	Positive scan with normal chest radiograph; start heparin Useful if perfusion is equivocal and chest radiograph or ventilation are normal May miss subsegmental PE
CMRI	Becoming more generally available; shows RV too
Pulmonary angiography	Essential for fragmentation or embolectomy Gold standard but invasive Involves radiation

CMRI, cardiac magnetic resonance imaging; PA, pulmonary artery; PE, pulmonary embolism; RV, right ventricle; SCT, spiral computed tomography; TOE, transesophageal echocardiography; TTE, transthoracic echocardiography.

for each trimester (see Figure 17.3) but more studies are still needed before these figures can be relied on.

Raised D-dimer levels are not specific but normal levels can be used to back up clinical assessment of the low probability to rule out PE and remove the need for imaging. Levels raised above the recently established norms in otherwise healthy pregnant women are highly suggestive of PE,[34,35] but more studies are still needed.

Diagnostic imaging (Table 17.5)

Echocardiography

Echocardiography is under-used as the most rapid diagnostic measure in emergency circumstances.[36] It is also non-invasive and does not involve radiation. Right ventricular dysfunction is found in about a third of all patients with acute PE (see Figure 17.4). The degree of dilatation and severity of systolic dysfunction give both therapeutic and prognostic guidance and are the single most important prognostic factor for in-hospital death.[37] They are usually immediately available in the accident and emergency department (A&E) to A&E staff, cardiologists or obstetricians faced with a patient in shock or with recent onset of puzzling symptoms, and their usefulness will increase further as hand-held machines come into more general use.

Although detection of right ventricular dysfunction lacks specificity, this is of much less importance in the largely healthy pregnant population than in the older suspect population with a higher incidence of co-morbidity. Rarely, echocardiography will reveal a clinically unsuspected cardiomyopathy, particularly peripartum cardiomyopathy with its high incidence of intraventricular thrombi that may present with pulmonary (or systemic) embolism.

Otherwise unexplained right ventricular dilatation, poor function and tricuspid regurgitation are frequently a surprise in patients with negative clinical findings who may have complained only of some shortness of breath, transient dizziness or faintness, and who do not appear to be in distress. Bowing of the ventricular septum towards the left ventricle in diastole indicates right ventricular volume overload.[38,39] Rarely, worm-like emboli swim in the right atrium to poke in and out of the tricuspid valve or extend into the ventricle or pulmonary artery.[40] The central pulmonary arteries are not seen in transthoracic views for which transesophageal imaging is needed.

Transesophageal echocardiography does not have the brilliant immediacy of transthoracic echocardiography but needs no preparation or cooperation from radiological colleagues to delay it. It shows the main pulmonary artery, the right and the proximal left pulmonary artery, and any thrombi or filling defects.[41]

Compression venous Doppler ultrasonography

Loss of venous compressibility indicates thrombosis. Augmentation of flow is absent or reduced during compression. This is the primary diagnostic test for DVT because it is non-invasive and totally safe for the fetus. The test is highly sensitive and specific for proximal DVT with thrombosis of femoral veins, but is not reliable for isolated iliac thrombosis (more prevalent during pregnancy) and ultrasound diagnosis of isolated calf vein thrombosis needs special expertise.[13,42]

About half of all patients with PE have no imaging evidence of DVT. Although a normal ultrasound examination therefore does not rule it out, its identification indirectly establishes the diagnosis of PE but false-positive results may be obtained in the third trimester as a result of compression of the iliofemoral veins by the uterus.

Real-time ultrasonography

The common femoral vein and popliteal vein can be visualized and intraluminal clots detected, although their echogenicity varies according to their age. Real-time imaging uses standard equipment, is easy, and can be repeated and combined with compression. It cannot detect isolated iliac vein thrombosis.

Contrast phlebography

This is reserved for investigation of equivocal results of ultrasound examination in patients with high clinical probability of DVT but with no evidence of PE. It is rarely indicated in pregnancy but the alternative may possibly be unnecessary heparin treatment.

Ventilation–perfusion scans

Perfusion lung scans

These are indicated as the primary test for PE. They are performed by injecting technetium-99m (^{99m}Tc) coupled to microaggregates of human albumin and scanning the distribution of radioactivity with a gamma camera. The radiation dose to the fetus is minimal. A normal scan rules out PE. Unfortunately an abnormal scan cannot confirm the diagnosis, although non-specific abnormalities are less frequent in pregnant patients than in an older age group. Large perfusion defects with a normal chest radiograph are likely to be the result of PE and make a ventilation scan unnecessary. The original classification stemming from the PIOPED trial has been revised[44] and was followed by the attempt in the PISAPED trial with the aim of eliminating equivocal results.[45]

Ventilation scans

These employ inhaled xenon-133 (^{133}Xe) or krypton-81m (^{81m}Kr). An abnormal perfusion scan followed by a normal ventilation scan is diagnostic of PE and reported as 'high probability of PE'. Matched abnormalities in perfusion and ventilation scans with an abnormal chest radiograph are likely to be caused by infection. One reason for abnormalities on the ventilation scan, especially when a scan is delayed, is the patchy atelectasis of embolized segments of lung that often follows in the next few days. The radiation dose is similar to that with a perfusion scan.

Doubt has been expressed as to whether the ventilation scan is any more useful than a chest radiograph in interpreting the perfusion scan.

Spiral computed tomography

With the development of more accurate scanners, spiral CT has increased in popularity as the primary imaging test for PE.[46,47] This preference is because ventilation–perfusion scans still produce so many equivocal results in older patients with co-morbidity, among whom reports of 'intermediate risk of PE' are frequent and frustrating. They are especially likely when the chest radiograph is abnormal. These limitations of ventilation–perfusion scans are much less of a problem in the younger and otherwise healthy pregnant population.

Spiral CT produces a definite positive or negative result but is less accurate in revealing segmental PE than central or lobar emboli. A normal study therefore cannot rule out isolated peripheral subsegmental PE or be the basis for withholding anticoagulant treatment.

The technique has the disadvantages of both exposure to radiation and a fetal dose of iodinated contrast, although the fetal radiation dose with spiral CT is lower than with ventilation–perfusion scanning and neonatal hypothyroidism has not been reported.

Magnetic resonance imaging

MRI with gadolinium enhancement now has similar accuracy to pulmonary angiography and CMRI also allows assessment of ventricular function. It avoids radiation and the use of radiographic contrast and imposes no risk, but is not usually immediately, or as yet generally, available.[48]

Both spiral CT and MRI can be extended to look for DVT but there is no point if imaging for PE has been positive. Neither CT nor MRI are needed if leg vein ultrasonography is positive.

Pulmonary angiography

Pulmonary angiography is safe during pregnancy with suitable abdominal screening, but is rarely indicated except as part of the interventional treatment of immediately life-threatening massive embolism. It is regarded as the gold standard but carries a mortality rate of about 0.5%, is technically demanding and often hard to interpret despite good image quality, for both of which the skills of a radiologist may be needed especially for out-of-hours emergency work. Safety and accuracy have been greatly increased by the use of selective injections, digital subtraction and magnification.[48–50] Anticoagulants may be withheld if pulmonary angiography is normal.[50,51]

Management

Patients in cardiogenic shock or hemodynamically unstable

Massive and subacute massive PE

The management of a patient with a high clinical probability of PE and who is in shock is aimed at restoring circulation and saving life (Table 17.6). The diagnosis needs to be confirmed and action taken with no time lost (Figure 17.5). If the diagnosis is confirmed by right ventricular dilatation shown on transthoracic echocardiography, percutaneous catheter fragmentation and thrombolysis (Figure 17.6) should be carried out immediately and without delay for other investigations.[18,31,52–54] It is usually successful if the embolism was truly acute. It

Table 17.6 Massive pulmonary embolism (emergency treatment to save life)

Cardiopulmonary resuscitation (CPR) if circulatory arrest
Elevate legs
Oxygen
Central intravenous line
Start heparin
Consider dobutamine infusion
Consider inhaled nitric oxide
Thrombolytic drug
Per catheter clot fragmentation and/or extraction

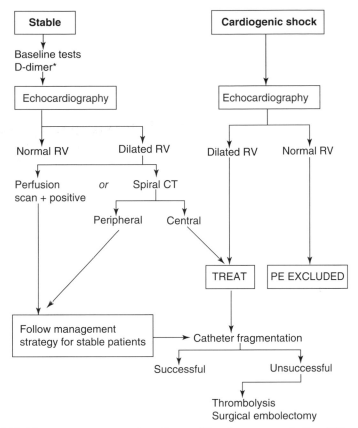

Figure 17.5 Management strategy in patients with pulmonary embolism (PE) again stressing the key role played by echocardiography. RV, right ventricle. [a]Reliability in pregnancy needs further confirmation.

will fail if the circulation has collapsed after apparent sudden onset, although all or most of the material has been gradually accreted through recurrent episodes.

A pigtail catheter should be introduced by the brachial route or central vein with the patient tilted head down. Fragmentation can be accomplished very swiftly and, if it is successful, blood pressure and consciousness are restored within minutes. The extreme emergency is over. The catheter is inserted via a brachial or central route so as to avoid dislodging any thrombus in the pelvis or vena cava, and to save the fetus from radiation if the patient is undelivered. Provided that the obstruction is caused by freshly arrived embolic material that is still lying centrally, it can usually be moved on with dramatic improvement. Formal angiography is not required but contrast is needed to guide the procedure and should be used as sparingly as possible.

If attempts to fragment central emboli and move them on are unsuccessful, per catheter embolectomy should be tried and, if all else fails, surgical embolectomy.

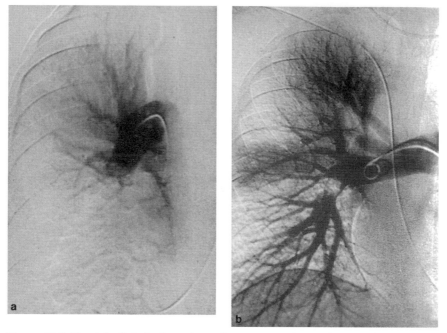

Figure 17.6 The right digital subtraction pulmonary arteriogram from a patient with massive pulmonary embolism (a) before and (b) after restoration of flow to the lower lobe by mechanical fragmentation. The pigtail catheter is clearly visible.

Other measures are adjuvant. The legs should be elevated and oxygen given. If consciousness has been lost chest compression will help to empty the right ventricle and be directly therapeutic if it dislodges thrombi and assists in moving them on. If the circulation is compromised and the right ventricle dilated, but the patient is conscious and not in shock, there is time for perfusion or spiral CT to assess the size and distribution of the clot burden.

A central line is inserted and unfractionated heparin is started. It is usual to give inotropes and vasopressors but, unless an effective circulation returns rapidly, an attempt should be made to fragment the emboli per catheter. Dobutamine is usually given even though endogenous neuroendocrine activation is likely to be providing maximum stimulation already. Dobutamine provides positive inotropic effect with pulmonary vasodilatation through its beta-adrenergic action. Inhaled nitric oxide may release pulmonary vasoconstriction and help to reduce right ventricular afterload.

Fluid loading is probably unhelpful and no more than 500 mL fluid should be given, more only if it appears to have been beneficial (as ventricular interdependence may cause further compromise of left ventricular filling). This can most rapidly be appreciated by following the effect of the infusion echocardiographically.

Thrombolytic treatment with recombinant plasminogen activator (rtPA) should be given only if the circulation remains compromised. This does not cross the placenta or directly injure the fetus but may cause bleeding and fetal risk. It can be started immediately after completion of mechanical fragmentation and given directly into the pulmonary arteries (although there is no proof of added efficacy by this route). Infusion of unfractionated heparin should follow.

Major PE

If echocardiography reveals right ventricular dysfunction, septal bowing and tricuspid regurgitation, but the circulation is not compromised, compensation is marginal and the patient should be regarded as unstable. The fetus is at risk if maternal output falls with exertional blood pressure dips. The patient is nursed in an intensive care or high dependency unit with oxygen, heparin and trial of dobutamine, but thrombolytic treatment is not indicated and recovery of right ventricular function is often swift over hours rather than days. A slower or no improvement suggests a subacute or acute on chronic pathogenesis with possible later need for elective surgical embolectomy if resolution fails.

Clinically stable patients

If the patient is hemodynamically stable with maintained blood pressure and cardiac output, anticoagulant treatment with heparin may be all that is required plus oxygen and pain relief. Absence of right ventricular dilatation on echocardiography adds reassurance but the risk of recurrent embolism continues until existing venous thrombus has been autolysed or organized. Now is the time for insertion of a prophylactic caval filter[18] if this is contemplated but the procedure, although improved, involves radiation, carries morbidity and is not always successful in preventing recurrence.

Continuing management

Intravenous unfractionated heparin should be given, aiming for an adjusted partial thromboplastin time (aPPT) between 1.5 and 2.5 times the control (anti-Xa activity 0.3–0.6 IU).[18] Control should be very tight because the therapeutic window is narrow. A changeover to low-molecular-weight heparin (LMWH) can be made after a week or so if the patient is stable and echocardiography shows that right ventricular function is restored. Follow-up ventilation–perfusion scanning can be delayed until the puerperium. LMWH is probably safe and effective but there are no data in pregnancy and it takes longer to reverse before delivery. After delivery a change can be made to warfarin (coumadin) which should be continued until the ventilation–perfusion scan is normal or there is no further improvement. Compression stockings should be worn through the rest of the pregnancy and early puerperium.

Patients who have suffered PE are at risk from recurrence until any thrombus in leg and pelvic veins has lysed, embolized or organized. Thrombolytic agents do not work immediately or completely, but patients who are destined to survive sometimes improve before thrombolytic activity has started through onward movement, compaction or shrinkage of embolized material. Heparin is not lytic and resorption of non-embolized material depends on endogenous lysis which is very active in the lungs. Patients who have suffered massive or major embolism are probably less likely to harbor unstable peripheral thrombus than patients suffering minor embolism, but are in a worse position to sustain another onslaught until resolution of the first. Further embolism from legs or pelvis remains a risk for the first few days and weeks.

Prevention of PE

Diagnosis of venous thrombosis

A full history is important because a positive history indicates the need to perform a full coagulation screen and to institute prophylactic measures in anyone with a personal or family history of unexplained thrombosis. This must be done before anticoagulants are started. Physical methods of prophylaxis include posture (sleeping semi-prone rather than supine in later pregnancy) and compression stockings. LMWH should be given to high-risk patients.

Prevention of PE relies on the prevention, rapid diagnosis and effective treatment of venous thrombosis. Accurate objective diagnosis is important because of the mortal risk from PE if DVT is untreated and also because long-term anticoagulant treatment in pregnancy carries risk to both mother and fetus, and a positive diagnosis has implications for prophylaxis in future pregnancies. Accurate diagnosis is mandatory (Table 17.7).

Clinical probability is assessed on medical history and clinical examination. Thrombosis is most frequent in the left femoral vein and calf antenatally. Distinction has to be made from benign pregnancy associated swelling, which is usually slowly progressive, painless and bilateral although occasionally rapid and unilateral even in the absence of thrombosis.

Perspective

Although thromboembolism is frequently missed it is still rare compared with the frequency with which it is suspected and the prevalence of high probability ventilation–perfusion scans in pregnant women with suspected PE is very low.

Table 17.7 Possible deep vein thrombosis (DVT)

High index of suspicion needed:
- half of patients with a PE do not have any sign of a DVT
- half of patients with an acutely swollen calf do not have a DVT

Investigation:
D-dimer: promising, needs more pregnancy data
- real-time venous ultrasonography: available, easy, non-invasive
- compression Doppler ultrasonography: needs expertise, non-invasive
- phlebography: invasive, involves radiation, painful, may cause DVT

Withholding anticoagulation in pregnant women with a low clinical probability of PE, negative leg Doppler and normal or non-diagnostic ventilation–perfusion scans is probably safe but simpler means of ruling out thromboembolism are needed. The reliability of a negative pregnancy level D-dimer in ruling out thromboembolism without the need for further investigation is promising but more data are awaited.

References

1 Rutherford S, Montoro M, McGehee W, Strong T. Thromboembolic disease associated with pregnancy: an 11 year review. *Am J Obstet Gynecol* 1991;**164**(suppl): 286.
2 Andersen BS, Steffensen FH, Sorensen HT, Nielsen G, Olsen J. The cumulative incidence of venous thromboembolism during pregnancy and puerperium—an 11 year Danish population based study of 63,300 pregnancies. *Acta Obstet Gynaecol Scand* 1998;**77**:170–3.
3 *Report on Confidential Enquiries into Maternal Deaths in the United Kingdom 1994–96.* London: HMSO, 1998.
4 Danilenko-Dixon DR, Heit JA, Silverstein MD et al. Risk factors for deep vein thrombosis and pulmonary embolism during pregnancy or post partum: a population based, case–control study. *Am J Obstet Gynecol* 2001;**184**:104–10.
5 Toglia MR, Weg JG. Venous thromboembolism during pregnancy. *N Engl J Med* 1996;**335**:108–13.
6 Hirsch DR, Mikkola KM, Marks PW et al. Pulmonary embolism and deep vein thrombosis during pregnancy or oral contraceptive use: prevalence of factor V Leiden. *Am Heart J* 1996;**131**:1145–8.
7 Peek MJ, Nelson RA, de Swiet M, Letsky EA. Activated protein C resistance in normal pregnancy. *Br J Obstet Gynaecol* 1997;**104**:1084–6.
8 Bauer KA. Hypercoagulability—a new co-factor in the protein C anticoagulant pathway. *Lancet* 1994;**330**:566–7.
9 Preston FE, Rosendaal FR, Walker ID et al. Increased fetal loss in women with heritable thrombophilia. *Lancet* 1996;**348**:913–16.
10 Carr MH, Towers VC, Eastenson AR, Pircon RA, Iriye BK, Adashek JA. Prolonged bed rest during pregnancy: does the risk of deep vein thrombosis warrant the use of routine heparin prophylaxis? *J Matern Fetal Med* 1997;**6**:264–7.
11 Weiner CP, Kwaan AC, Xu C et al. Antithrombin III deficiency in women with hypertension during pregnancy. *Obstet Gynecol* 1985;**65**:301–6.
12 Lindqvist P, Dahlback B, Marsal K. Thrombotic risk during pregnancy: a population study. *Obstet Gynecol* 1999;**94**:595–9.
13 Kyrle PA, Eichinger S. Deep vein thrombosis. *Lancet* 2005;**365**:1111–202.
14 Khamashta MA, Mackworth-Young C. Antiphospholipid (Hughes') syndrome—a treatable cause of recurrent pregnancy loss. *BMJ* 1997;**314**:244.
15 Den Heyer M, Koster T, Blom HJ et al. Hyperhomocysteinaemias a risk factor for deep vein thrombosis. *N Engl J Med* 1996;**334**:759–62.
16 Rosendaal FR. Risk factors for venous thrombosis disease. *Thromb Haemost* 1999;**82**:610–19.
17 Prandoni P, Lensing AW, Coigo A et al. The long term clinical course of acute deep venous thrombosis. *Arch Intern Med* 1996;**125**:1–7.

18 Task Force on Pulmonary Embolism, European Society of Cardiology. Guidelines on diagnosis and management of acute pulmonary embolism. *Eur Heart J* 2000;**21**: 1301–36.

19 The PIOPED Investigators. Value of the ventilation–perfusion scan in acute pulmonary embolism. Results of the prospective investigation of pulmonary embolism diagnosis. *JAMA* 1990;**263**:2753–9.

20 Sergysels R. Pulmonary gas exchange abnormalities in pulmonary embolism. In Morpurgo M (ed.), *Pulmonary Embolism*. New York: Marcel Dekker, 1994: pp 89–96.

21 Colman NC. Pathophysiology of pulmonary embolism. In Leclerk JR (ed.), *Venous Thromboembolic Disorders*. Philadelphia: Lea Febiger, 1991: pp 65–73.

22 Coon WW, Coller FA. Clinicopathologic correlation in thromboembolism. *Surg Gynecol Obstet* 1959;**109**:259–69.

23 Chan WS, Ray JG, Murray S et al. Suspected pulmonary embolism in pregnancy. *Arch Intern Med* 2002;**162**:1170–5.

24 Stein PD, Terrin ML, Hales CA et al. Clinical, laboratory, roentgenographic and electrocardiographic findings in patients with acute pulmonary embolism and no pre-existing cardiac or pulmonary disease. *Chest* 1991;**100**:598–603.

25 Stein PD, Henry JW, Miller AC. Arterial blood gas analysis in the assessment of suspected acute pulmonary embolism. *Chest* 1996;**109**:78–81.

26 Amarenco P. Patent foramen ovale and the risk of stroke: smoking gun guilty by association? *Heart* 2005;**91**:441–7.

27 Konstantinides S, Geibel A, Kasper W, Olschewski M, Blumel L, Just H. Patent foramen ovale is an important predictor of adverse outcome in patients with major pulmonary embolism. *Circulation* 1998;**97**:1946–51.

28 Gei AF, Vadhera RB, Hankins GD. Embolism during pregnancy: thrombus, air and amniotic fluid. *Anesthesiol Clin North Am* 2003;**21**:16.

29 Berkowitz KD, Goldstein DP. Gestational trophoblastic disease. *Cancer* 1995;**76**: 2079–85.

30 Kearon C. Diagnosis of pulmonary embolism. *Can Med Assoc J* 2003;**168**:1–22.

31 Kucher N, Luder CM, Dornhofer T, Windecker S, Meier B, Hess OM. Novel management strategy for patients with suspected pulmonary embolism. *Eur Heart J* 2003;**24**: 366–76.

32 Nijkeuter M, Geleijns J, de Roos A, Meinders AE, Huisman MV. Diagnosing pulmonary embolism in pregnancy: rationalising fetal radiation exposure in radiological procedures. *J Thromb Haemost* 2004;**2**:1857–8.

33 Ang CK, Tan TH, Walters A, Wood C. Postural influence on maternal capillary oxygen and carbon dioxide tension. *BMJ* 1969;**4**:201–3.

34 Hernandez J, Hambleton G, Kline JA. D-dimer concentrations in normal pregnancy. *Acad Emerg Med* 2004;**11**:526–7.

35 Morse M. Establishing a normal range for D-dimer levels through pregnancy to aid in the diagnosis of pulmonary embolism and deep vein thrombosis. *J Thromb Haemost* 2004;**2**:1202.

36 Cheriex EC, Sreeram N, Eussen Y, Pieters FA, Wellens HJ. Cross sectional Doppler echocardiography as the initial technique for the diagnosis of acute pulmonary embolism. *Br Heart J* 1994;**72**:52–7.

37 Wolfe MW, Lee RT, Feldstein ML, Parker JA, Come PC, Goldhaber SZ. Prognostic significance of right ventricular hypokinesis and perfusion lung scan defects in pulmonary embolism. *Am Heart J* 1994;**127**:1371–5.

38 Mc Connell MV, Solomon SD, Rayan M, Come PC, Goldhaber RT. Regional right ventricular dysfunction detected by echocardiography in acute pulmonary embolism. *Am J Cardiol* 1996;**78**:469–73.

39 Kasper W, Geibel A, Tiede N et al. Distinguishing between acute and subacute massive pulmonary embolism by conventional and Doppler echocardiography. *Br Heart J* 1993;**70**:352–6.

40 Chapoutot L, Nazerollas P, Metz D et al. Floating right heart thrombi and pulmonary embolism: diagnosis, outcome and therapeutic management. *Cardiology* 1996;**87**: 169–74.

41 Pruszczyk P, Torbicki A, Pacho R et al. Non-invasive diagnosis of suspected severe pulmonary embolism: transoesophageal echocardiography vs spiral CT. *Chest* 1997; **112**:722–8.

42 Kearn C, Julian JA, Newman E, Ginsberg JS, for the McMaster Diagnostic Imaging Practice Guidelines Initiative. Non-invasive diagnosis of deep vein thrombosis. *Ann Intern Med* 1998;**128**:663–77.

43 Chan WS, Ray JG, Murray S, Coady GE, Coates G, Ginsberg JS. Suspected pulmonary embolism in pregnancy: clinical presentation, result of lung scanning and subsequent maternal and pediatric outcomes. *Arch Intern Med* 2002;**162**:1170–5.

44 Sostman HD, Colman RE, DeLong DM, Newman GE, Paine S. Evaluation of revised PIOPED criteria for ventricular perfusion scintigraphy in patients with suspected pulmonary embolism. *Radiology* 1994;**193**:103–7.

45 The PISA-PED Investigators. Value of perfusion lung scan in the diagnosis of pulmonary embolism: results of the prospective study of acute pulmonary embolism diagnosis (PISA-PED). *Am J Respir Crit Care Med* 1996;**154**:1387–93.

46 Doyle NM, Ramirez MM, Mastrobattista JM, Monga M, Wagner LK, Gardner MO. Diagnosis of pulmonary embolism: a cost-effectiveness analysis. *Am J Obstet Gynecol* 2004;**191**:1019–23.

47 Mayo JR, Remy-Jardin M, Muller NL et al. Pulmonary embolism: prospective comparison of spiral CT with ventilation/perfusion scintigraphy. *Radiology* 1997;**205**: 447–52.

48 Goodman LR, Lipchik RJ, Kuzo RS et al. Subsequent pulmonary embolism after a negative pulmonary angiogram—prospective comparison with scintigraphy. *Radiology* 2000;**215**:535–42.

49 Johnson MS, Stine SB, Shah H, Harris VJ, Ambrosius WT, Trerotola SO. Possible pulmonary embolus: evaluation with digital subtraction versus cut-film angiography—prospective study in 80 patients. *Radiology* 1998;**207**:131–8.

50 Oudkerk M, van Beek EJ, Wielopolski P et al. Comparison of contrast enhanced magnetic resonance angiography and conventional pulmonary angiography for the diagnosis of pulmonary embolism: a prospective study. *Lancet* 2002;**359**:1643–7.

51 de Swiet M. Management of pulmonary embolus in pregnancy. *Eur Heart J* 1999;**20**:1378–85.

52 Brady AJB, Crake T, Oakley CM. Percutaneous catheter fragmentation and distal dispersion of proximal pulmonary embolus. *Lancet* 1991;**338**:1186–9.

53 Mazeika PK, Oakley CM. Massive pulmonary embolism in pregnancy treated with streptokinase and percutaneous catheter fragmentation. *Eur Heart J* 1994;**15**: 1281–3.

54 Sofocleous CT, Hinrichs C, Bahramipour P, Barone A, Abujudeh H, Contractor D. Percutaneous management of life-threatening pulmonary embolism complicating early pregnancy. *J Vasc Interv Radiol* 2001;**12**:1355–6.

CHAPTER 18

Hypertensive disorders of pregnancy

Alexander Heazell, Philip N Baker

Hypertensive disorders of pregnancy are the most common medical problem encountered in the second half of pregnancy, affecting about 6–10% of pregnancies.[1] Although there are many different causes of hypertension in pregnancy, the most clinically important condition is pre-eclampsia, affecting between 1 and 3% of pregnancies.[2] Pre-eclampsia is associated with increased maternal and fetal morbidity and mortality.[3] As there is no effective intervention for pre-eclampsia, except delivery, pre-eclampsia is responsible for about a half of induced pre-term deliveries, with the associated consequences of premature birth.

At present, the precise cause of pre-eclampsia is unknown, although it is understood to be a disorder of widespread endothelial dysfunction. It is hypothesized that decreased invasion and subsequent remodeling of maternal spiral arteries in the first trimester lead to reduced placental perfusion, and release of factors into the maternal circulation, resulting in endothelial cell damage (Figure 18.1).[4–6] As every organ has a blood supply, pre-eclampsia should be regarded as a multi-system disease, which may affect each patient differently (Tables 18.1 and 18.2). Therefore, the management of pre-eclampsia involves far more than the treatment of hypertension alone.

In normal pregnancy the maternal blood pressure decreases in the first half of pregnancy, rising to pre-pregnancy levels or higher from about 30 weeks' gestation. Hypertension in pregnancy is defined as a blood pressure >140/90 mmHg on two separate occasions, at least 4 hours apart, or a single diastolic reading >110 mmHg.[7] If this occurs before 20 weeks' gestation, it is presumed to be chronic hypertension. If new hypertension occurs after 20 weeks' gestation without proteinuria, it is termed 'pregnancy-induced hypertension'.[7] Pre-eclampsia is defined as new onset hypertension with proteinuria (>300 mg/24 h or ++ on urine dipstick) in the absence of a urinary tract infection after 20 weeks' gestation.[8] If a patient with pre-existing hypertension develops proteinuria (>300 mg/24 h or ++), this is termed superimposed pre-eclampsia (Table 18.3). Eclampsia is defined as a tonic–clonic seizure occurring in the presence of pre-eclampsia.

Much of the antenatal care in the UK is directed towards the identification of pre-eclampsia. As there is currently no reliable screening test to identify women

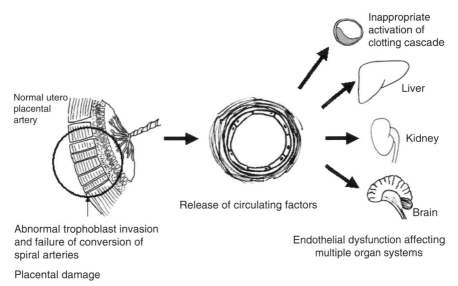

Figure 18.1 Proposed pathophysiology of pre-eclampsia.

who will go on to develop pre-eclampsia, regular screening of blood pressure and urine is carried out throughout pregnancy, because this has been shown to reduce perinatal mortality sevenfold. In addition, women at risk of developing hypertension in pregnancy should be identified. The incidence of pre-eclampsia is increased in primigravidae (or first pregnancy with that partner), multiple pregnancies, women with a first-degree relative with hypertension in pregnancy, and at extremes of reproductive age.[2,6,9,10] Important risk factors in a patient's past medical history include: chronic renal disease, chronic hypertension (especially if poorly controlled), diabetes mellitus and thrombophilia.[11–14] Patients with a positive past medical history should be classified as a high-risk pregnancy, and managed in a specialist high-risk obstetric clinic, being seen more frequently than 'low-risk' patients. Patients who have had previous pre-eclampsia should also be managed as a high-risk pregnancy because the risk of recurrence of some form of pre-eclampsia is between 20 and 40% depending on the population studied.[15]

It is important to note that pre-eclampsia is a heterogeneous condition, and the diagnosis may be made from the presence of clinical features, such as those above, in combination with the presence of hypertension and proteinuria (see Table 18.1). Patients may also have biochemical and/or hematological abnormalities that may be found on further investigation (see Table 18.2).

Despite widespread abnormalities in the cardiovascular system, cardiologists are rarely involved in the management of hypertensive disorders of pregnancy, except in severe or resistant hypertension or in other unusual circumstances, e.g. secondary hypertension resulting from coarctation of the aorta. Most cardiologists therefore have little experience in the routine management of

Table 18.1 Clinical features of pre-eclampsia

Central nervous system
Eclamptic convulsions
Cerebral hemorrhage, intraventricular or subarachnoid
Cerebral infarction: microinfarction or macroinfarction (e.g. cortical blindness caused by
    infarction of occipital cortex)

Coagulation system
Thrombocytopenia
Microhemangiopathic hemolysis
HELLP syndrome (hemolysis, elevated liver enzymes, low platelets)
Disseminated intravascular coagulation

Eyes
Retinal detachment
Retinal edema

Kidney
Acute tubular necrosis
Acute cortical necrosis
Unspecified renal failure

Liver
Rupture of hepatic capsule
Infarction
Jaundice
Decreased synthesis of soluble clotting substances
HELLP syndrome

Respiratory system
Pulmonary edema
Laryngeal edema
Adult respiratory distress syndrome

hypertension in pregnancy. This may be a particular problem in pre-pregnancy counseling for women with hypertension, prophylaxis for pre-eclampsia, and the use of pharmacological agents in pregnancy, or in the follow-up of patients who have had pre-eclampsia. Therefore, this chapter addresses hypertension in pregnancy with particular respect to these areas.

Blood pressure measurement in pregnancy

The measurement of blood pressure in pregnancy is subject to the same problems as in normal patients, such as: selection of appropriate cuff size, observer error and bias, and blood pressure variability, all of which may affect the final documented reading. However, in pregnancy there are specific concerns relating to the position of the patient. The blood pressure is lower in the second half of pregnancy in patients lying supine. This is because the gravid uterus obstructs

Table 18.2 Abnormalities that may be found on investigation indicating pre-eclampsia

Maternal
Elevated urea and creatinine[a, b]
Elevated liver function tests[a] (aspartate transaminase, alanine transaminase)
Hemolysis[a]
Hyperuricemia[a]
Hypocalcemia
Increased packed cell volume[a]
Proteinuria[a]
Raised antithrombin III in plasma
Raised fibronectin in plasma
Raised von Willebrand's factor in plasma
Thrombocytopenia[a]

Fetal
Intrauterine growth restriction
Abnormal umbilical artery Doppler flow
Abnormal fetal cardiac trace (as measured by cardiotocography)

[a]Tests commonly used in the UK.

[b]Urea and creatinine both fall during pregnancy as a result of hemodilution; values should be compared with 'normal' ranges for pregnancy.

Table 18.3 Classification of hypertensive disorders in pregnancy

Chronic hypertension
Pregnancy-induced hypertension (gestational hypertension)
Pre-eclampsia
Pre-eclampsia superimposed on chronic hypertension

the venous return from the lower limbs and reduces cardiac pre-load. Therefore blood pressure should be measured in the left lateral or sitting position. As a result of difficulties in maintaining the sphygmomanometer cuff at the level of the heart in the left lateral position, sitting is the preferred position.

In the UK (although not in the USA) the fourth Korotkoff sound (K4), rather than the fifth (K5), was previously recommended for the measurement of diastolic blood pressure. This was because of concern that K5 may be audible at zero cuff pressure. However, a study of 250 patients found the diastolic blood pressure was always >50 mmHg.[16] K5 is nearer to intra-arterial diastolic blood pressure than K4, and can be recognized more consistently than K4.[17] K5 is now recommended for the measurement of diastolic blood pressure in pregnancy in the UK.

'White coat hypertension', in which the blood pressure is excessively high because of the clinical environment, is as much of a problem in pregnancy as in non-pregnant women, if not more. Its impact is minimized by devices that allow blood pressure to be measured frequently and outside the hospital, such as 24-hour ambulatory monitoring.[8]

Automatic blood pressure devices, either ambulatory or static, are widely used in antenatal clinics, delivery units and high-dependency areas, and need to be calibrated specifically for pregnancy and specifically for pre-eclampsia. Many of the machines in current use have not been validated. In pre-eclampsia, in particular, the physical characteristics of blood vessels are altered. The pattern of pressure changes between systole and diastole analyzed by oscillometric machines is altered and the algorithm used to calculate diastolic pressure is no longer accurate. In severe pre-eclampsia, machines that rely on oscillometric measurement may underestimate diastolic blood pressure by 15 mmHg compared with conventional sphygmomanometry; this may lead to inadequate treatment of hypertension. Even machines using a microphone to detect Korotkoff's sounds are not immune to this problem. We recommend the SpaceLabs 90207 and SpaceLabs Scout as the only automatic blood pressure machines that have been shown to be accurate in severe pre-eclampsia to date.[18]

Prevention of pre-eclampsia

The possibility of prevention of pre-eclampsia is particularly important, because delivery of the infant remains the only effective treatment for the condition. There are two main groups of women at risk of pre-eclampsia: those who have had hypertension in a previous pregnancy and those who have a medical condition such as hypertension or renal disease that predisposes patients to pre-eclampsia.

Early trials with antiplatelet agents, in particular low-dose aspirin 60–150 mg/day, were encouraging, suggesting a 70% reduction in risk.[19,20] In contrast, larger trials such as CLASP (Collaborative Low-dose Aspirin Study in Pregnancy) showed no overall reduction in risk; however, further analysis of the CLASP data did suggest that early onset pre-eclampsia might be reduced by as much as 50%, which is significant because it is early onset pre-eclampsia (before 34 weeks) that is associated with the highest perinatal morbidity.[21] Subsequent meta-analysis of 32 trials of anti-platelet therapy found a 15% reduction in risk of developing pre-eclampsia; this benefit was independent of gestation on entry to the trial or dose of aspirin administered.[22] The most common dose of aspirin used in the UK is 75 mg/day, which should ideally be taken during the first trimester, because this is when underlying pathological changes of pre-eclampsia commence.

Several dietary measures have been used in an attempt to reduce the risk of pre-eclampsia. There is no beneficial effect of a reduction in salt intake or magnesium supplementation.[23,24] However, calcium supplementation of at least 1 g/day appears to result in a reduction of the risk of hypertension and pre-eclampsia of 19% and 30%, respectively.[25] These effects seem to be most marked in women with a high risk of pre-eclampsia. Supplementation of antioxidants, such as vitamins C and E, has been shown in a study of 283 high-risk women to reduce incidence of pre-eclampsia from 26% to 8%.[26] A large multicenter, placebo-controlled, randomized trial is being undertaken in the UK and is expected to report results in 2006.

A Cochrane meta-analysis of antihypertensive treatment before conception or during pregnancy concluded that there was a reduction in the number of patients presenting with severe hypertension, but there was no reduction in the risk of developing pre-eclampsia, or in the fetal or neonatal outcomes.[27] Therefore, patients who are known to be hypertensive before pregnancy should be investigated in the usual way, and treatment should be commenced to achieve optimal blood pressure before pregnancy. No antihypertensive drugs have been shown conclusively to be teratogenic, although angiotensin-converting enzyme (ACE) inhibitors may be related to skull defects and renal dysfunction.[28] Therefore, the choice of drugs to be used before pregnancy may be made irrespective of any consideration of a future pregnancy. However, if the patient wishes to conceive, it is better to control blood pressure with agents that are suitable for use throughout pregnancy, rather than have to change drugs in the first trimester, which may lead to suboptimal control of hypertension during placental development. There are no levels of blood pressure above which pregnancy cannot be countenanced. Patients should be counseled about the risks of pre-eclampsia and the possible prophylactic therapy.

Management of hypertension in pregnancy

There are two important differences between the management of hypertension in pregnancy and the management of hypertension outside pregnancy. Most cases of hypertension outside pregnancy are idiopathic or 'essential', i.e. follow a chronic course, with the major purpose of treatment being to prevent long-term complications such as stroke and myocardial infarction. A few patients present outside pregnancy with acute severe hypertension, which must be treated immediately because of the risk of hypertensive encephalopathy or cerebral hemorrhage, but this is now uncommon. It is realized that acute lowering of blood pressure in the non-pregnant state has major risks to the individual. However, hypertension in pregnancy normally resolves post partum, so there is no justification for treatment of hypertension to prevent long-term complications. Importantly, pre-eclampsia carries acute risks of eclampsia and cerebral hemorrhage; the latter complication is the cause of most of the maternal mortality in the disease.[3] In contrast to the non-pregnant state, acute lowering of blood pressure is often necessary in severe pre-eclampsia.

The most important difference between the management of hypertension outside pregnancy and that in pregnancy is the multisystem nature of pre-eclampsia, and the cardiovascular consequences of endothelial dysfunction, including prothrombotic tendency, reduced intravascular volume and increased endothelial permeability. Pre-eclampsia is extremely varied in its presentation, and hypertension may even be mild or absent in patients who otherwise have severe manifestations of the condition. It is essential that other features of the syndrome must be looked for and managed appropriately (see Tables 18.1 and 18.2). The presence of these features is variable and different aspects of the pre-eclamptic process may progress at different speeds. Progression is, however, relentless and no intervention has been shown to halt the condition except delivery.

As a result of this varied presentation, division of hypertensive disorders of pregnancy and pre-eclampsia into mild, moderate and severe disease is complicated and may not reflect clinical presentation. Therefore, the whole clinical picture, including maternal symptoms, signs, investigations and fetal well-being, must be assessed, before determining whether the patient has mild, moderate or severe disease. As a result of the focus of this chapter, assessment of fetal well-being and the timing of delivery are not discussed in depth.

Patients who have asymptomatic hypertension with no proteinuria, or no abnormalities of renal, liver or clotting function, and whose blood pressure remains <150 mmHg systolic and <95 mmHg diastolic, can be successfully managed as outpatients, preferably when day-unit facilities are available, where a clinician can commence and monitor response to antihypertensive medication. Over 40% of patients who initially develop hypertension alone, will go on to develop pre-eclampsia.[29] Therefore, these patients should be kept under regular surveillance with regular blood pressure measurement, assessment of proteinuria, full blood count, and renal, liver and clotting function.

Patients with blood pressure >160/100 mmHg without proteinuria should immediately be assessed by an obstetrician or day-care unit. If proteinuria is present admission will be required.[30] Patients should be managed in hospital, not because hospital admission or bedrest affects the progression of pre-eclampsia, but because admission allows intensive monitoring of mother and fetus, namely 4-hourly blood pressure measurement, 24-hour urine collection, full blood count, renal, liver and clotting function, and fluid balance monitoring. As the only present 'treatment' to halt the development of pre-eclampsia is delivery, the purpose of this intensive monitoring is twofold: first, to assess the need for, institute and monitor the response to antihypertensive medication for maternal safety, and so that the pregnancy may be continued to maximal fetal maturity, and second, because close observation of blood pressure, organ function and fetal well-being enables early recognition of the need for delivery.

The specific aims of antihypertensive therapy are to prevent maternal cerebrovascular accident or eclampsia, and to prolong pregnancy to enable corticosteroids to be administered to aid fetal lung maturity if the fetus is <34 weeks. Maternal blood pressure does not require to be lowered to 'normal' levels, because this may further compromise placental function. A target blood pressure should be approximately 140/90 mmHg.

Management of mild-to-moderate hypertension

The Cochrane database meta-analysis of all trials of antihypertensive drugs for mild-to-moderate hypertension suggested that treatment of lower degrees of blood pressure (where there is no acute maternal risk) does not improve the fetal outcome, but reduces the incidence of severe hypertension.[27] However, patients with chronic hypertension, who are at high risk of developing pre-eclampsia, are likely to be receiving antihypertensives at the beginning of pregnancy and have been excluded from most of the trials in the Cochrane database. There is equivocal evidence to suggest that pregnancy can be prolonged by expectant management of pre-eclampsia, with careful blood pressure control and appropriate biochemical and hematological investigations, because the control of blood pressure does not prevent deterioration of pre-eclampsia or the perinatal morbidity.[31,32] Therefore, an important factor about expectant management is the gestation of the infant. Expectant management may be appropriate for a woman presenting at 26 weeks, whereas at 38 weeks there is little to be gained by continuation of the pregnancy.

Methyldopa

Despite limited efficacy as a hypotensive agent, methyldopa is still the most commonly used drug for long-term control of blood pressure in pregnancy. It has been shown to improve fetal outcome when compared with placebo and there are long-term follow-up data at 7 years that show no detriment to the offspring in the methyldopa-treated group.[33,34] Recently, methyldopa has been reported to be the only antihypertensive *not* to have effects on the fetoplacental circulation,[35] although this may reflect its limited antihypertensive effect. The usual dose range is 250 mg to 1 g three times a day. At high doses the sedative and depressant effects of methyldopa are marked. Methyldopa should not be used if there is a substantial risk of maternal depression when a beta-blocking agent or calcium antagonist may be more suitable.

Beta-blocking drugs

Beta blockers such as labetalol (an alpha and beta blocker) are well established in clinical practice in the UK. Administration of beta blockers has been associated with a reduction in the incidence of severe hypertension, probably via the reduction in maternal cardiac output and decreased peripheral resistance. Other beta blockers have been tested, such as oxprenolol, which has been compared with methyldopa, and atenolol compared with placebo. These have had varied success in the reduction of the risk of the development of pre-eclampsia.[36,37] However, there are concerns that beta blockers, particularly atenolol, may lead to the development of intrauterine growth restriction as a result of decreased uteroplacental perfusion, because there is a reduction in fetal weight and placental weight after atenolol therapy.[38] It is not clear whether the risk of growth retardation is specific to atenolol. As atenolol does not have intrinsic sympathomimetic activity (unlike oxprenolol) or mixed alpha and beta-antagonist activity (labetalol), the pharmacological profile of each individual beta blocker may be important. Despite the relatively mild beta-antagonist effects of labetalol, this drug should not be used in patients who are asthmatic.

Nifedipine

Nifedipine is the only calcium antagonist for which there is any extensive experience in pregnancy, and this is anecdotal rather than in the context of a robust clinical trial. A retrospective study has shown that it is a useful antihypertensive agent,[39] either alone or together with methyldopa or labetalol. Nifedipine has been shown to be effective in lowering maternal blood pressure and reducing cerebral artery vasospasm.[40] The use of long-acting nifedipine preparations is particularly useful in enhancing compliance, and in women with labile blood pressure.

Diuretics

Diuretics were formally used extensively for the 'treatment' or prevention of pre-eclampsia. Meta-analysis has shown that they reduce edema but have no impact on perinatal survival.[41] Diuretics are theoretically contraindicated because the circulating blood volume is already contracted in severe pre-eclampsia and any further reduction might impair placental perfusion. Diuretics also raise the concentration of serum urate that is used to monitor the progress of pre-eclampsia (see Table 18.2). For these reasons, and because they are ineffective hypotensive agents, diuretics are not used to control blood pressure in pregnancy.

ACE inhibitors

These drugs should not be used after the first trimester. They cause renal failure in the fetus, which is shown before delivery as oligohydramnios and after delivery as oliguria and anuria.[42] The condition can be fatal for the fetus; both captopril and enalapril have been implicated.

Management of severe hypertension

A blood pressure >170/110 mmHg results in direct endothelial damage, and is just below the level of blood pressure (180–190/120–130 mmHg) at which cerebral autoregulation fails, leading to increased risk of cerebral hemorrhage.[43] There is also increased risk of placental abruption or asphyxia.[43] Therefore, blood pressure of 170/110 mmHg requires urgent management. At present intravenous hydralazine or labetalol is the most common antihypertensive used in this setting, although there is insufficient evidence at present to suggest which is the more effective.[44] However, clinicians should use a drug with which they are familiar, because the side-effect profiles of these agents may mimic symptoms of pre-eclampsia (e.g. headache).[45] It is essential that the maternal blood pressure be reduced to a safe level, without causing a precipitate decrease in blood pressure, which may reduce uteroplacental perfusion, and in turn lead to fetal hypoxia. Therefore, the fetal heart rate should be continuously monitored during intravenous antihypertensive therapy. The management of severe acute hypertension should be undertaken where one-to-one care can be provided, and there are facilities for regular blood pressure monitoring at least every 15 minutes.

Hydralazine

Hydralazine is the drug that has previously been used most commonly for blood pressure control in acute severe hypertension. Intravenous boluses (10–20 mg over 10–20 minutes) will lower the blood pressure to a safe level.[46] While the intravenous bolus dose is being given blood pressure should be checked every 5 minutes. The drug may then be given by intravenous infusion between 1 and 5 mg/h. Side effects of hydralazine include headache, flushing, dizziness and palpitations.

Labetalol

Labetalol is a combined alpha- and beta-adrenergic antagonist, and has become the most frequently used antihypertensive for acute severe hypertension. Initially, 200 mg can be given orally. If there is no response to oral therapy, a bolus dose of 50 mg can be given intravenously over 1 minute. This is followed by an infusion of 20 mg/h, which may be increased in increments of 20 mg/h, up to a maximum of 160 mg/h. Patients with a history of asthma or cardiac disease should not be given labetalol because of its beta-blocking component.

Nifedipine

The calcium antagonist nifedipine is effective for oral control of acute severe hypertension. The sublingual form of nifedipine should not be used in pregnancy, because there may be a precipitate fall in blood pressure leading to fetal hypoxia.[47] In severe acute hypertension 10 mg of the standard preparation (not long acting) may be given. Side effects include headache, dizziness and palpitations. Recent studies have shown that co-administration of nifedipine and magnesium sulfate does not potentiate either agent, calming initial concerns that co-administration may lead to profound hypotension.[48,49]

Anticonvulsant drugs

Patients who have severe pre-eclampsia are at increased risk of eclamptic seizures, which are detrimental to both mother and fetus. In the USA parenteral magnesium sulfate has long been used to control seizures. Lucas et al. showed that magnesium sulfate was considerably better than phenytoin for seizure prophylaxis.[50] A randomized placebo-controlled trial of 10 110 women with hypertension and proteinuria found a 58% lower risk of eclamptic seizures in women given magnesium sulfate compared with placebo.[51] There was no effect on fetal mortality, although there was a reduction in the incidence of placental abruption. In a subsequent meta-analysis of this and other randomized studies of magnesium sulfate in seizure prophylaxis, the relative risk of having an eclamptic seizure was 0.33 for patients receiving magnesium sulfate compared with placebo.[52] In addition magnesium sulfate was found to be more effective than phenytoin in the prevention of eclampsia.[53]

Magnesium sulfate (10%) is given as a 4 g loading dose intravenously over 10 minutes, followed by intravenous infusion of 1 g/h for 24 h; this should be continued until after delivery of the baby. Provided that the respiratory rate is

>16/minute, the urine output is >25 ml/h and deep tendon reflexes (knee/elbow) are present, there is no need for estimation of magnesium concentrations in the blood. If tendon reflexes become absent (magnesium about 5 mmol/l), the magnesium sulfate should be discontinued. If there is cardiorespiratory arrest (magnesium > 10 mmol/l), the patient's airway and breathing should be managed, cardiopulmonary resuscitation (CPR) should be commenced, the infusion stopped and 10 ml 10% calcium gluconate given intravenously.

Fluid balance

Women with severe pre-eclampsia require strict control of their fluid balance. They may have increased extracellular tissue fluid, evident as edema and depleted intravascular volume resulting from increased endothelial permeability. If women become fluid overloaded, this will be lost into the tissue space, and can result in pulmonary edema. Therefore, patients should be catheterized, with hourly urine output recorded as well as fluid intake, which should not exceed 80 ml/h or 1 mg/kg. If the patient has a low urine output, a careful assessment of fluid status is required, with consideration of invasive central venous pressure/pulmonary capillary pressure monitoring. If there are no signs of pulmonary edema, a fluid challenge of 250 ml colloid should be given. If signs of pulmonary edema are present 20 mg furosemide should be given intravenously. In patients with severe disease, invasive arterial or central venous pressure, monitoring should be considered. Rarely, pulmonary capillary wedge pressure is required to direct either volume infusion or reduction of cardiac preload or afterload.[54]

Other essential features of the management of severe pre-eclampsia such as the correction of coagulopathy, and the timing and route of delivery are beyond the scope of this chapter.

Eclampsia

Although eclampsia may develop from severe pre-eclampsia, 11% of patients who had an eclamptic seizure had neither proteinuria nor significant hypertension at the time of the first fit and 43% did not have the combination of these abnormalities. Eclampsia can occur in the antenatal (38%), intrapartum (18%) or postpartum (44%) periods.[55] In the UK, the incidence of eclampsia is 1 in 2000 deliveries. The mortality rate of eclampsia is approximately 2%.[55] The priorities of management are the maintenance of airway, breathing and circulation, and the termination of the convulsion.

Magnesium sulfate is clearly superior to either phenytoin or diazepam in preventing further seizures, with relative risks of 67% and 52% respectively.[56] There were also trends towards better maternal and fetal outcomes. Therefore all those concerned with the management of eclampsia must become familiar with the use of magnesium sulfate. A loading dose of 4 g 10% magnesium sulfate is given either intravenously or intramuscularly and, if no intravenous access is available, an infusion of 1 g/h to prevent further seizures. Observation of respiratory rate and deep tendon reflexes is required as described above.

Secondary hypertension in pregnancy

The earlier in pregnancy that hypertension presents, especially if before 20 weeks of gestation, the more likely it is to be unrelated to the pregnancy. As in the non-pregnant state, most cases of hypertension in early pregnancy have no obvious cause (essential hypertension) and a cause can be found in less than 5%. However, some forms of secondary hypertension have specific problems that must be considered and excluded from the differential diagnosis.

Pheochromocytoma

Almost every maternal mortality report has a death from pheochromocytoma. The condition can mimic all the features of pre-eclampsia and undiagnosed it has a mortality rate of 50%.[57] As in the non-pregnant state most cases lack the typical features, all patients with severe hypertension in pregnancy should be screened for pheochromocytoma by whatever method is used locally—direct measurement of catecholamines or their metabolite, vanillylmandelic acid. As methyldopa interferes with many biochemical screens for pheochromocytoma, the need to screen for this must be considered before starting treatment. If the tests suggest pheochromocytoma, treatment should be started immediately with alpha- and beta-adrenergic blockade. Phenoxybenzamine and propranolol can be used notwithstanding any concern about the use of beta-blocking agents in pregnancy. Once effective alpha- and beta-blockade have been established the maternal risk should be eliminated.[58] The tumor may be localized antenatally by ultrasonography or magnetic resonance imaging (MRI) which is considered safe in pregnancy. If the tumor has been localized with confidence, it may be removed by a combined approach at the time of delivery or subsequently.[58] If it has not been localized before delivery (more likely with lesions outside the adrenal glands) delivery is safe under combined alpha- and beta-adrenergic blockade. The tumor can then be localized and removed after delivery.

Coarctation of the aorta

Most patients with substantial coarctation have the lesion repaired before pregnancy. If this has not been done, there is an increased risk of dissection of the aorta as a result of the increased cardiac output of pregnancy.[59] Patients with coarctation should have their blood pressure scrupulously controlled by beta-adrenergic blockade notwithstanding any possible risks to the fetus. Beta blockade is preferred because it reduces cardiac contractility and therefore the shear stress on the aorta (see Chapter 4).

Renal disease

Renovascular hypertension has no specific problems in pregnancy but this is not true of renal parenchymal disease. Hypertension and renal impairment interact in a way that is not well understood to increase the risks of superimposed pre-eclampsia and acute and chronic fetal distress, e.g. in renal disease the presence of hypertension increases the incidence of intrauterine growth restriction from 2% to 16% and of pre-term delivery from 11% to 20%.[60] Fetal loss is increased tenfold in women with chronic renal dysfunction.[61] Additional investigation of renal function is required, because of the increased demands placed on the maternal kidneys, which is normally compensated in pregnancy by an increased glomerular filtration rate. A proportion of women will have an irreversible decline in renal function during pregnancy.[62]

Essential hypertension

This is the diagnosis in most women presenting before 20 weeks. It is now realized that essential hypertension itself does not put the fetus at risk, although antihypertensive treatment can result in fetal compromise. The only risk is of developing superimposed pre-eclampsia; in women with essential hypertension requiring treatment before pregnancy, the risk of developing pre-eclampsia is about 20%, compared with 4% in those without hypertension. The purpose of management of patients with essential hypertension early in pregnancy is to prevent the development of life-threatening hypertension.

Very rarely, severe hypertension early in pregnancy may persuade doctors that the pregnancy should be terminated because continuing the pregnancy will put the mother's life at significant risk.

Postnatal care of the hypertensive patient

Hypertensive disorders of pregnancy usually improve after delivery of the infant. However, treatment should not be discontinued abruptly because this carries a risk of rebound hypertension. There are no antihypertensive drugs that are unsuitable for breastfeeding women. Women who had hypertension in pregnancy, especially if there was severe hypertension, should be reviewed 6 weeks after delivery for assessment of blood pressure and urine. By this time, about 90% of women will be normotensive. The remaining 10% will require routine investigation of hypertension to ensure that there is no underlying cause, such as pheochromocytoma, or underlying cardiovascular disease, such as left ventricular hypertrophy.

Women who have had pre-eclampsia are twice as likely as those who have had normal pregnancies to develop ischaemic heart disease in the 20 years after the pregnancy.[63] In addition, women with any hypertensive disorder of pregnancy are at increased risk of the metabolic syndrome and hypertension as short a time as 7 years after the development of pre-eclampsia.[64] This may be the result of common features of both pre-eclampsia and metabolic syndrome, such as hyperinsulinemia, hyperlipidemia and altered vascular function.[65] Further prospective research is required to determine the link between pre-eclampsia and the metabolic syndrome. Nevertheless, women who develop hypertensive disorders in pregnancy require education about their lifetime risks of cardiovascular disease, and this opportunity should be taken to reduce cardiovascular risk factors, such as diet and body mass index. Women who have had a hypertensive disorder of pregnancy require long-term follow-up of their cardiovascular risk factors, to reduce their risk of future cardiovascular disease.

References

1 Brown MA, Buddle ML. What's in a name? Problems with the classification of hypertension in pregnancy. *J Hypertens* 1997;**15**:1049–54.
2 Myers JE, Brockelsby J. The epidemiology of pre-eclampsia. In: Baker PN, Kingdom JCP (eds), *Pre-eclampsia: Current perspectives on management.* Parthenon: London, 2004.
3 CEMACH. *Why Mothers Die 2000–2002.* London: RCOG Press, 2004.
4 Pijnenborg R, Anthony J, Davey DA et al. Placental bed spiral arteries in the hypertensive disorders of pregnancy. *Br J Obstet Gynaecol* 1991;**98**:648–55.
5 Meekins JW, Pijnenborg R, Hanssens M et al. A study of placental bed spiral arteries and trophoblast invasion in normal and severe pre-eclamptic pregnancies. *Br J Obstet Gynaecol* 1994;**101**:669–74.
6 Walker JJ. Pre-eclampsia. *Lancet* 2000;**356**:1260–5.
7 National High Blood Pressure Education Program Working Group. Report on high blood pressure in pregnancy. *Am J Obstet Gynecol* 2000;**183**:S1–S22.
8 Higgins JR, de Swiet M. Blood-pressure measurement and classification in pregnancy. *Lancet* 2001;**357**:131–5.
9 Trupin LS, Simon LP, Eskenazi B. Change in paternity: a risk factor for preeclampsia in multiparas. *Epidemiology* 1996;**7**:240–4.
10 Saftlas AF, Olson DR, Franks AL et al. Epidemiology of preeclampsia and eclampsia in the United States, 1979–1986. *Am J Obstet Gynecol* 1990;**163**:460–5.
11 Murakami S, Saitoh M, Kubo T et al. Renal disease in women with severe preeclampsia or gestational proteinuria. *Obstet Gynecol* 2000;**96**:945–9.
12 Siddiqi T, Rosenn B, Mimouni F et al. Hypertension during pregnancy in insulin-dependent diabetic women. *Obstet Gynecol* 1991;**77**:514–19.
13 Kupferminc MJ, Eldor A, Steinman N et al. Increased frequency of genetic thrombophilia in women with complications of pregnancy. *N Engl J Med* 1999;**340**:9–13.
14 Samadi AR, Mayberry RM, Reed JW. Preeclampsia associated with chronic hypertension among African–American and White women. *Ethn Dis* 2001;**11**:192–200.
15 Sibai BM, Mercer B, Sarinoglu C. Severe preeclampsia in the second trimester: recurrence risk and long-term prognosis. *Am J Obstet Gynecol* 1991;**165**(5 Pt 1):1408–12.
16 Shennan A, Gupta M, Halligan A et al. Lack of reproducibility in pregnancy of Korotkoff phase IV as measured by mercury sphygmomanometry. *Lancet* 1996;**347**:139–42.
17 Brown MA, Buddle ML, Farrell T et al. Randomised trial of management of hypertensive pregnancies by Korotkoff phase IV or phase V. *Lancet* 1998;**352**:777–81.
18 Shennan A, Halligan A, Gupta M et al. Oscillometric blood pressure measurements in severe pre-eclampsia: validation of the SpaceLabs 90207. *Br J Obstet Gynaecol* 1996;**103**:171–3.
19 Beaufils M, Uzan S, Donsimoni R et al. Prevention of pre-eclampsia by early antiplatelet therapy. *Lancet* 1985;**1**:840–2.

20 Wallenburg HC, Dekker GA, Makovitz JW et al. Low-dose aspirin prevents pregnancy-induced hypertension and pre-eclampsia in angiotensin-sensitive primigravidae. *Lancet* 1986;**1**:1–3.
21 CLASP: a randomised trial of low-dose aspirin for the prevention and treatment of pre-eclampsia among 9364 pregnant women. CLASP (Collaborative Low-dose Aspirin Study in Pregnancy) Collaborative Group. *Lancet* 1994;**343**:619–29.
22 Duley L, Henderson-Smart D, Knight M, King J. Antiplatelet drugs for prevention of pre-eclampsia and its consequences: systematic review. *BMJ* 2001;**322**:329–33.
23 Duley L, Henderson-Smart D, Meher S. Altered dietary salt for preventing pre-eclampsia, and its complications. *The Cochrane Database of Systematic Reviews* 2005(4):CD005548.
24 Makrides M, Crowther CA. Magnesium supplementation in pregnancy. *The Cochrane Database of Systematic Reviews* 2001(4):CD000937.
25 Atallah AN, Hofmeyr GJ, Duley L. Calcium supplementation during pregnancy for preventing hypertensive disorders and related problems. *The Cochrane Database of Systematic Reviews* 2002(1):CD001059.
26 Chappell LC, Seed PT, Briley AL et al. Effect of antioxidants on the occurrence of pre-eclampsia in women at increased risk: a randomised trial. *Lancet* 1999;**354**:810–16.
27 Abalos E, Duley L, Steyn DW et al. Antihypertensive drug therapy for mild to moderate hypertension during pregnancy. *The Cochrane Database of Systematic Reviews* 2001(2):CD002252.
28 Burrows RF, Burrows EA. Assessing the teratogenic potential of angiotensin-converting enzyme inhibitors in pregnancy. *Aust N Z J Obstet Gynaecol* 1998;**38**:306–11.
29 Barton JR, O'Brien JM, Bergauer NK et al. Mild gestational hypertension remote from term: progression and outcome. *Am J Obstet Gynecol* 2001;**184**:979–83.
30 Milne F, Redman C, Walker J et al. The pre-eclampsia community guideline (PRECOG): how to screen for and detect onset of pre-eclampsia in the community. *BMJ* 2005;**330**:576–80.
31 Sibai BM, Gonzalez AR, Mabie WC et al. A comparison of labetalol plus hospitalization versus hospitalization alone in the management of preeclampsia remote from term. *Obstet Gynecol* 1987;**70**(3 Pt 1):323–7.
32 Hall DR, Odendaal HJ, Steyn DW. Expectant management of severe pre-eclampsia in the mid-trimester. *Eur J Obstet Gynecol Reprod Biol* 2001;**96**:168–72.
33 Redman CW. Fetal outcome in trial of antihypertensive treatment in pregnancy. *Lancet* 1976;**2**:753–6.
34 Cockburn J, Moar VA, Ounsted M et al. Final report of study on hypertension during pregnancy: the effects of specific treatment on the growth and development of the children. *Lancet* 1982;**1**:647–9.
35 Houlihan DD, Dennedy MC, Ravikumar N et al. Anti-hypertensive therapy and the feto-placental circulation: effects on umbilical artery resistance. *J Perinat Med* 2004;**32**:315–19.
36 Gallery ED, Saunders DM, Hunyor SN et al. Randomised comparison of methyldopa and oxprenolol for treatment of hypertension in pregnancy. *BMJ* 1979;**1**:1591–4.
37 Rubin PC, Butters L, Clark DM et al. Placebo-controlled trial of atenolol in treatment of pregnancy-associated hypertension. *Lancet* 1983;**1**:431–4.
38 Butters L, Kennedy S, Rubin PC. Atenolol in essential hypertension during pregnancy. *BMJ* 1990;**301**:587–9.
39 Constantine G, Beevers DG, Reynolds AL et al. Nifedipine as a second line antihypertensive drug in pregnancy. *Br J Obstet Gynaecol* 1987;**94**:1136–42.

40 Serra-Serra V, Kyle PM, Chandran R et al. The effect of nifedipine and methyldopa on maternal cerebral circulation. *Br J Obstet Gynaecol* 1997;**104**:532–7.

41 Collins R, Yusuf S, Peto R. Overview of randomised trials of diuretics in pregnancy. *BMJ (Clin Res Ed)* 1985;**290**:17–23.

42 Barr M Jr. Teratogen update: angiotensin-converting enzyme inhibitors. *Teratology* 1994;**50**:399–409.

43 Redman CW, Roberts JM. Management of pre-eclampsia. *Lancet* 1993;**341**:1451–4.

44 Duley L, Henderson-Smart DJ, Meher S. Drugs for treatment of very high blood pressure during pregnancy. *The Cochrane Database of Systematic Reviews* 2006(1): CD001449.

45 Heazell AEP, Mahomoud S, Pirie AM. The treatment of severe hypertension in pregnancy: a review of current practice and knowledge in West Midlands maternity units. *J Obstet Gynaecol* 2004;**24**:897–8.

46 Paterson-Brown S, Robson SC, Redfern N et al. Hydralazine boluses for the treatment of severe hypertension in pre-eclampsia. *Br J Obstet Gynaecol* 1994;**101**:409–13.

47 Impey L. Severe hypotension and fetal distress following sublingual administration of nifedipine to a patient with severe pregnancy induced hypertension at 33 weeks. *Br J Obstet Gynaecol* 1993;**100**:959–61.

48 Scardo JA, Vermillion ST, Hogg BB et al. Hemodynamic effects of oral nifedipine in preeclamptic hypertensive emergencies. *Am J Obstet Gynecol* 1996;**175**: 336–8; discussion 338–40.

49 Magee LA, Miremadi S, Li J et al. Therapy with both magnesium sulfate and nifedipine does not increase the risk of serious magnesium-related maternal side effects in women with preeclampsia. *Am J Obstet Gynecol* 2005;**193**:153–63.

50 Lucas MJ, Leveno KJ, Cunningham FG. A comparison of magnesium sulfate with phenytoin for the prevention of eclampsia. *N Engl J Med* 1995;**333**:201–5.

51 Altman D, Carroli G, Dulay L et al. Do women with pre-eclampsia, and their babies, benefit from magnesium sulphate? The Magpie Trial: a randomised placebo-controlled trial. *Lancet* 2002;**359**:1877–90.

52 Duley L, Gulmezoglu AM, Henderson-Smart DJ. Magnesium sulphate and other anticonvulsants for women with pre-eclampsia. *The Cochrane Database of Systematic Reviews* 2006(3):CD000025.

53 Duley L, Henderson-Smart D. Magnesium sulphate versus phenytoin for eclampsia. *The Cochrane Database of Systematic Reviews* 2006(3):CD000128.

54 Clark SL, Greenspoon JS, Aldahl D et al. Severe preeclampsia with persistent oliguria: management of hemodynamic subsets. *Am J Obstet Gynecol* 1986;**154**:490–4.

55 Douglas KA, Redman CW. Eclampsia in the United Kingdom. *BMJ* 1994;**309**:1395–400.

56 The Eclampsia Trial Collaborative Group. Which anticonvulsant for women with eclampsia? Evidence from the Collaborative Eclampsia Trial. *Lancet* 1995;**345**: 1455–63.

57 Lamming GD, Symonds EM, Rubin PC. Phaechromocytoma in pregnancy: still a cause of maternal death. *Clin Exp Hypertens* 1990;**9**:57–68.

58 Harper MA, Murnaghan GA, Kennedy L et al. Phaeochromocytoma in pregnancy. Five cases and a review of the literature. *Br J Obstet Gynaecol* 1989;**96**:594–606.

59 Deal K, Wooley CF. Coarctation of the aorta and pregnancy. *Ann Intern Med* 1973;**78**:706–10.

60 Surian M, Imbasciati E, Cosci P et al. Glomerular disease and pregnancy. A study of 123 pregnancies in patients with primary and secondary glomerular diseases. *Nephron* 1984;**36**:101–5.

61 Jungers P, Chauveau D, Choukroun G et al. Pregnancy in women with impaired renal function. *Clin Nephrol* 1997;**47**:281–8.

62 Jones DC, Hayslett JP. Outcome of pregnancy in women with moderate or severe renal insufficiency. *N Engl J Med* 1996;**335**:226–32.

63 Smith GC, Pell JP, Walsh D. Pregnancy complications and maternal risk of ischaemic heart disease: a retrospective cohort study of 129,290 births. *Lancet* 2001;**357**: 2002–6.

64 Forest JC, Girouard J, Masse J et al. Early occurrence of metabolic syndrome after hypertension in pregnancy. *Obstet Gynecol* 2005;**105**:1373–80.

65 Pouta A, Hartikainen AL, Sovio U et al. Manifestations of metabolic syndrome after hypertensive pregnancy. *Hypertension* 2004;**43**:825–31.

CHAPTER 19

Management of labour and delivery in the high-risk patient

Kirk D Ramin

Labour and delivery are a unique time and bring with them a degree of anxiety, apprehension, and fear for the gravid woman with cardiovascular disease and her obstetrician. Roughly 0.2–3% of pregnant women suffer some degree of cardiac disease and account for more than 25% of all maternal deaths.[1–3] Marked changes in maternal hemodynamics occur during pregnancy: a 40% rise in blood volume, increases in uterine blood flow (low resistance shunt) to 500 ml/min at term, and marked falls in both pulmonary and systemic vascular resistance (Table 19.1).[4–7] In addition, the contracting uterus autotransfuses 300–500 ml/contraction in labour and 500–1000 ml of total blood in the immediate postpartum period.[5,8–10] Cardiac output rises 3–3.5 l/min during the second stage and the immediate postpartum period.[6,9,11] Average blood loss for a singleton vaginal delivery is 500 ml, and for cesarean delivery and vaginal twins it is >1000 ml.[5,12] Anemia, pre-eclampsia, chorioamnionitis, tocolytic therapy and hemorrhage can complicate labour and delivery by adding markedly to the increases in cardiac demand.

Taken together these factors necessitate the establishment of a management team consisting of an obstetrician, cardiologist, anesthesiologist and pediatrician to ensure a favorable outcome for the gravida with cardiac disease. The collaboration of this team is paramount, given that it is estimated that over a half of all maternal deaths could be eliminated by changes in patient, provider and system factors.[13–16] It must be kept in mind that as most of the hemodynamic changes occur before the end of the first trimester, lack of cardiovascular reserve may show itself even at this stage.

In addition to establishing a management team, several general measures should be instituted when managing all gravid women with heart disease (Table 19.2), including pain control, strict input and output, continuous ECG monitoring, oxygen supplementation and intravenous filters if a shunt is present. In addition, attention to patient positioning in the semi-recumbent/left lateral tilt, fetal monitoring, thrombosis and (in high-risk patients) infective endocarditis prophylaxis (Table 19.3) are recommended. Confusion often surrounds the use of prophylactic antibiotics and leads to their excessive and unnecessary use. The American College of Cardiology and the American Heart Association have

Table 19.1 Maternal hemodynamic changes during labour and delivery

Maternal blood volume[5,6]	+40%
Uterine blood flow (term)[7]	500 ml/min
Autotransfusion (labour)[8,10]	300–500 ml
Autotransfusion (post partum)[5]	1000 ml
Cardiac output (change[a]) (l/min)[6,9,11]	
Latent phase	+1.10
Accelerating phase	+2.46
Decelerating phase	+2.17
Second stage	+3.50
Postpartum (immediate)	+3.10
Blood loss (ml)[5,12]	
Vaginal delivery	500 ml
Vaginal delivery (twins)	1000 ml
cesarean delivery	1000 ml

[a]Compared with late third trimester values.

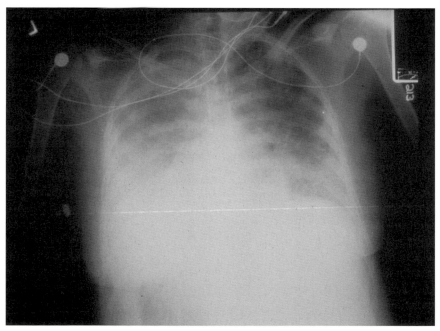

Figure 19.1 Chest X-ray showing pulmonary edema in a pregnant woman with cardiac disease.

Table 19.2 General management principles of cardiac lesions in labour and delivery

Management team
Cardiology
Obstetrics
Pediatrics
Anesthesia

Patient care
Strict input and output
Continuous ECG monitoring
Control hemorrhage
Oxygen supplementation
Fetal monitoring
Arterial line
Semi-recumbent positioning
Left lateral tilt
Adequate pain control
Intravenous line filters
Thrombosis prophylaxis
Infective endocarditis prophylaxis
Delivery by 39 completed weeks **if possible**
Earlier delivery indicated with pre-eclampsia or **halted fetal growth**
Postpartum surveillance

made it clear that prophylaxis is recommended in women with moderate and high-risk lesions in the setting of possible bacteremia (Table 19.3).[17] The challenge to the practicing obstetrician and cardiologist is predicting, from first principles, which individual delivery will involve 'complications'.

Potential adverse consequences of each of the individual cardiac lesions are outlined in detail in Table 19.4. Unfortunately, many patients present with composite lesions such as mitral valve prolapse with tricuspid valve regurgitation, or mitral valve stenosis (usually rheumatic) with *right* ventricular failure. In the latter case, the challenge is to maintain cardiac output given the limited ability to fill the *left* ventricle, while balancing the need to avoid volume in an overloaded left atrium. These situations require an experienced team, thorough echocardiographic evaluation and sometimes the use of inotropic cardiac agents. Although tachyarrhythmias may complicate any of the given cardiac lesions, they are especially prominent in the setting of atrial enlargement. These conditions commonly include atrial septal defect (ASD), mitral insufficiency and myocardial infarction. Atrial arrhythmias should be treated with digoxin, which is also a positive inotrope (see Chapter 16). However, class III amiodarone should be avoided if possible because of its risk of fetal hypothyroidism.[18] For ventricular tachyarrhythmias, beta blockers remain the mainstay of therapy. These medications, when used during gestation, can and should be continued throughout labour and the postpartum period.

Table 19.3 Antibiotic prophylaxis for the prevention of infective endocarditis[17]

Cardiac lesion	Prophylaxis – uncomplicated delivery	Prophylaxis – infective endocarditis	Regimen
Negligible risk			
Mitral valve prolapse without regurgitation	None	None	None
Prior rheumatic fever – no valve dysfunction	None	None	None
Kawasaki's disease – no valve dysfunction	None	None	None
Pacemaker	None	None	None
Prior coronary bypass surgery	None	None	None
Moderate risk			
Mitral valve prolapse with regurgitation	None	Recommended	Ampicillin 2 g i.v./i.m. or Amoxicillin 2 g p.o. 1 h before or vancomycin 1 g i.v. over 1–2 h
Acquired valve dysfunction	None	Recommended	
Unrepaired ASD, VSD, PDA	None	Recommended	
Hypertrophic cardiomyopathy	None	Recommended	
High risk			
Prosthetic valves	Discretionary	Recommended	Ampicillin 2 g i.v./i.m. plus gentamicin 1.5 mg/kg i.v. (max. 120 mg) load
Prior infective endocarditis	Discretionary	Recommended	
Cyanotic malformation	Discretionary	Recommended	Followed 6 h later by ampicillin 1 g i.v. or amoxicillin 1 g p.o.
Surgically corrected systemic pulmonary shunts	Discretionary	Recommended	Penicillin allergies: vancomycin 1 g i.v. over 1–2 h; gentamicin 1.5 mg/kg i.v. (max. 120 mg)

Table 19.4 Adverse consequences of cardiac lesions in labour

ASD	Atrial fibrillation
	Supraventricular tachycardia
	Atrial flutter
	Right ventricular failure
Non-restrictive VSD	Pulmonary hypertension
	Arrhythmias
	Congestive heart failure
	Thrombosis
Large PDA	Pulmonary hypertension
	Thrombosis
Eisenmenger syndrome	**Increased** cyanosis
	Thrombosis
Coarctation of aorta	Dissection
	Congestive heart failure
	Cerebral vascular accident
Tetralogy of Fallot (uncorrected)	Cyanosis
	Erythrocytosis
	Right ventricular hypertension
	Thrombosis
Pulmonic stenosis	Right ventricular failure
Ebstein's anomaly	Right-sided enlargement
Mitral stenosis	Right ventricular failure
	Pulmonary edema
Mitral insufficiency	Atrial fibrillation
Aortic stenosis	Fixed cardiac output
	Pulmonary edema
	Angina
Hypertrophic cardiomyopathy	**Pulmonary edema**
Marfan or Ehlers–Danlos syndrome or Takayasu's aortitis	Aortic dissection
Myocardial infarction	Arrhythmias
	Congestive heart failure

ASD, atrial septal defect; PDA, patent ductus arteriosus; VSD, ventricular septal defect.

The hypercoagulable state of pregnancy, lower extremity venous stasis and bedrest during the second and third trimesters combine to increase the risk of thrombosis, which should be countered by prophylactic pneumatic compression stockings or low-molecular-weight heparin (LMWH). Cyanotic heart lesions are the most susceptible to thrombosis (see Table 19.2). Controversy

Table 19.5 Special management considerations in the critically ill gravidas

Aortic dissection/rupture risk	
Marfan syndrome	Epidural
Ehlers–Danlos syndrome	Beta-adrenergic blockade-pressure
Coarctation	Elective cesarean delivery (preferred)
Takayasu's aortitis	Assisted vaginal delivery
Fixed cardiac output	
Avoid hypovolemia	Central hemodynamic monitoring
Aortic stenosis	Epidural—maintain filling pressures
Hypertrophic cardiomyopathy	Assisted vaginal delivery
Pulmonary hypertension	Cesarean delivery — epidural or general analgesia
	Aggressive use of pulmonary vasodilators in pulmonary hypertension
Avoid pulmonary edema	Beta-adrenergic blockade—tachycardia
Mitral stenosis	Epidural
	Central hemodynamic monitoring
	Maintain wedge pressure 14–20 mmHg
	Assisted vaginal delivery
	Elevate head of bed immediately after delivery
Shunt lesions	'F' series prostaglandin contraindicated
Eisenmenger syndrome	Sympathetic agent contraindicated
Tetralogy of Fallot (unrepaired)	Intravenous line filters
	Monitor systemic saturation
	Vaginal delivery preferred
	Aggressive use of pulmonary vasodilators[a]
	Aggressive blood loss management
	Labour—opioid epidural
	Cesarean indicated—monitored recovery for 10 days has been recommended

[a]A note on pulmonary vasodilators: employ inhaled nitric oxide (iNO) alongside prostacyclin analogues—iNO via facemask or nasal cannula to final alveolar concentrations of 5–40 p.p.m. and iloprost diluted in 0.9% NaCl at 20 μg/2 ml up to six times daily, *or* prostacyclin infusion of 1–10 ng/kg per min up to 60 μg/h.[29–32]

surrounds the appropriate management of patients with mechanical valve replacement. The benefits of warfarin with its superior efficacy over heparin have to be weighed against the risk of warfarin embryopathy[19–22] (see Chapters 7 and 9). Lastly, patients with Marfan syndrome, Ehlers–Danlos syndrome, coarctation of the aorta (even after repair) or Takaysau's aortitis are at the greatest risk for aortic dissection or rupture (Table 19.4).

Management of gravid women at risk of aortic rupture or dissection is outlined in Table 19.5. The use of sympathetic blockade with epidural analgesia can reduce systemic vascular resistance and increase venous pooling, and beta-adrenergic blocking agents reduce blood pressure and heart rate. These actions combine to reduce stress on the aortic wall during labour and delivery. Propranolol has been used extensively and does not inhibit the progress of labour.[23] Elective cesarean delivery is preferred but, if vaginal delivery is elected, vacuum or forceps assistance is recommended.

With respect to the fixed cardiac output lesions, two primary categories of adverse outcomes exist: those in which hypovolemia should be avoided (pulmonary hypertension, aortic stenosis and hypertrophic cardiomyopathy) and those in which pulmonary edema is a primary risk (mitral stenosis, aortic stenosis, hypertrophic cardiomyopathy).

Among these fixed cardiac output lesions, the tenets of managing those in which hypovolemia is of highest risk may involve central hemodynamic monitoring with judicious use of epidural, being careful to maintain filling pressure. cesarean delivery should be limited to obstetric indications with epidural or general anesthesia and avoidance of spinal analgesia. Finally, efforts to minimize vasovagal autonomic responses with assisted vaginal delivery should be considered, with caution taken to minimize blood loss (e.g. vacuum).

The second category of limited output cardiac lesions requires focus on reduction of risk of pulmonary edema balanced against adequate cardiac output. These are the women in whom beta-adrenergic blockade is critical and central hemodynamic monitoring useful in accurately maintaining pulmonary wedge pressures at 14–20 mmHg. Experienced clinicians generally employ the use of epidural analgesia, assisted vaginal delivery and elevation of the head of the bed immediately after delivery.

We should now address those women with Eisenmenger syndrome. During the antepartum period, the decreased systemic vascular resistance increases both the likelihood and the degree of right-to-left shunting. Pulmonary perfusion decreases, resulting in hypoxemia with maternal and then fetal deterioration. Every effort should be made to maintain a stable maternal cardiovascular state with maximum oxygenation, and to avoid hypotension. Central monitoring adds risk but not information in patients whose pulmonary and systemic pressures are linked through a non-restrictive ventricular septal defect (Eisenmenger complex). Full information is obtained from systemic blood pressure and oxygen saturation. A central venous line adds approximate cardiac output. Experience has been that abdominal delivery under general anesthesia may secure a lesser degree of cardiovascular stress and metabolic demand, minimize right-to-left shunting by removing physical effort and maintain best fetal condition.[24,25] However, given that our understanding of the pathophysiology surrounding those instances of acute decompensation among Eisenmenger syndrome patients is incompletely understood, the issues surrounding preference for vaginal versus cesarean delivery remain unsettled.

In a recent report of 13 pregnancies in 12 women with Eisenmenger syndrome, there were three maternal deaths (23%)—two during gestation and one post partum.[25] In this series, a relatively good outcome was attributed to bedrest after the second trimester, oxygen therapy, heparin prophylaxis and planned cesarean section under general anesthesia. Seven pregnancies were successful. One of the babies had a VSD.

Composite maternal mortality in Eisenmenger syndrome ranges from 30% to 60%.[25–27] In the classic literature review of Eisenmenger syndrome and pregnancy, Gleicher and colleagues reported a 39% mortality rate associated with vaginal delivery and a 75% mortality rate with cesarean delivery.[26] Eisenmenger syndrome, associated with VSD, appears to carry a higher mortality risk than that associated with patent ductus arteriosus or ASD. In addition to hypovolemia and hemorrhage, thromboembolic disease has been associated with up to 43% of all maternal deaths.[26] Prophylactic peripartum heparin therapy was associated with increased maternal mortality in an early paper,[28] but it is believed that heparin therapy, oxygen therapy and bedrest improve maternal and fetal outcomes. No large and well-orchestrated trials have been done to support or refute this claim because, fortunately, the numbers are too small.[25] Sudden death in the postpartum period has been reported to occur up to 6 weeks after delivery. Observation of these deaths suggests a 'vasovagal' attack associated with systemic vasodepression, and maintenance or elevation of pulmonary vascular resistance to pre-pregnant values (see Chapter 5). Delivery in these women signals the paramount potential for preferential ejection from the right ventricle directly into the aorta, bypassing the lungs. The management team's task begins with the end of the pregnancy.

References

1 Kuczkowski KM. Labour analgesia for the parturient with cardiac disease: what does an obstetrician need to know? *Acta Obstet Gynecol Scand* 2004;**83**:223–33.
2 De Swiet M. Cardiac disease. In: *Why Mothers Die 1997–1999. The Confidential Enquiries into Maternal Deaths in the United Kingdom.* London: Royal College of Obstetricians and Gynecologists, 2001: p. 153.
3 Chang J, Elam-Evans LD, Berg CJ et al. Pregnancy related mortality surveillance—United States, 1991–1999. *MMWR* 2003;**52**:1.
4 Clark SL, Cotton DB, Lee W et al. Central hemodynamic assessment of normal term pregnancy. *Am J Obstet Gynecol* 1989;**161**:1439.
5 Pritchard JA. Changes in blood volume during pregnancy and delivery. *Anesthesiology* 1965;**26**:393.
6 Peck TM, Arias F. Hematologic changes associated with pregnancy. *Clin Obstet Gynecol* 1979;**22**:785.
7 Metcalfe J, Romney SL, Ramsey LJ et al. Estimation of uterine blood flow in normal human pregnancy at term. *J Clin Invest* 1955;**34**:1632.
8 Adams, JQ, Alexander AM. Alterations in cardiovascular physiology during labour. *Obstet Gynecol* 1958;**12**:542.
9 Kjeldsen J. Hemodynamic investigations during labour and delivery. *Acta Obstet Gynecol Scand Suppl* 1979;**89**:1.
10 Hendricks ECM, Quilligan EJ. Cardiac output during labour. *Am J Obstet Gynecol* 1958;**76**:969.
11 Ueland K, Metcalfe J. Circulating changes in pregnancy. *Clin Obstet Gynecol* 1975;**18**:41.

12 Ueland K. Maternal cardiovascular dynamics. VII. Intrapartum blood volume changes. *Am J Obstet Gynecol* 1976;**126**:671.

13 Berg CJ, Atrash HK, Koonon LM, Tucker M. Pregnancy-related mortality in the United States, 1987–1990. *Obstet Gynecol* 1996;**88**:161–7.

14 Hoyert DL, Danel I, Jully P. Maternal mortality, United States and Canada, 1982–1997. *Birth* 2000;**27**:4–11.

15 Nannini A, Weiss J, Goldstein R, Fogerty S. Pregnancy-associated mortality at the end of the twentieth century: Massachusetts, 1990–1999. *J Am Med Women's Assoc* 2002;**57**:140–3.

16 Geller SE, Rosenberg D, Cox SM, Brown M, Simonson L, Driscoll CA, Kilpatrick SJ. The continuum of maternal morbidity and mortality: factors associated with severity. *Am J Obstet Gynecol* 2004;**191**:939–44.

17 ACC/AHA guidelines for the management of patients with valvular heart disease: A report of the ACC/AHA Task Force on Practice Guidelines. *J Am Coll Cardiol* 1998;**32**:1486–588.

18 Page RL. Treatment of arrhythmias in pregnancy. *Am Heart J* 1995;**130**:871–6.

19 APPCR Panel and Scientific Roundtable. Anticoagulation and enoxaparin use in patients with prosthetic heart valves and/or pregnancy. *Clinical Cardiology Consensus Reports* 2002;**3**(9).

20 Golby AJ, Bush EC, DeRook FA, Albers GW. Failure of high dose heparin to prevent recurrent cardioembolic strokes in a pregnant patient with mechanical cardiac valve prosthesis. *Cardiology* 1992;**42**:2204.

21 Salazar E, Izaguirre R, Verdejo J et al. Failure of subcutaneous heparin to prevent thromboembolic events in pregnant patients with mechanical cardiac valve prosthesis. *Cardiology* 1996;**27**:1698.

22 Vitale N, DeFeo M, De Santo LS et al. Dose dependent fetal complication of warfarin in pregnant women with mechanical heart valves. *J Am Coll Cardiol* 1995;**33**:1637.

23 Mitani A, Oettinger M, Abinader EG. Use of propranolol in dysfunctional labour. *Br J Obstet Gynaecol* 1975;**82**:651–5.

24 Lumley J, Whitwam JG, Morgan M. General anaesthesia in the presence of Eisenmenger's syndrome. *J Anaesth Analg Curr Res* 1977;**56**: 543–7.

25 Avila WS, Grinberg M, Snitcowsky R et al. Maternal and fetal outcomes in pregnant women with Eisenmenger's syndrome. *Eur Heart J* 1995;**16**:460.

26 Gleicher N, Midwall J, Hochberger D, Jaffin H. Eisenmenger syndrome in pregnancy. *Obstet Gynecol Surv* 1979;**34**:721–41.

27 Szekely P, Julian DG. Heart disease in pregnancy. *Curr Probl Cardiol* 1979;**4**:1.

28 Pitts JA, Crosby WM, Basta LL. Eisenmenger's syndrome in pregnancy. Does heparin prophylaxis improve the maternal mortality rate? *Am Heart J* 1977;**93**:321.

29 Lam GK, Stafford RE, Thorp J et al. Inhaled nitric oxide for primary pulmonary hypertension in pregnancy. *Obstet Gynecol* 2001;**98**:895–8.

30 Monnery L, Nanson J, Charlton G. Primary pulmonary hypertension in pregnancy: a role for the novel vasodilators. *Br Anaesth* 2001; **87**:295.

31 Stewart R, Tuazon D, Olson G, Duarte, AG. Pregnancy and primary pulmonary hypertension: successful outcome with epoprostenol therapy. *Chest* 2001;**119**:973.

32 Weiss BM, Maggiorini M, Jenni R et al. Pregnant patient with primary pulmonary hypertension: inhaled pulmonary vasodilators and epidural anesthesia for delivery. *Anesthesiology* 2000;**92**:1191.

CHAPTER 20

Anesthesia and the pregnant cardiac patient

Gurinder Vasdev

The latest edition of the Confidential Enquiry into Maternal and Child Health (CEMACH) report has shown the greatest rise in maternal mortality among pregnant women with cardiac disease.[1] These are some of the most challenging cases in obstetric practice. Anesthesia services are required for pregnant women who need non-obstetric surgery, obstetric surgery, *in utero* fetal surgery and vaginal delivery.[2,3] The physiological stress of pregnancy and parturition on the pregnant cardiac patient necessitates the early involvement of anesthesia services. A well-executed anesthetic should minimize the adverse physiological effects of parturition on maternal pathophysiology and respond rapidly to emergency situations. This requires additional trained personnel and judicious use of invasive cardiac monitors.

Timing of the delivery is critical and needs a multi-specialty approach to ensure that appropriate resources are available. In cases where pregnant women do not have sufficient cardiac reserve to compensate for the hemodynamic changes associated with a 'stat cesarean section', alternative delivery options need to be pre-empted.[4] Anesthesia care for the pregnant cardiac patient includes preoperative evaluation, conscious sedation, general anesthesia, central neuraxial conduction anesthesia and postoperative care, including intensive care.[5] The focus of this chapter is to review the effects of anesthesia on women with cardiac disease.

Risk to mother

The major risk to the pregnant woman is the additional cardiac reserve needed to meet the demands of pregnancy ($\uparrow$ intravascular volume, $\uparrow$ risk of thromboembolism, $\uparrow$ cardiac output or CO, $\uparrow$ heart rate or HR, $\uparrow$ O_2 consumption and $\downarrow$ pulmonary vascular resistance or PVR). Limitation of a viable pregnancy is related to the nature of the cardiac disease. The secondary concern arises from the patient's ability to cope with the stress of labour and the risk of acute decompensation. Risk is associated with severity of disease and obstetric complications.[6] In addition to the usual perioperative risk factors, cardiac pregnant patients have a significantly increased rate of critical events from dysrhythmia, hemorrhage and thromboembolism. Intervention with uterine artery balloon catheters is beneficial for those women who are likely to bleed, e.g. those with placenta accreta.[7]

For most patients, uterine contraction can be achieved with oxytocin ($\downarrow$ systemic vascular resistance or SVR, $\uparrow$ HR, $\uparrow$ PVR) and methylergonovine ($\uparrow$ SVR) but cardiovascular side effects may be deleterious in certain cardiac patients. For pregnant women who will not tolerate blood loss, the mode of delivery becomes even more important. One needs to compare the risks of postpartum hemorrhage with vaginal delivery against the expected additional blood loss (500–1000 mL) associated with an elective cesarean section. Preoperative testing for cardiac reserve is beneficial and helpful to determine the potential for success of pregnancy and guide the choice of which invasive hemodynamic monitor may be appropriate. Termination of pregnancy may be indicated in women with severe disease, e.g. Eisenmenger syndrome.

Anesthesia-related maternal mortality is primarily related to difficult airway management in emergency situations. However, in the operating room anesthesiologists must manage bleeding and embolic complications. Maternal deaths from hemorrhage, thromboembolism and cardiac disease now represent a significant number of all pregnancy-related deaths.[1] Providing anesthesia services for these patients is not restricted to tertiary care centers, as analysis of the CEMACH report revealed that many of the deaths associated with cardiac disease occurred when the presence of cardiac disease was unknown. Thus early screening may not pick up women who will decompensate later in pregnancy. Staff in obstetric units should monitor pregnant women for the development of cardiac disease throughout their pregnancies and have a lower threshold for initiating cardiac evaluation.[1]

Anesthetic management

General principles of anesthesia

Anesthesia requires the patient to be unaware of or insensitive to painful stimuli. This is primarily achieved using general anesthetic medications or local anesthetics.

General anesthesia

This results in decreased oxygen consumption. Cardiovascular effects are dependent on the drugs used, the dose and rate of administration (Table 20.1). The greatest cardiovascular stress occurs with endotracheal tube placement. Severe hypertension can arise at the time of intubation.[8] The options to blunt the hypertensive response to intubation without increasing the dose of induction agent include rapidly acting opiates (e.g. remifentanil, nitroglycerin), beta blockade and lidocaine.[9] General anesthesia blocks the protective laryngeal reflexes, so the airway needs to be secured with a cuffed endotracheal tube to prevent aspiration of gastric contents. A rapid sequence induction can lead to cardiovascular instability, especially in emergency situations. Awake fiberoptic

Table 20.1 The effect of common anesthetic agents on normal pregnant patients. Use of vasoactive medications will either decrease or enhance these effects

	Heart rate	Stroke volume	SVR
Induction agents			
Ketamine	↑	↑	•↑
Pentothal	→↑	→↓	↓
Propofol	↓	↓	↓↓
Midazolam	→	→	→
Fentanyl	↓	→	→↓
Etomidate	→	→	→
Volatile agents			
N_2O	↑	→	↑ (PVR)
Sevoflurane	→	↓	→
Isoflurane	↑	↓	↓
Desflurane	↑	↓	→
Muscle relaxants			
Atracurium	→		
Pancuronium	↑		
Vaccinium	↓		
Succinyl choline	→		
Obstetric drugs			
Oxytocin	↑↑	→	↓↓
Methylergonovine	→	↓	↑↑
Misoprostol	→↑		↓ (↑ PVR)
Carboprost	–	–	(↑ PVR)
Reversal agents			
Atropine	↑↑↑	↑	–
Glycopyrrolate	↑↑	→	–
Neostigmine	↓↓	→	–

intubation after topical oral application of 2% lidocaine solution is another option.[10] Patient positioning to avoid aortocaval compression can be achieved by using a 15°, left uterine displacement wedge.[11] The use of muscle relaxants necessitates the use of positive pressure ventilation, which in turn may have a deleterious effect on cardiac function (↓ venous return, ↑ PVR, ↑ HR). Intravenous access devices should have air filters to avoid paradoxical embolism, especially in patients with right-to-left shunts.

Sedation
This is beneficial for minor procedures, but the depth of sedation needs to be carefully monitored. The pregnant woman should not lose her protective airway reflexes or become under-ventilated. Diazepam has been associated historically with fetal cleft lip when administered in the first trimester; however, the

evidence for cause and effect is weak.[12] Propofol, midazolam and fentanyl have been used without any fetal problems. Sedation works best for first and second trimesters. In the third trimester, significant reduction in the functional residual capacity of the lungs and risk of aspiration complicate the ease of administration of sedative agents.[13]

Central neuraxial anesthesia

This is suitable for lower body surgery, cesarean section and vaginal delivery. These blocks are achieved using a spinal, epidural or combined spinal–epidural anesthetic technique. All these techniques have been successfully used in women with cardiac disease. By using low concentrations of bupivacaine and lipophilic opiates, the patient's hemodynamics can be well controlled.[9] Sympathectomy and bradycardia are the major hemodynamic sequelae of central neuraxial blocks. Preloading the patient with a balanced salt solution is only moderately helpful and has the potential to overload the patient.[14] Local anesthetics administered through an epidural catheter have the slowest onset of action, and this technique may be beneficial to limit the degree of sympathectomy and allow time for the judicious use of pressors. All direct and indirect acting pressors will affect uterine perfusion, which can result in fetal acidosis, but, by limiting the dose of pressor to maintain maternal cardiac output, fetal acidosis will be limited because the uterine vessels are maximally dilated. Uterine vessels do not autoregulate and depend on maternal cardiac output. Direct acting alpha agonists (e.g. phenylephrine) are preferred because they have minimal effect on maternal tachycardia.[15] The risk of spinal hematoma is increased with a central neuraxial block technique if the woman is anticoagulated.[16]

Miscellaneous blocks

These blocks (e.g. pudendal paracervical wound infiltration) and wound irrigation with local anesthetics decrease the demand for parenteral opiates.

Non-obstetric surgery

Two percent of all pregnant women will have some form of non-obstetric surgery (e.g. cholecystectomy, appendectomy, trauma) during their pregnancy.[17] Elective surgery can often be postponed until after delivery, and essential surgery is best reserved for the second trimester when the risk of teratogenesis and preterm labour is minimized.[18] Anesthesia for these patients is conducted with respect to the underlying cardiac disease. Aortocaval compression becomes significant after 20 weeks' gestation. The risk of aspiration after 18 weeks' gestation requires a secured airway with a cuffed endotracheal tube. The routine use of non-particulate antacids, metoclopramide and H_2-receptor blockers is controversial.[19,20] Laparoscopic surgery on pregnant women (usually in the first and second trimester) is possible. However, the underlying cardiac disease can decompensate with the hemodynamic effects of a pneumoperitoneum

($\downarrow$ venous return, $\uparrow$ SVR, $\uparrow$ HR, $\uparrow$ Pao_2), and there is a high risk of paradoxical air embolism. Surgeons need to minimize inflation pressures.[21]

In addition to the routine American Society of Anesthesiology monitors (ECG, Fio_2, temperature, end-tidal CO_2 partial pressure [$PE\text{Tco}_2$], non-invasive blood pressure [NIBP], ECG, O_2 alarm), invasive monitors (arterial line, central venous pressure [CVP], pulmonary artery [PA] catheter, transesophageal echocardiography [TEE]) are indicated by the nature and severity of the underlying cardiac disease. For those patients with multiple cardiac anomalies, anesthesia should be tailored for the most critical. Postoperative care may involve admission to the intensive care unit (ICU) for monitoring and ensuring that facilities for delivery are available should preterm labour occur.

Cardiac pregnant patients may need cardiac surgery during pregnancy. Anesthesia technique is determined by the nature of the cardiac disease. The risks of cardiopulmonary bypass (CPB) on the fetus can be limited by using surgical techniques that minimize operation time and by use of near normothermia. CPB flow rates need to be maintained at a higher level to take into account the increased oxygen consumption of the fetus.[22] Anesthesia for maternal cardioversion after 18 weeks' gestation needs airway protection to prevent aspiration.

Fetal monitoring is generally recommended when there is a viable fetus (>28 weeks), but it has not changed fetal outcome.[23] All drugs that cross the blood–brain barrier will affect the fetus. Fetal myocardium has a stiff ventricular mass and relies on increased heart rate to maintain cardiac output. Any vagotonic medications can decrease fetal cardiac output and oxygenation. Preterm labour is associated with non-obstetric surgery; suitable monitoring needs to be implemented because many women may not feel contractions secondary to postoperative analgesics. The use of local anesthetic blocks for postoperative analgesia decreases opiate requirements and may be beneficial in limiting respiratory depression. Early ambulation and deep vein thrombosis prophylaxis are recommended.

Management of pregnancy

Patients with congenital heart disease should be advised of the risks associated with pregnancy and delivery. Occasionally, these patients present to obstetric practice despite repeated warnings of danger. These are some of the more challenging situations to manage. With the advent and widespread use of echocardiography, the assessment of the pregnant cardiovascular system has become much easier. Depending on the type of lesion, the effects of labour and delivery need to be considered. Patients with more advanced cardiac disease require more frequent multidisciplinary follow-up. The delivery plan needs to account for the anesthetic and obstetric risk associated with elective versus emergency surgical delivery. In the cases where the obstetric risks associated with an emergency delivery are high (e.g. induction, maternal age, abnormal lie and diabetes), an elective cesarean section should be considered.

Anticoagulation in pregnancy

Most women with valvular disease, chronic atrial fibrillation or a history of thromboembolism will be on anticoagulant therapy. The longer duration of action of low-molecular-weight heparin and difficulty in assessing anticoagulation effect become a challenge when managing labour and delivery, especially when regional anesthesia is indicated.[24] Whenever possible, the woman should be switched to unfractionated heparin. Before placing a central neuraxial conduction block (especially epidural catheter placement), coagulation assessment will help decrease the small but dangerous risk of spinal hematoma.[16]

Antibiotic prophylaxis

It is recommended that pregnant women with structural heart disease have prophylaxis for infective endocarditis. The timing of administered antibiotic should be such that peak tissue levels are achieved at the time of incision or delivery. Airway instrumentation is associated with transient bacteremia.[25] Regional blocks have a low risk of bacteremia if strict aseptic techniques are used.

Specific anesthetic management options (Table 20.2)

Anesthetic management of acyanotic congenital heart disease

Atrial septal defects (ASDs) are one of the most common congenital lesions and, unless there is severe pulmonary hypertension, patients usually tolerate pregnancy well (see Chapter 4). For the management of labour, vaginal delivery is preferred and an epidural is placed early in the course of labour; it can decrease the degree of shunt by decreasing left-sided pressure.[26] Using a low concentration and volume of local anesthetic, combined with preservative-free opiates, the height of the block can be carefully titrated. Radial arterial line placement is beneficial. Pushing in the second stage (Valsalva) may result in an elevation of left- and right-sided pressures. The epidural can be loaded in the sitting position with a higher concentration of local anesthetic to increase the chances of caudal spread (for a saddle block). The sympathectomy from the epidural decreases the risk of congestive heart failure and can minimize the effects of Valsalva. Open glottic pushing has some merit but most often obstetric assistance is needed to deliver the head.[27] Ergometrine maleate should be used cautiously to avoid elevations in left ventricular pressure. Carboprost tromethamine (Hebamate) or 15-methyl-prostaglandin $F_{2\alpha}$ can be used as an adjunct to oxytocin to enhance myometrial contraction.

Management of cyanotic heart disease

Central cyanosis is clinically apparent once 5 g/dL of unsaturated arterial hemoglobin is present; in pregnancy dilutional anemia may mask these signs. In pregnant women with central generalized cyanosis, fetal demise occurs in about 50% of pregnancies (see Chapter 5). Evidence for progression of disease

Table 20.2 Classification of congenital heart disease

Congenital heart disease without shunt
Left-sided lesions: aortic stenosis, coarctation of the aorta, mitral stenosis
Right-sided lesions: pulmonary stenosis, Ebstein's anomaly, idiopathic pulmonary artery
dilation.
Congenital heart disease with shunt
Acyanotic left-to-right shunt
Persistent ductus arteriosus
Atrial septal defect (ASD)
Anomalous pulmonary venous drainage with or without ASDs
Ventricular septal defect (VSD)
Cyanotic disease with right-to-left shunt
Decreased pulmonary blood flow (PA pressures normal or decreased)
VSD and pulmonary stenosis
Tetralogy of Fallot
ASD and pulmonary stenosis
Elevated PA pressure
Large patent ductus arteriosus
Large VSD (non-restrictive)
Large ASD
Cyanotic with increased pulmonary blood flow
Truncus arteriosus
Transposition of the great vessels

and/or decompensation by the physiological demands of pregnancy are manifested as congestive heart failure, preterm labour, poor neonatal growth and occasionally an abrupt precipitation of cardiac dysrhythmia.[28] Aggravation of pre-existing cyanosis is caused by decreased pulmonary artery blood flow secondary to a fall in systemic vascular resistance, decreased right ventricular function (e.g. tetralogy of Fallot, tricuspid stenosis), increasing oxygen demand and increase in right-to-left shunt. Limited options are available to the anesthesiologist to optimize right ventricular function. Intervention, such as balloon valvuloplasty, can be useful in certain conditions (see Chapter 21). To achieve the goals of anesthesia there is significant risk of maternal death. For labour and delivery the risks of a sympathectomy versus positive pressure ventilation on maternal hemodynamics need to be addressed. Both general anesthesia and regional anesthesia have been used successfully. There is no evidence to support one being better than the other, but the current trend is to use regional anesthesia whenever possible. Systemic vasodilation should be avoided because it increases right-to-left shunting, reducing Sao_2, and may cause a fall in blood pressure.[9]

Pulmonary hypertension and Eisenmenger syndrome

Eisenmenger syndrome occurs when pulmonary hypertension results from a large left-to-right shunt (e.g. ventricular septal defect or VSD) and the high PVR reverses the shunt, causing cyanosis (see Chapter 5). The primary anesthetic principles involve trying to lower the PVR, preserving cardiac output and maintaining SVR. General anesthesia with surgical delivery has historically been recommended because of the relative prevention of hemodynamic instability and ability to ventilate the lungs optimally. However, regional techniques have been described and successful outcomes reported for both spinal and epidural anesthesia with judicious use of ephedrine to obviate the effects of sympathectomy.[29] In patients with pulmonary hypertension, pulmonary vasodilators (nitric oxide and prostacyclin) have been used successfully without fetal compromise. Pulmonary artery catheters are not necessary if there is free communication between systemic and pulmonary circuits, which links the pressures. Sao_2 is inversely related to PVR. The risk of pulmonary artery rupture and the risk of precipitating arrhythmias need to be weighed against the need for monitoring PVR. Maternal mortality is primarily related to hemodynamic instability and not anesthesia and tends to occur some days after delivery[30] (see Chapter 5).

Valvular lesions

Aortic and mitral regurgitation

These lesions are usually well tolerated in pregnancy. As CVP and pulmonary capillary wedge pressure (PCWP) increase in pregnancy and SVR decreases, the degree of regurgitation diminishes. This vasodilatory effect is secondary to the dilatation of the placental circulation, which increases as pregnancy progresses. Patients are usually delivered vaginally with an epidural or combined spinal–epidural block. Women are encouraged **not** to push because transient increases in SVR are best avoided. Epidural anesthesia must be reliable; any patchy blocks need to be addressed before the second stage of labour. Arterial and CVP monitoring may be useful only in symptomatic women. Optimal preload and afterload reduction with normal or slightly elevated heart rate should be maintained.[31]

Mitral stenosis

The incidence is decreasing in developed countries. Management of symptomatic women includes aggressive treatment of atrial fibrillation and antithrombotic therapy where heparin is indicated. Intractable heart failure or hemoptysis may be an indication for urgent intervention.

Balloon valvuloplasty is well tolerated and is indicated if the PCWP rises suddenly during the pregnancy and the anatomy is favorable. Anesthetic management aims to maintain PCWP at or below 20 mmHg by optimizing preload and keeping the slow heart rate. Most of these patients are in sinus rhythm and benefit markedly from beta-blocking drugs (see Chapter 7). With a monitored arterial line, regional anesthesia has been shown to be safe.[6] Increases in heart rate, rapid changes in SVR and increases in CVP preclude pushing during vaginal delivery, so carefully titrated lumbar epidural or combined spinal–epidural block is indicated with the usual precaution of anticoagulation therapy and changes in SVR. If the women are in New York Heart Association (NYHA) functional class III or IV, they do not tolerate blood loss well. In these patients an elective cesarean section under general anesthesia may be a reasonable option.

For surgical delivery, careful attention to patient position is key. A steep Trendelenberg position increases left atrial pressure and the head-up position decreases venous return.[11] Balloon-tipped pulmonary artery catheters are seldom used. The use of methergine needs careful consideration because it elevates SVR and oxytocin should be used cautiously as a result of its effects on SVR and PCWP, and its predisposition to cause reflex tachycardia. Patients with mitral stenosis may be beta blocked, so epidurals should be very carefully loaded because precipitous hypotension may occur. The maintenance of sinus rhythm is very important. Digoxin and diltiazem are well tolerated in pregnancy.[28] Calcium channel blockers are associated with uterine atony. This can easily be reversed with intravenous calcium chloride. The rate of injection needs to be carefully titrated to avoid any hypertensive response.

Aortic stenosis

This is a rare condition in pregnancy because most of these patients have had either an aortic valve replacement or balloon valvuloplasty. However, for those who present with severe stenosis, pregnancy may not be tolerated (see Chapter 4). Ventricular hypertrophy can result in subendocardial ischemia and arrhythmia if there is a fall in the SVR. Signs of fluid depletion and hypotension should be carefully monitored using CVP and arterial cannulation. Rapid infusion of intravenous oxytocin can result in significant hypotension.[32] Anesthetic management using regional or general anesthesia has been used with good outcome.[33] A combined spinal–epidural technique allows for a more controlled spinal injection with lower volumes. Intrathecal narcotics are helpful in providing analgesia,[34] give a more rapid and profound block, and have been used successfully for both cesarean section and vaginal delivery. Careful afterload control with phenylephrine is beneficial, with few fetal effects. Patients with severe stenosis do not tolerate blood loss or tachycardia well.[35] This problem needs to be addressed in the delivery plan.

Prosthetic heart valves

Pregnant patients with artificial heart valves sometimes have other structural heart disease (which is often but not always corrected at the time of surgery). Problems in labour and delivery usually occur from impaired ventricular function or an outgrown or too small prosthesis or from associated cardiac abnormalities. The type of replacement valve may be important. Bioprostheses have been widely available since 1980, and have the advantage of not needing anticoagulant treatment unless the patient is in atrial fibrillation, but the disadvantage of shorter durability in younger patients. Most pregnant patients whom we encounter currently have bioprostheses. However, those with mechanical valves may occasionally present in a tertiary care center. The risks of artificial valves are primarily infection (endocarditis) and thromboembolism. Anticoagulant therapy is often difficult secondary to the thrombophilia caused by the pregnant state. (See Chapter 9 for a full discussion of anticoagulant care and of the advantages and disadvantages of tissue versus mechanical prostheses.) Regional anesthesia may be beneficial for the underlying cardiac disease; however, there is an increased risk of spinal hematoma.[16] The risk of endocarditis necessitates the need for prophylactic antibiotics. Administration of antibiotics should coincide with peak levels at the time of incision or delivery.

For vaginal delivery, low-molecular-weight heparin should have been changed to unfractionated heparin infusion because of its short duration of action and reversibility with protamine in cases of emergency. Heparin infusion is discontinued on the labour floor and a period of time allowed for the heparin to metabolize before placement of regional anesthesia. Once a regional anesthetic has been established, some centers will restart the heparin infusion without a bolus. Heparin infusion is switched off before the second stage of labour. Mechanical valves for the most part are protected for about 12–24 hours off anticoagulation, provided that there is no demonstrable source of thrombus. There is some urgency to get these patients delivered so that anticoagulation can be restarted. Labour augmentation with oxytocin is frequently employed and is associated with an increased incidence of operative delivery.

Cardiomyopathies

Hypertrophic cardiomyopathy

Women with hypertrophic cardiomyopathy usually tolerate pregnancy well (see Chapter 13) because the left ventricle seems to adapt normally to the needs of pregnancy. Fatalities are rare in pregnancy but sudden death has been described in a patient who was taking verapamil, which should be changed to a beta blocker, and vasodilator drugs should be avoided. The main patients at risk are those with severe diastolic dysfunction who are at risk from fluid overload; sudden pulmonary edema may also occur in the third stage as a result of autotransfusion from the contracting uterus. The management of most of these patients includes the use of beta-blocking agents to limit left ventricular obstruction. The patients are managed as patients with aortic stenosis, because substantial decreases in SVR (e.g. spinal anesthesia and hemorrhage) may be associated with worsening of the outflow obstruction.

Adequate diastolic filling time is important to maintain cardiac output and tachycardia should be avoided. Anesthesia options for these patients depend on the degree of outflow obstruction and NYHA class; cesarean section under general anesthesia may be indicated.[6] Classically, halothane is used for these patients, but, with the decline in its use, it is not readily available in many obstetric anesthesia units. Sevoflurane has suitable cardiovascular effects and may be used instead. The key is to prevent a decrease in SVR and an increase in contractility of the hypertrophied septum. Phenylephrine is used to maintain perfusion pressure; however, in high doses this will decrease placental perfusion and hence general anesthesia should be cautiously administered. Dilute slow infusions of oxytocin are well tolerated and methergine may also be used.

Restrictive cardiomyopathy

Restrictive cardiomyopathy is very rare in pregnancy. Anesthetic management principles are similar to those of cardiac tamponade.[36] The main goal is to maintain cardiac output. Preload needs to be closely monitored and tachycardia should be treated to allow more time for diastolic filling. Such patients do not tolerate an abrupt drop in SVR. For those who come to near term, surgical delivery with a balanced general anesthetic is generally recommended. CVP and arterial line monitoring are beneficial.

Dilated cardiomyopathy

Dilated cardiomyopathy is recognized by systolic dysfunction and should be treated as heart failure. Pregnancy is rarely seen because it is contraindicated if the condition is recognized, unless it is very mild. Peripartum cardiomyopathy (PPCM) is an unexplained dilated cardiomyopathy that develops in the last month of pregnancy or within 5 months of delivery in previously healthy women. It has an estimated incidence of 1 in 4000 pregnancies. Symptoms in pregnant women with dilated cardiomyopathy often develop insidiously and can be confused with normal fatigue and shortness of breath associated with the third trimester or sleepless nights after delivery. The goal is to obtain the maximal fetal maturity with the least impact on maternal morbidity. This is an exceedingly fine line because many patients will suddenly decompensate, making emergency cesarean section and subsequent management very difficult, especially if the patient has myocardial ischemia (see Chapter 14).

Access to bypass or ventricular assist devices may be needed in obstetric disasters. Occasionally steroids can help patients with PPCM to reduce inflammation secondary to either viral or autoimmune processes. This has an added advantage in helping fetal lung maturity. Sometimes even patients with mild ventricular impairment need to be delivered preterm. Cesarean sections are often indicated by maternal disease (inductions can be prolonged and the effects of fluid retention poorly tolerated). Regional techniques are appropriate for these patients.[37] If vaginal delivery is induced, these patients cannot undergo Valsalva and afterload reduction with an epidural can help tremendously. Hemabate and methergine should be used with great caution because elevation in the SVR can further impede ventricular function. An arterial line is useful for both vaginal and cesarean section delivery. Aggressive management of afterload is key to prevent ventricular failure but angiotensin-converting enzyme (ACE) inhibitors and angiotensin receptor blockers cannot be used until after delivery; until then reliance has to be on hydralazine and nitrates.

Ischemic heart disease and myocardial infarction

Efforts to reduce maternal oxygen demand will help in the management of ischemic and infarcted pregnant women. Depending on the severity of the illness, early or emergency delivery should be planned.[38] Anesthesia services will be involved in providing sedation for angiogram, angioplasty and stenting or even coronary artery bypass surgery (see Chapter 15). Sedation should be administered cautiously to avoid hypotension and hypoventilation. If a prolonged procedure is anticipated, endotracheal intubation and light general anesthetic may be more appropriate (with left uterine displacement indicated). In the case of poor cardiac function balloon counterpulsation is helpful in optimizing cardiac output. Arrhythmias can be challenging to treat as a result of the fetal effects of many of the agents. Most probably the fetus will need to be delivered with general anesthesia in an operating room with bypass facilities. Postoperative management in the coronary care unit requires the availability of drugs to deal with postpartum hemorrhage because these patients will be on anticoagulants and nitroglycerin, which cause uterine relaxation.

Other conditions

Rare cases of pulmonary valve disease, coarctation of the aorta, aortic aneurysm, Marfan syndrome and pheochromocytomas need intervention or surgery in pregnancy. Anesthetic management is dependent on the predominant impact of the particular cardiac anomaly, and on what needs to be done — hemodynamic, endocrine or safeguard of a fragile aorta.

Conclusion

Heart disease in pregnancy is increasing because of the number of older primiparous women, morbid obesity and the number of congenital heart patients surviving to reproductive age. The CEMACH report[1] revealed that most maternal deaths occurred in pregnant women where cardiac disease was unknown. Anesthetic management of these patients includes participation in pre-pregnancy evaluation and surveillance for cardiac disease, and the determination of optimal delivery to minimize maternal and fetal burden. This can be accomplished only by close communication among the obstetrician, cardiologist, cardiac surgeon, anesthesiologist, intensivist and neonatologist. It is vital to devise a plan that covers all possible obstetric complications. Managed electively, anesthesia contributes to the safety of mother and baby and successful outcome in most conditions. Postoperative monitoring and ICU resources are needed to ensure safe resolution of operative hemodynamic changes. Most of the anesthesia literature emphasizes that anesthesia techniques need to be tailored to the individual needs of the patient and the unique circumstances that they present.

References

1 Malhotra S, Yentis SM. Reports on Confidential Enquiries into Maternal Deaths: management strategies based on trends in maternal cardiac deaths over 30 years. *Int J Obstet Anesth* 2006;**15**:223–6.
2 Goodman S. Anesthesia for nonobstetric surgery in the pregnant patient. *Semin Perinatol* 2002;**26**:136–45.

3 Cauldwell CB. Anesthesia for fetal surgery. *Anesthesiol Clin N Am* 2002;**20**:211–26.

4 Robson SC, Dunlop W, Hunter S et al. Haemodynamic changes associated with caesarean section under epidural anaesthesia. *Br J Obstet Gynaecol* 1989;**96**:642–7.

5 Yentis SM, Robinson PN. Definitions in obstetric anaesthesia: how should we measure anaesthetic workload and what is 'epidural rate'? *Anaesthesia* 1999;**54**:958–62.

6 Gomar C, Errando CL. Neuroaxial anaesthesia in obstetrical patients with cardiac disease. *Curr Opin Anesthesiol* 2005;**18**:507–12.

7 Ojala K, Perala J, Kariniemi J et al. Arterial embolization and prophylactic catheterization for the treatment for severe obstetric hemorrhage. *Acta Obstet Gynecol Scand* 2005;**84**:1075–80.

8 Atlee JL, Dhamee MS, Olund TL, George V. The use of esmolol, nicardipine, or their combination to blunt hemodynamic changes after laryngoscopy and tracheal intubation. *Anesth Analg* 2000;**90**:280–5.

9 Dob DP, Yentis SM. Practical management of the parturient with congenital heart disease. *Int J Obstet Anesth* 2006;**15**:137–44.

10 Jenkins SA, Marshall CF. Awake intubation made easy and acceptable. *Anaesth Intensive Care* 2000;**28**:556–61.

11 Danilenko-Dixon DR, Tefft L, Cohen RA et al. Positional effects on maternal cardiac output during labour with epidural analgesia. *Am J Obstet Gynecol* 1996;**175**:867–72.

12 Czeizel A. Lack of evidence of teratogenicity of benzodiazepine drugs in Hungary. *Repr Toxicol* 1987;**1**:183–8.

13 Quan WL, Chia CK, Yim HB. Safety of endoscopical procedures during pregnancy. *Singapore Med J* 2006;**47**:525–8.

14 Kubli M, Shennan AH, Seed PT, O'Sullivan G. A randomised controlled trial of fluid pre-loading before low dose epidural analgesia for labour. *Int J Obstet Anesth* 2003;**12**:256–60.

15 Ngan Kee WD, Khaw KS. Vasopressors in obstetrics: what should we be using? *Curr Opin Anesthesiol* 2006;**19**:238–43.

16 Vandermeulen E. Anaesthesia and new antithrombotic drugs. *Curr Opin Anesthesiol* 2005;**18**:353–9.

17 Kuczkowski KM. The safety of anaesthetics in pregnant women. *Expert Opin Drug Safety* 2006;**5**:251–64.

18 Cohen-Kerem R, Railton C, Oren D et al. Pregnancy outcome following non-obstetric surgical intervention. *Am J Surg* 2005;**190**:467–73.

19 Calthorpe N, Lewis M. Acid aspiration prophylaxis in labour: a survey of UK obstetric units. *Int J Obstet Anesth* 2005;**14**:300–4.

20 Imarengiaye CO, Ekwere IT. Acid aspiration prophylaxis and caesarean delivery: time for another close look. *J Obstet Gynaecol* 2005;**25**:357–8.

21 Steinbrook RA. Anaesthesia, minimally invasive surgery and pregnancy. *Best Pract Res Clin Anaesthesiol* 2002;**16**:131–43.

22 Crowhurst JA. Anaesthesia for non-obstetric surgery during pregnancy. *Acta Anaesthesiol Belg* 2002;**53**:295–7.

23 ACOG Committee Opinion Number 284, August 2003: Nonobstetric surgery in pregnancy. *Obstet Gynecol* 2003;**102**:431.

24 Stirrup CA, Lucas DN, Cox ML et al. Maternal anti-factor Xa activity following subcutaneous unfractionated heparin after Caesarean section. *Anaesthesia* 2001;**56**:855–8.

25 Goldstein S, Wolf GL, Kim SJ et al. Bacteraemia during direct laryngoscopy and endotracheal intubation: a study using a multiple culture, large volume technique. *Anaesth Intensive Care* 1997;**25**:239–44.

26 Ucbing A, Steer PJ, Yentis SM, Gatzoulis MA. Pregnancy and congenital heart disease. *BMJ* 2006;**332**:401–6.

27 McKeon VA, O'Reilly M. Nursing management of second stage labour. *Online J Knowl Synth Nurs* 1997;**4**:4.

28 Gowda RM, Khan IA, Mehta NJ et al. Cardiac arrhythmias in pregnancy: clinical and therapeutic considerations. *Int J Cardiol* 2003;**88**:129–33.

29 Bonnin M, Mercier FJ, Sitbon O et al. Severe pulmonary hypertension during pregnancy: mode of delivery and anesthetic management of 15 consecutive cases. *Anesthesiology* 2005;**102**:1133–7; discussion 5A–6A.

30 Martin JT, Tautz TJ, Antognini JF. Safety of regional anesthesia in Eisenmenger's syndrome. *Reg Anesth Pain Med* 2002;**27**:509–13.

31 DeLaRosa J, Sharoni E, Guyton RA. Pregnancy and valvular heart disease. *Heart Surg Forum* 2002;**6**:E7–9.

32 Davies GA, Tessier JL, Woodman MC et al. Maternal hemodynamics after oxytocin bolus compared with infusion in the third stage of labour: a randomized controlled trial. *Obstet Gynecol* 2005;**105**:294–9.

33 Suntharalingam G, Dob D, Yentis SM. Obstetric epidural analgesia in aortic stenosis: a low-dose technique for labour and instrumental delivery. *Int J Obstet Anesth* 2001;**10**:129–34.

34 Deschamps A, Kaufman I, Backman SB, Plourde G. Autonomic nervous system response to epidural analgesia in labouring patients by wavelet transform of heart rate and blood pressure variability. *Anesthesiology* 2004;**101**:21–7.

35 Lewis NL, Dob DP, Yentis SM. UK registry of high-risk obstetric anaesthesia: arrhythmias, cardiomyopathy, aortic stenosis, transposition of the great arteries and Marfan's syndrome. *Int J Obstet Anesth* 2003;**12**:28–34.

36 Webster JA, Self DD. Anesthesia for pericardial window in a pregnant patient with cardiac tamponade and mediastinal mass. *Can J Anaesth* 2003;**50**:815–18.

37 Okutomi T, Saito M, Amano K et al. Labour analgesia guided by echocardiography in a parturient with primary dilated cardiomyopathy. *Can J Anaesth* 2005;**52**:622–5.

38 Liu SS, Forrester RM, Murphy GS et al. Anaesthetic management of a parturient with myocardial infarction related to cocaine use. *Can J Anaesth* 1992;**39**:858–61.

CHAPTER 21

Cardiac percutaneous intervention and surgery during pregnancy

Patrizia Presbitero, Giacomo Boccuzzi, Felice Bruno

Cardiac conditions that need percutaneous intervention or surgery during pregnancy are very rare because usually they are diagnosed and treated before pregnancy. However, as a result of the important hemodynamic changes in the maternal cardiovascular system during pregnancy, some previously undiagnosed conditions can be unmasked or can rapidly deteriorate even in patients who had been well and stable in the non-pregnant state.

Indications for intervention

1 Worsening of previous cardiac conditions that had previously been missed or underestimated: this can occur particularly in mitral and aortic valve disease. The pressure gradient across a narrowed valve may increase greatly during pregnancy because of the rise in cardiac output. As a result of the higher metabolism of pregnancy, a possible acceleration of the disease process can occur. It is well known that progressive calcification of bioprostheses (either porcine or bovine) can occur during pregnancy (although possibly not more rapidly than outside pregnancy in young adults). Sudden dilatation of the aortic root in patients with Marfan syndrome is rare but can occur and is very worrying. These conditions have to be closely followed clinically and with echocardiography in order to optimize the time for possible interventional treatment.
2 Occurrence of sudden life-threatening complications: acute myocardial infarction, aortic dissection, infective endocarditis, prosthetic valve thrombosis or discovery of an atrial myxoma. In these cases it is very important not to delay intervention because the fetal risk is related to the maternal state.

Percutaneous intervention

Over the last 20 years, interventional cardiology has emerged as a new therapeutic tool and an effective alternative to surgical therapy in several cardiac diseases, particularly valve stenosis and coronary artery disease.[1] Therefore, if the disease can be treated by both percutaneous and surgical procedures, percutaneous intervention should be chosen because it carries less risk to mother and fetus. Lack of knowledge of the 'real' fetal risk of radiation and contrast medium is overstated and not a reason to choose surgery.

The effects of radiation on the fetus depend on the maternal radiation dose and the gestational age at which exposure occurs. The maximal permissible dose of radiation to the pregnant woman has been set at 0.5 rad, but some authors have suggested that 10 rad exposure is safe. If the radiation fetal dose is in excess of 25 rad, elective pregnancy termination should be recommended because the risk of an adverse outcome is high. The effect of radiation during pregnancy can be divided into three main phases. Irradiation during the preimplantation period (0–9 days) tends to cause death rather than anomalies. The effects appear to be 'all or none'. The incidence of spontaneous embryo re-sorption during the first 2 weeks of gestation is approximately 25–50% and a dose of 10 rad is estimated to increase that number by 0–1%. During the period of active organogenesis (9–42 days), radiation causes severe structural anomalies. A dose of 200 rad will produce a 100% incidence of congenital abnormalities, whereas a dose of 10 rad results in a 1% increase in malformations over a baseline of 5–10%.

During the second and third trimester, risks are primarily related to the development of childhood leukemia and other malignancies. It has been estimated that a dose of 1 rad increases the risk of childhood cancer by 2 cases per 100 000 births to a total of 6 cases in 100 000 live births. Although the development of most organs is complete by 9–12 weeks, the brain continues to grow and thus remains sensitive to the effects of radiation. Some reports have correlated radiation exposure to mental handicap and microcephaly. It has been calculated that cardiac catheterization causes a mean skin dose of 47 rad per examination, and a mean radiation exposure to the chest of 1.1 rad, and to the unshielded abdomen of 0.15 rad. When there is direct exposure of the maternal pelvis to radiation, <20% of the dose reaches the fetus because of tissue attenuation. Shielding the gravid uterus from direct radiation, shortening of fluoroscopic time and delaying the procedure until, at least, completion of the period of major organogenesis (>12 weeks after menses) will minimize the radiation exposure. The risk of fetal hypothyroidism, from the use of iodine contrast, is present after 25 weeks of gestation when the thyroid becomes active. This risk changes on the basis of the amount of contrast used during the procedure.

The best time for performing percutaneous intervention procedures is considered to be the fourth month, during which period organogenesis has been completed, the fetal thyroid is still inactive and the volume of the uterus is still small, so that there is a greater distance between the fetus and the chest than in the following months.[1] [2]

Percutaneous mitral balloon valvotomy

Mitral valve stenosis, almost always of rheumatic origin, is the most common (90%) and important cardiac valvular problem during pregnancy, particularly in developing countries. Most of the women with severe, but also those with moderate, mitral valve stenosis have worsening of their symptoms in the second or third trimester of pregnancy. Percutaneous balloon mitral valvotomy (PBMV) or valve repair/replacement during pregnancy should be considered in patients with moderate or severe mitral valve stenosis and persistent symptoms despite optimal medical therapy.[3–5] Open mitral valvotomy or valve replacement during pregnancy is rarely necessary and has virtually disappeared from the surgical repertoire because young women have pliable valves without too much calcification that are suitable for percutaneous balloon valvotomy. This technique has taken over from surgical closed mitral valvotomy which has been carried out safely with excellent results since the 1950s. PBMV, since the initial description by Inoue in 1984, has been shown to be successful in large studies of patients with symptomatic mitral stenosis. The mechanism of balloon mitral valvotomy—commissural splitting—is similar to that of surgical valvotomy. This procedure has given good results, especially in young patients with non-calcified, thin valves without subvalvular thickening or significant mitral regurgitation. Dilatation of the stenotic mitral valve results in immediate hemodynamic improvement.

The mitral gradient generally decreases from 33% to 50% of its initial value, and the cross-sectional area doubles. Both pulmonary capillary wedge pressure and pulmonary artery pressure decrease immediately, with the latter dropping further during the week after valvuloplasty. There are potential complications associated with this procedure, including atrial perforation resulting from transseptal puncture, cardiac tamponade, arrhythmias, embolism, mitral regurgitation and hypotension. Mortality in the more recent series is reported to be 0.5%. Mitral regurgitation is the most common complication. In published reports its incidence varies from 0% to 50%. Severe regurgitation is, however, uncommon, and will occur only when there is structural damage to the mitral valve. The development or increase in the grade of mitral regurgitation is predicted by the presence of regurgitation and the severity of stenosis before the procedure. In patients with pliable valves, the development of mitral regurgitation is less frequent. Creation of a significant atrial septal defect secondary to septal dilatation has been reported to vary from 5% to 20% and is hemodynamically insignificant in all patients. The long-term effect of these shunts is unknown, but it seems that most atrial septal defects close within 24 h.[1,4–6]

Since 1988, 250 women are reported to have had PBMVs in pregnancy. In women with severe mitral stenosis and well-documented immediate clinical and hemodynamic results, the mean gradient across the stenotic mitral valve declined from a mean value of 21 to 5 mmHg and the mitral valve area increased from a mean value of 0.9 to 2.1 cm^2. There have been no reports of serious maternal complications and only two fetal deaths. The reported incidence of mitral regurgitation is low, and in most cases it was only trivial or mild.

Balloon inflation generally causes transient maternal hypotension and a transient decrease in fetal heart rate. Both parameters return to baseline within a few seconds of balloon deflation, with no serious fetal distress noted. During balloon mitral valvotomy, the supine position is necessary. This may cause maternal hypotension that can be alleviated by intravenous fluid infusion. The recumbent position causes pressure of the gravid uterus on the pelvic vessels, which may obstruct the passage of catheters. The use of fluoroscopy during the procedure carries the risk of fetal radiation exposure (discussed above). In the pregnant patient the procedure has been performed with both the single- and the double-balloon technique. Nowadays the use of the single-balloon catheter procedure has reduced the fluoroscopy time. Transesophageal ultrasonography or even simple transthoracic ultrasonography (when a good echo window in the supine position can be achieved) can be used during percutaneous balloon valvotomy in order to minimize radiation exposure.[4-7]

At present, patients with severe mitral stenosis in functional New York Heart Association (NYHA) class III/IV and favorable valvular anatomy are the best candidates for percutaneous mitral valvotomy. In asymptomatic patients with mitral stenosis, the risk of maternal death during pregnancy and delivery is very low. However, deterioration in hemodynamic conditions can be expected and emergency valvotomy may become necessary. A simple 'rule of thumb' is an increase of one NYHA functional class any time during pregnancy. In these cases a 'prophylactic' percutaneous mitral valvotomy should be considered, provided that there is a satisfactory echocardiographic score (<8). The indication for balloon mitral valvotomy should not be expanded because of the pregnant status. In cases with an echocardiographic score >8, surgery should be considered.

Balloon mitral valvotomy in the pregnant patient is a technically complex procedure that needs to be done quickly by an expert team. As a result of the possibility of a need for subsequent emergency surgery, it should be done only in centers that have extensive experience with this procedure and have a cardiac surgery department on-site.

Percutaneous aortic balloon valvotomy

Severe aortic valve stenosis is rare during pregnancy because both the congenital bicuspid form is more commonly found in men and patients have percutaneous or surgical valvotomy in childhood and before conception. During pregnancy, as a result of the increase in cardiac output, the transvalvular gradient may double its basal value and clinical deterioration can develop. Intervention is indicated only in severe symptomatic aortic valve stenosis and the echocardiographic features alone are not enough to decide on management.[8-10]

Percutaneous aortic balloon valvotomy is a procedure in which one or more balloons are placed across the stenotic aortic valve and inflated. The aim is to relieve the stenosis, presumably by separation of the fused commissures or fracturing calcified deposits within the valve leaflets, or by stretching of the annulus. Early changes after successful valvotomy include a moderate reduction in the transvalvular pressure gradient and an often dramatic improvement in symptoms. However, the post-procedure valve area rarely exceeds 1.0 cm^2.

Nine cases of balloon aortic valvotomy during pregnancy have been reported in the literature with significant reduction of valve gradient, hence enabling the pregnancy to continue.[1,11] As it is only a palliative procedure, allowing deferral of valve replacement until after delivery, the aim, particularly in the case of thick and calcified aortic valves, is just to obtain a modest increase in the aortic valve area, avoiding important aortic insufficiency. Balloon size to aortic annulus of 1 : 1 is recommended. The most frequently used technique is the retrograde approach (arterial approach), although the antegrade one (venous approach) has been described. In women with significant aortic regurgitation as well as in those with heavily calcified valves, surgery is the obligatory alternative,[12] knowing that cardiopulmonary bypass carries a risk with maternal and fetal mortality rates of 1.5% and 9.5%, respectively.

Coronary artery disease

Acute myocardial infarction (AMI) in pregnancy is a rare event that occurs in 1 in 20 000–30 000 deliveries, with a mortality rate ranging from 21–37% in past series to 7% in the most recent ones.[13–14] With the current trend, at least in western countries, for child-bearing at an older age and the ongoing effects of cigarette smoking, stress and cocaine use, the occurrence of AMI during pregnancy is expected to increase. Most commonly, AMI happens during the third trimester, peripartum and puerperal period. It has been noted to occur more in multigravidas and is most commonly located in the anterior wall. Risk factors for AMI in young women generally include: a family history of coronary disease, familial hyperlipoproteinemia, low levels of high-density lipoprotein (HDL), high levels of low-density lipoprotein (LDL), or both, diabetes mellitus, cigarette smoking and previous use of oral contraceptives. The most likely mechanisms underlying this event are: coronary dissection, atherosclerotic disease, thrombosis and coronary artery spasm.[13–15]

Other possible causes are paradoxical embolism coming from the venous system (it is well known that pregnancy is associated with a fourfold increase in venous thrombosis) in patients with a patent foramen ovale. There are several reports of spontaneous coronary artery dissection during pregnancy and the puerperium. More than two-thirds of cases present in the postpartum period, usually within 2 weeks of delivery. Multiparity and advanced age were found to be associated with spontaneous coronary artery dissection. The arterial wall changes (smooth muscle cell proliferation, impaired collagen synthesis, alterations in the protein and acid mucopolysaccharide content of the media) under hormonal influence are the basis of the pathogenesis of aortic as well as coronary dissection.

The increased risk of thrombosis during pregnancy is a result of profound alterations in the coagulation and fibrinolytic system. During pregnancy there are increases in procoagulant factors, such as von Willebrand's factor, factor VIII, factor V and fibrinogen, which occur together with an acquired resistance to the endogenous anticoagulant, activated protein C, and a reduction in protein S, the co-factor for protein C. These changes are accompanied by impaired fibrinolysis through increases in plasminogen activator inhibitors 1 and 2, the latter being produced by the placenta. These changes represent physiological preparation for the hemostatic challenge of delivery.[16]

Direct coronary angiography is recommended as the first step in patients with AMI, allowing a correct diagnosis and therapeutic strategy. Primary percutaneous balloon angioplasty represents, nowadays, the treatment of choice in any case of acute occlusion of a coronary vessel during pregnancy. Heparin and aspirin are mandatory during the procedure. In cases of massive coronary thrombosis and in life-threatening conditions the use of intracoronary thrombolytic therapy or a IIb/IIIa inhibitor should be considered as adjunctive therapy even if only limited data are available. Percutaneous transluminal coronary angioplasty (PTCA) with stenting is the therapy of choice in single-vessel dissection. In cases of left main dissection and multi-vessel involvement, coronary artery bypass grafting should be considered even if extensive coronary stenting can be performed safely. The most important objective in a young pregnant woman with AMI is avoidance of treatment delay. Rapidly irreversible myocardial damage in these patients is the result of lack of preconditioning ischemia. Immediate access to a cardiac interventional department is mandatory in order to ensure optimal management.

Pulmonary valve and arteries intervention

Mild, moderate and moderately severe right ventricular outflow tract obstruction are very well tolerated during pregnancy, as shown in previous series in which no deaths and a low incidence of complications have been reported.[17] However, severe forms of pulmonary valve stenosis, for some reason not treated during childhood, and even moderate ones with impaired right ventricular function and/or symptoms, may require percutaneous pulmonary balloon valvuloplasty during pregnancy. Percutaneous balloon pulmonary valvotomy with splitting of the valve commissures has been shown to be safe and effective, and the mortality and morbidity associated with it appear to be minimal. Four successful cases of percutaneous balloon pulmonary angioplasty in pregnant women have been reported in the literature.[1,17] In all these cases the valve gradient was halved and the pregnancy continued uneventfully. As happens outside pregnancy, arrhythmias and transient right bundle-branch block can occur during intervention. Any resulting pulmonary regurgitation is not severe and does not appear to be a clinically relevant problem and, as in childhood, does not require surgical intervention.

The need to dilate pulmonary arteries during pregnancy is exceptional. We performed stenting of a right pulmonary artery in a 38-year-old pregnant woman with right pulmonary artery stenosis at the site of an old Waterston shunt. The stenosis was moderate with a gradient of 40 mmHg, but it was a twin pregnancy, which imposes much more strain on the right ventricle and the patient was in heart failure. The percutaneous intervention was carried out at the eighth month so that she could deliver without problems.

Percutaneous intervention in cyanotic heart disease

Cyanosis is a worrying condition during pregnancy on account of both the mother and the fetus, so correction of the underlying condition, or at least improvement in the cyanosis, is mandatory before pregnancy if possible.[1,18] Some interventions can be performed with caution, even during pregnancy, in order to improve the pregnancy outcome. Figure 21.1 shows a patient with single ventricle, tight pulmonary stenosis and an old Blalock–Taussig shunt who was extremely hypoxic at the third month of pregnancy because of a tight stenosis in her left shunt. This was enlarged using a wall stent through the left Blalock with a rise in O_2 saturation up to 90%. However, at 6 months she developed heart failure because the shunt was too big, and pre-term delivery was necessary at 7 months (Figure 21.2). Other interventional procedures can be performed safely during pregnancy such as bronchial artery embolization for massive hemoptysis or shunt closure.

Surgery

Early reports indicated that the mortality risk for the mother was higher than outside pregnancy and that fetal mortality rate was up to 20–30%. Nowadays,

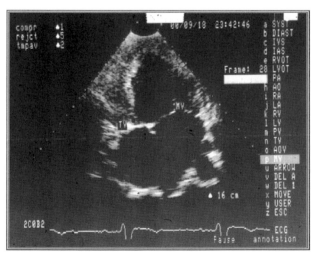

Figure 21.1 Echocardiogram of a cyanotic pregnant woman (single ventricle, tricuspid atresia, pulmonary stenosis).

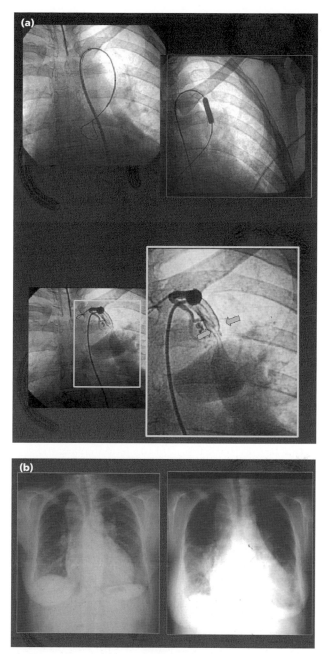

Figure 21.2 Angiogram in same patient shown in Figure 21.1. a) Showing severe left Blalock stenosis treated with a wall stent (arrows). b) Chest X-ray of the patient before and 6 months after percutaneous intervention (see text).

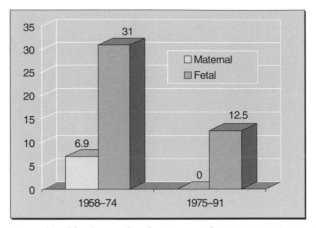

Figure 21.3 Maternal and fetal mortality during open-heart surgery in two periods of time in a large series.

open heart surgery does not carry greater risk to the mother's life than outside pregnancy (unless performed as an emergency because risk depends on the maternal condition and surgery is not performed electively in pregnancy) and ranges in the few series available from 0% to 1.5% (Figure 21.3).[1,19] The fetal death rate is between 9 and 15% and results partially from non-pulsatile blood flow and hypotension associated with cardiopulmonary bypass, which can adversely affect placental blood flow. Furthermore, all open heart operations are necessarily carried out under full anticoagulation with heparin, which does not pass the placental barrier to the fetus but can lead to placental separation from retroplacental bleeding. In addition, platelet aggregates cause microemboli and the risk to the fetus increases with longer duration of bypass.

Finally, much of the fetal risk relates to the maternal state before and at the conclusion of the operation—her heart rate, blood pressure, output and oxygenation—because all this affects uteroplacental perfusion and jeopardizes fetal safety. It is very important that the mother arrives for the operation in a good condition and not too late. The anesthetist should try to minimize the induction time and to stabilize the swings in heart rate and blood pressure that may occur during intubation. Cardiopulmonary bypass must be performed at high flow and high pressure, with normothermia (hypothermia decreases placental blood flow and may cause fetal bradycardia and lead to intrauterine death), and a perfusion index of 3.0 during cardiopulmonary bypass with the shortest possible cross-clamping time.

Continuous fetal monitoring is essential during induction, throughout the operation and postoperatively. Fetal distress is indicated by slowing of the fetal heart. If this occurs, prompt steps should be taken to try to improve the delivery and quality of blood to the fetus.

For all these possible fetal problems during maternal cardiopulmonary bypass, if the fetus is viable and well (beyond 28–30 weeks) and there had been time to prepare the fetal lungs, the best option is to deliver the child by cesarean section and then to proceed to maternal cardiac intervention. If the fetus is not viable the best time to perform surgery is early in the second trimester because in the first trimester abortion and, later on, pre-term labour can result. It is usually possible to delay the intervention until the midtrimester in valve diseases, with rest and medical treatment, because the hemodynamic burden is less important in the first few months of pregnancy.

Nowadays an emergency need for surgery can occur in valve diseases, particularly for sudden degeneration or rupture of bioprosthetic valves or thrombus formations on mechanical valves. Thrombolysis can be performed when thrombus is present on the valve or in the left atrium or ventricle. However, when the thrombus is too big the risk of embolization is thought to be high and surgical removal is safer.

Particular interest is raised in Marfan syndrome because of the risk of aortic dissection during pregnancy. Twenty-five years ago, based on case reports, this risk was evaluated at around 50%, but, most recently, on the basis of a few series and two prospective studies the risk has been found to be between 2 and 8%—very similar to the risk in a childless group of women of similar age.[20,21] It has also been demonstrated that the aortic root, with the exception of a few cases, does not dilate during pregnancy more than it does outside pregnancy, when the risk of dissection increases with an aortic root diameter of 45 mm or more. In the presence of such root dimensions a patient has to be followed very carefully with monthly echocardiograms. Other factors have to be taken into account in evaluating the risk of dissection in a patient with Marfan syndrome, such as family history of dissection, presence of mitral or aortic incompetence, age at pregnancy, presence of hypertension and multiparity.[22] Intervention should be planned only if a sudden increase of 5–10 mm in the aortic root is recorded. Aortic dissection during pregnancy can occur not only in Marfan syndrome but also in patients with unoperated coarctation of the aorta either undiagnosed or with a residual gradient after operation, in patients with bicuspid aortic valve or, indeed, in previously apparently healthy young women.

Aortic dissection should be suspected in the presence of severe chest pain, occurrence of new aortic regurgitation, or pain radiating through to the back or down into the abdomen or iliac fossae. After confirmation of the diagnosis by transesophageal echocardiography, emergency aortic root replacement is needed for type A dissection. Figure 21.4 shows the important achievement reached in the last two decades in decreasing maternal and fetal mortality during the operation for type A aortic dissection during pregnancy. Forty women were operated on in the time period 1983–2002 in two prestigious institutions: there was no maternal mortality in 20 patients operated on in the last 7 years and fetal mortality rate dropped from 50% to 10%. In repairing aortic dissection, avoiding hypothermia precludes an open distal aortic repair, which is preferable. A good compromise may be the use of antegrade cerebral perfusion for brain protection

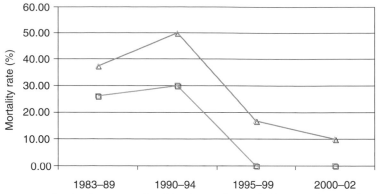

Figure 21.4 Reduction in maternal and fetal mortality in the last two decades for surgery for a type A aortic dissection. (From Immer et al.[24] with permission.)

and moderate hypothermia (28°C) as described by Bachet and Guilmet.[23] After 30 weeks of gestation, immediate cesarean section followed directly by cardiac surgery seems to be the most promising option to save the mother and the child: cardiopulmonary bypass can be utilized simultaneously during cesarean section (femoral or axillary cannulation). In patients with type B dissection, conservative treatment is recommended with rest and beta-blocking drugs. However, a high incidence of fetal loss is reported, probably as a result of a partial occlusion of the internal iliac artery or the uterine arteries, decreasing placental blood flow. Complications of type B dissection such as rupture or malperfusion require immediate surgical intervention or positioning of an endoprothesis.

References

1 Presbitero P, Prever SB, Brusca A. Interventional cardiology in pregnancy. *Eur Heart J* 1996;**17**:182–8.
2 Timins JK. Radiation during pregnancy. *N J Engl Med* 2001;**98**:29–33.
3 Bonow RO, Carabello B, de Leon AC. ACC/AHA guidelines for management of patients with valvular heart disease: a report of the American College of Cardiology American Heart Association Task Force on Practice Guidelines. *J Am Coll Cardiol* 1998;**32**:1486–588.
4 Reimold SC, Rutherford MB. Valvular heart disease in pregnancy. *N Engl J Med* 2003;**349**:52–9.
5 Silversides CK, Colman JM, Sermer M et al. Cardiac risk in pregnant women with rheumatic mitral stenosis. *Am J Cardiol* 2003;**91**:1382–5.
6 de Souza JAM, Martinez EE, Ambrose JA et al. Percutaneous balloon mitral valvuloplasty in comparison with open mitral valve commissurotomy for mitral stenosis during pregnancy. *J Am Coll Cardiol* 2001;**37**:900–3.
7 Cheng TO. Percutaneous Inoue balloon valvuloplasty is the procedure of choice for symptomatic mitral stenosis in pregnant women. *Catheter Cardiovasc Interv* 2000; **50**:418.

8 Myerson SG, Mitchell AR, Omerod OJ, Banning AP. What is the role of balloon dilatation for severe aortic stenosis during pregnancy? *J Heart Valve Dis* 2005;**14**:147–50.
9 Radford DJ, Walters DL. Balloon aortic valvotomy in pregnancy. *Aust NZ J Obstet Gynaecol* 2004;**44**:577–9.
10 Bhargava B, Agarwal R, Yadav R. Percutaneous balloon aortic valvuloplasty during pregnancy: use of the Inoue balloon and the physiologic antegrade approach. *Cathet Cardiovasc Diagn* 1998;**45**:422–5.
11 Banning AP, Pearson JF, Hall RJ. Role of balloon dilatation of the aortic valve in pregnant patients with severe aortic stenosis. *Br Heart J* 1993;**70**:544–5.
12 Ben Ami M, Battino S, Rosenfeld T et al. Aortic valve replacement during pregnancy. A case report and review of the literature. *Acta Obstet Gynaecol Scand* 1990;**69**:651–3.
13 Roth A, Elkayam U. Acute myocardial infarction associated with pregnancy. *Ann Intern Med* 1996;**125**:751–62.
14 Ladner HE, Danielsen B, Gilbert WM. Acute myocardial infarction in pregnancy and the puerperium: a population study. *Obstet Gynecol* 2005;**105**:480–4.
15 Maeder M, Ammann P, Angehrn W, Rickli H. Idiopathic spontaneous coronary artery dissection: incidence, diagnosis and treatment. *Int J Cardiol* 2005;**101**:363–9.
16 Greer IA. Thrombosis in pregnancy: maternal and foetal issues. *Lancet* 1999;**353**:1258–65.
17 Oakley C, ed. Acyanotic congenital heart disease. In: *Heart Disease in Pregnancy*. London: BMJ Publishing Group, 1997: pp 19–51.
18 Presbitero P, Somerville J, Stone S et al. Pregnancy in cyanotic congenital heart disease. Outcome of mother and fetus. *Circulation* 1994;**89**:2673–6.
19 Oakley C, ed. 1997; Cardiac intervention and surgery during pregnancy. In: *Heart Disease in Pregnancy*. London: BMJ Publishing Group, 1997: pp 397–400.
20 Rossiter JP, Repke JT, Morales AJ, Murphy EA, Pyeritz RE. A prospective longitudinal evaluation of pregnancy in the Marfan syndrome. *Am J Obstet Gynecol* 1995;**173**:1599–606.
21 Meijboom LJ, Vos FE, Timmermans J, Boers GH, Zwinderman AH, Mulder BJ. Pregnancy and aortic root growth in the Marfan syndrome: a prospective study. *Eur Heart J* 2005;**26**:914–20.
22 Child AH. Pregnancy management in Marfan syndrome and other connective tissue disorders. In: Oakley C (ed.), *Heart Disease in Pregnancy*. London: BMJ Publishing Group, 1997: pp 153–62.
23 Bachet J, Guilmet D. [Current treatment of acute dissections of the ascending aorta.] *Arch Mal Coeur Vaiss* 1997;**90**(12 suppl):1769–80.
24 Immer FF, Bansi AG, Immer-Bansi AS et al. Aortic dissection in pregnancy: analysis of risk factors and outcome. *Ann Thorac Surg* 2003;**76**:309–14.

CHAPTER 22
Genetic counseling

Michael A. Patton

This chapter is intended to act as a quick reference for doctors who are faced with a pregnant woman with heart disease who asks the question 'What is the risk that my baby will have a heart problem?'. In most cases, a risk figure is available, and appropriate investigations of the baby are suggested. However, in the case of some rare genetic syndromes, sequencing a gene to identify a mutation in a specific family may take many months and it would be better to have the opportunity of seeing these patients before they plan their pregnancy.

Genetic counseling is not just a case of providing a risk figure and arranging the necessary scans. It may involve making the diagnosis of a genetic disorder and certainly involves providing accurate and up-to-date information. One definition of genetic counseling is that it is: 'An educational process that seeks to assist affected and/or at risk individuals to understand the nature of the genetic disorder, its transmission and the options open to them in management and family planning.'[1] In other words, what do the family understand about the condition and what will they do with the risk figure that they have been given? Do they perceive the risk as being high or low? If a problem is detected, is it amenable to surgery and, if so, when? Will special arrangements have to be made with regard to the delivery of the baby? Will the baby be affected to the same degree as the parent, or might it be more severely affected? If a severe problem were detected in the fetus, would they wish to consider having a termination of pregnancy? Figure 22.1 shows the appearance of the normal fetal heart at 18–20 weeks' gestation, using ultrasonography.

Some of these issues can be dealt with adequately by both the cardiologist and obstetrician involved in the case. Others may require referral to your local clinical genetics unit, especially if the family tree is complex or special investigations are required.

Risk calculation

In genetic counseling, it is standard practice to provide a figure for the risk of recurrence, usually expressed either as odds or percentages. There are a number of different types of risk estimation used in practice, but, for the purposes of this chapter, the two main types are Mendelian and empirical risks. Mendelian risks relate to those disorders known to be caused by a single gene and with a clear

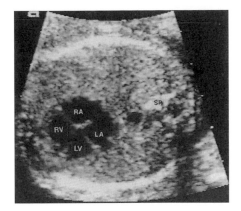

Figure 22.1 Transverse section through the fetal chest at the level of the heart, showing a normal four chamber view. RA, right atrium; LA, left atrium; RV, right ventricle; LV, left ventricle. (Reproduced by permission of JS Carvalho, Royal Brompton Hospital, London, UK.)

mode of inheritance. Thus the offspring risk for those conditions known to be dominantly inherited, such as Marfan syndrome, is 50%. The offspring risk when a parent has an autosomal recessive disorder, such as Ellis–van Creveld syndrome, is likely to be negligible. This is because, in autosomal recessive conditions, for the child to be affected it must receive an abnormal gene from both the mother and the father. The chance that the partner of an affected woman is also a carrier of a rare recessive gene is obviously small, unless the parents are related or consanguineous, in which case the risks to a child may be quite high.

Empirical risk figures are risks based on observed data, from family studies, rather than theoretical predictions based on an understanding of the mode of inheritance. This type of figure is used for most of the more common non-Mendelian disorders, such as neural tube defects, cleft lip and palate, and most isolated congenital heart defects.

Mendelian disorders

The first task, when advising a mother with congenital heart disease about risks to her offspring, is to determine if she has an isolated cardiac defect or whether there are associated features suggesting a single gene or Mendelian disorder. Examples of some of the important single gene disorders that can be associated with congenital heart disease, along with their mode of inheritance, are given in Table 22.1, and described in greater detail in the appropriate section below.

Holt–Oram syndrome

The combination of skeletal abnormalities of the upper limb with congenital heart disease, usually secundum atrial septal defect (ASD), was first reported in 1960 by Holt and Oram.[2] It is an autosomal dominant condition with extremely variable expression in terms of both skeletal and cardiac defects.

Commonly the thumbs are involved and show either hypoplasia, triphalangism or complete absence. The radius, ulna and humerus may be abnormal,

Table 22.1 Mendelian disorders associated with heart disease

Disorder	Inheritance
Holt–Oram syndrome	Autosomal dominant
Noonan syndrome	Autosomal dominant
LEOPARD syndrome	Autosomal dominant
Marfan syndrome	Autosomal dominant
Long QT (Romano–Ward) syndrome	Autosomal dominant
Jervell–Lange–Nielsen syndrome	Autosomal recessive
Supravalvar aortic stenosis	Autosomal dominant
Ellis–van Creveld syndrome	Autosomal recessive
Kartagener syndrome	Autosomal recessive

and an inability to supinate and pronate the hand is common. Upper limb pho-comelia occasionally occurs. The lower limbs are not affected.

ASD is the cardiac anomaly identified in over two-thirds of cases. However, persistent ductus arteriosus, coarctation of the aorta, ventricular septal defect, transposition of the great vessels and prolapsed mitral valve have all been reported in families in which other members have more typical features.[3]

Occasionally no congenital heart lesion is present, but arrhythmias or more minor ECG abnormalities are the only cardiac finding.

Mental handicap or learning disorder is not a feature of the Holt–Oram syndrome. Detailed ultrasonography, including fetal echocardiography, should be offered at about 18–20 weeks of pregnancy, so that the extent of the limb abnormalities, if present, can be identified and their prognosis and management discussed. Secundum ASD, the most common cardiac abnormality in Holt–Oram syndrome, is not detectable in the fetus, but other less common cardiac lesions should be excluded. The gene causing Holt–Oram syndrome is the *TBX5* gene located on chromosome 12.[4]

Noonan syndrome

This is a relatively common dysmorphic syndrome associated with congenital heart disease, usually pulmonary stenosis. It is an autosomal dominant disorder, but around half of the cases are sporadic and result from new mutations. The facial features are often more marked in childhood and may be more difficult to recognize in adult life. The cell-signaling gene *PTPN11* on chromosome 12 has been found to be the causative gene in over half of affected patients and can provide confirmation of the clinical diagnosis.[5]

The cardinal features of Noonan syndrome are short stature, a broad or webbed neck, and pectus excavatum or carinatum, associated with down-slanting palpebral fissures, ptosis, low-set posteriorly rotated ears and a low posterior hairline.[6] Cryptorchidism, commonly bilateral, occurs in 60% of affected boys and may require corrective surgery. Affected girls do not have genital abnormalities. Mild learning difficulties may be a feature in around 10% of children with Noonan syndrome. Abnormalities in the intrinsic clotting cascade may lead to postoperative bleeding.

Congenital heart lesions occur in most patients. Pulmonary stenosis is the most common cardiac defect and is surgically correctable. In about 10% of patients hypertrophic cardiomyopathy may occur and may be associated with heart failure in infancy.

Prenatal testing by chorionic villous sampling is available if a mutation has been confirmed in the family. Otherwise detailed fetal echocardiography is indicated in any pregnancy when one or other parent has Noonan syndrome, or when parents have had a previous child with the condition.

LEOPARD syndrome

The name of this syndrome is an acronym for multiple **L**entigines, **E**CG abnormalities, **O**cular hypertelorism, **P**ulmonary stenosis, **A**bnormalities of the genitalia, **R**etardation of growth and sensorineural **D**eafness. It is a diagnosis that should be considered in patients with a combination of any of the above features with multiple lentigines. It is inherited as an autosomal dominant with variable expression, and mild mental handicap can be a feature.

Mutations in the same gene as the gene for Noonan syndrome have now been found in this disorder, and it appears that it may overlap with Noonan syndrome. Genetic referral may be helpful in undertaking further investigation.[7]

A variety of cardiac findings have been reported. ECG abnormalities may show axis deviations, unilateral or bilateral hypertrophy or conduction abnormalities, such as prolonged P–R interval, hemiblock, bundle-branch block or complete heart block. Pulmonary stenosis may be either valvar or infundibular, and other cardiac defects such as aortic stenosis, mitral stenosis and obstructive cardiomyopathy are less common.

Fetal echocardiography is indicated, to exclude a severe congenital heart lesion, if either parent has LEOPARD syndrome.

Marfan syndrome

This connective tissue disorder has been described in detail in Chapter 10. It is inherited as an autosomal dominant, and so an affected parent has a 50% chance of passing it on to offspring. The gene that causes Marfan syndrome has been isolated—the fibrillin gene on chromosome 15.[8] If no mutation can be identified, then linkage studies may be helpful if there are several affected family members. Prenatal ultrasonography, including fetal echocardiography, is not particularly helpful, because most of the clinical features of the condition are not necessarily present in the fetus or neonate. Affected parents who wish to discuss the possibility of prenatal diagnosis should be referred for genetic advice, preferably before starting their family, so that the feasibility of genetic tests can be considered and arranged.

Long QT (Romano–Ward) syndrome

This condition, in which syncopal attacks associated with a long Q–T interval (but not with deafness—see Jervell–Lange–Nielsen syndrome below) occur, is inherited in an autosomal dominant manner, with a 50% risk to offspring.[9] In theory, prenatal diagnosis is possible by fetal electrocardiography with enhanced resolution for T-wave analysis. In practice, most affected families opt for diagnosis in the neonatal period by ECG and appropriate medical or surgical treatment. There is considerable genetic heterogeneity and several causative ion channel genes have been identified.[10]

Jervell–Lange–Nielsen syndrome

The features of Jervell–Lange–Nielsen syndrome are a prolonged Q–T interval, leading to syncopal attacks, associated with congenital, or at least early onset, severe sensorineural deafness.[11] This latter feature permits differentiation from Romano–Ward syndrome and, as the condition is autosomal recessive, risks for the offspring are low.

Supravalvar aortic stenosis

This anomaly can occur as a sporadic condition, but familial cases, in which it is inherited as an autosomal dominant with variable expression, have been reported.[12] Supravalvar pulmonary stenosis is a common associated finding. In view of its variability, even within families, risks for offspring of an affected parent are difficult to assess, and may require cardiological assessment of other relatives to establish whether a case is truly sporadic or likely to be associated with a dominant gene. If other family members are known to be affected, the offspring risk is likely to be 50%.

Prenatal diagnosis by fetal echocardiography is difficult, but it is worth excluding other congenital heart defects. Most cases can be diagnosed postnatally by appropriate investigations and are amenable to surgical correction.

Supravalvar aortic stenosis and peripheral pulmonary artery stenoses are both seen with additional abnormalities in Williams syndrome, which is a disorder with characteristic coarse facial features, developmental delay, behavioral problems, hypercalcemia and sensitivity to sound (hyperacusis). Most cases of Williams syndrome are associated with a submicroscopic deletion involving the elastin gene on the long arm of chromosome 7.[13] Most genetic laboratories will offer a specific chromosome test using fluorescent *in situ* hybridization for Williams syndrome. Williams syndrome usually arises as a new deletion and does not recur in future pregnancies.

Ellis–van Creveld syndrome

Ellis–van Creveld syndrome is also known as chondroectodermal dysplasia. The characteristic features are postaxial polydactyly, short-limbed dwarfism, dysplastic nails, and a congenital heart defect, usually a large atrial septal defect.[14]

This condition is inherited as an autosomal recessive, and thus after one affected child there will be a 25% recurrence risk. However, the risk for the offspring of an affected individual is low.

There are two genes for Ellis–van Creveld syndrome, which are located side by side on the short arm of chromosome 4.[15]

Kartagener syndrome

Kartagener syndrome is characterized by bronchiectasis, recurrent sinusitis, dextrocardia with or without other heart defects, and other evidence of partial or complete situs inversus.[16] Diagnosis may require electron microscopic examination of cilia morphology, which consistently shows a reduced number of inner and outer dynein arms. Generally it is considered to be an autosomal recessive condition, with a low risk to offspring. There are three potential gene loci but the gene for dynein protein on chromosome 9 appears to be the most common in European populations.[17]

Chromosomal abnormalities

Chromosome imbalance frequently leads to abnormalities in cardiac development and often other malformations and learning disorder. Thus any child or adult with a congenital heart lesion associated with dysmorphic features and learning disorder should have their chromosome karyotype checked to exclude a chromosome abnormality. There are some well-recognized associations, e.g. atrioventricular septal defect is commonly seen in Down syndrome (trisomy 21) and coarctation of the aorta is the characteristic abnormality in girls with Turner syndrome (45X).

There is now a wider range of cytogenetic tests using molecular probes to identify abnormalities that would not have been visible with standard chromosome analysis. The technique of fluorescence *in situ* hybridization (FISH) will detect new chromosome deletion syndromes such as Williams syndrome (see above) and DiGeorge syndrome where a microdeletion on chromosome 22 has been found. Newer techniques using DNA microarrays or 'gene chips' may advance the analysis of chromosomes even further.

Deletions of chromosome 22q had been described clinically in various ways before the chromosome deletion was recognized. Thus the terms 'velocardiofacial syndrome' or 'Shprintzen syndrome' are also used in the literature. The characteristic features of 22q deletions or DiGeorge syndrome are cardiac abnormalities, especially ventricular septal defects and Fallot's tetralogy, with cleft palate or palatal insufficiency, characteristic facies, mild learning difficulties, hypoparathyroidism and immunodeficiency.[18] It has also been associated with psychiatric problems including schizophrenia. In most cases, DiGeorge syndrome occurs as a sporadic condition, but it can be inherited as an autosomal dominant and the phenotype can be variable, e.g. a mildly affected parent with just a cleft palate and ventricular septal defect may have a child with learning disorder and severe congenital heart disease. Microdeletions involving chromosome 22q have also been found in occasional families with apparently dominant inheritance of isolated congenital heart lesions.

Congenital heart disease

Congenital heart disease occurs in between 0.5 and 1% of all births. Most cases (probably about 90%) are of unknown etiology and are considered to result from multifactorial or 'polygenic' inheritance. Only about 3% of cases follow simple Mendelian inheritance. Chromosomal disorders and environmental causes account for the rest.

If environmental exposure is the cause of heart disease in the mother, the risk to the offspring is lower than the risk for polygenic inheritance. An example is exposure to rubella, which is an unusual cause of persistent ductus arteriosus and other congenital heart lesions since the introduction of mass immunization programs, but may be a more prevalent cause in older age groups.

Genetic advice is most often requested by parents who have had one child with congenital heart disease. However, with improvements in management and surgery in recent years, many survivors are now reaching reproductive age and requesting genetic counseling with regard to risks to offspring. A number of studies have now been completed,[19–21] which provide information about offspring risks taking into account the sex of the affected parent as well as the precise anatomical lesion present in the parent. However, the number of participants in these studies is generally small, and may not be representative, and the figures vary widely between studies. It would appear that the risks are higher for the offspring of affected women than of affected men, for reasons that are not understood. When a recurrence does occur, the lesion is identical to that in the affected parent in only about half the cases, which needs to be taken into account when counseling. Parents need to appreciate that a child may have a fatal or untreatable lesion as opposed to one that is amenable to surgery, and that prognosis should be discussed at the time of detection of the problem. Figure 22.2 shows an atrioventricular septal defect on fetal echocardiography.

Table 22.2 gives general recurrence risks when the precise anatomical lesion is unknown and Table 22.3 gives offspring risks, according to affected parent, for a number of the more common congenital heart defects. Both tables have been modified from those published in Peter Harper's textbook *Practical Genetic Counselling*.[22]

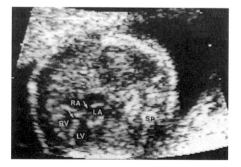

Figure 22.2 Transverse section through the fetal chest at the level of the heart, which shows an atrioventricular septal defect with a common atrioventricular valve. The arrows point to the atrial and ventricular components of the defect. RA, right atrium; LA, left atrium; RV, right ventricle; LV, left ventricle. (Reproduced by permission of JS Carvalho, Royal Brompton Hospital, London, UK.)

Table 22.2 General recurrence risks in congenital heart disease

	Percentage risk
Population incidence	0.5–1
Sibling of isolated case	2–3
Half-sibling or second-degree relative	1–2
Offspring of isolated case:	
Mother	5
Father	2–3
Two affected siblings (or sibling and parent)	10
More than two affected first-degree relatives	50

Table 22.3 Offspring risks for specific congenital heart lesions

Lesion	Mother affected	Father affected
Ventricular septal defect	9.5	2.5
Atrial septal defect	6	1.5
Persistent ductus arteriosus	4	2
Fallot's tetralogy	2.5	1.5
Atrioventricular septal defect	14	1
Pulmonary stenosis	6.5	2
Aortic stenosis	18	5
Coarctation of aorta	4	2.5

Based on multiple studies, collated by Nora et al.[23]

Pulmonary hypertension

Primary pulmonary hypertension usually occurs as a sporadic condition, with a predominance of women, but occasional families showing autosomal dominant inheritance have been reported.[24] It has been found to be caused by the BMPR2 gene on chromosome 2.[25]

Autoimmune disorders

Autoimmune disorders have been discussed in Chapter 11. Most of them are not inherited as single gene disorders, but often show familial aggregations. However, they may have a direct clinical effect on the fetus as, for example, in systemic lupus erythematosus (SLE). SLE is an autoimmune disorder with a marked female predominance. The heart is involved in up to 25% of cases, in the form of pericarditis with or without pericardial effusion. Cardiac symptoms do not necessarily predominate, the disease being a multisystem disorder, but affected women can have significant obstetric problems, including recurrent miscarriages, pre-term labour and an exacerbation of symptoms during pregnancy. Offspring of affected mothers may have complete heart block requiring supportive treatment in the neonatal period. These problems appear to result from the passage of autoantibodies across the placenta.

Cardiomyopathies

Hypertrophic cardiomyopathy is frequently inherited as an autosomal dominant disorder. The onset of symptoms is usually in early adult life rather than in childhood. It may cause sudden arrhythmia. Early diagnosis can lead to effective treatment. There are now a number of genes identified including cardiac beta-myosin heavy chain gene, the cardiac troponin T gene, and the alpha-tropomyosin gene.[26,27] Fetal echocardiography will not recognize the adult-onset cardiomyopathies and prenatal diagnosis will depend on identifying the causative mutation in the family. Preconceptual referral to a specialized center would be recommended.

   Idiopathic dilated cardiomyopathy is also a heterogeneous group of disorders, but occasionally may show an inherited pattern. Most families are consistent with autosomal dominant inheritance, although occasional families with autosomal recessive inheritance and X-linked inheritance have been reported.[28,29] The variability in expression may also make counseling difficult. Review of the family history may help elucidate the inheritance pattern, but in small families it is often considered best to offer echocardiographic screening of all first-degree relatives to detect occult disease.

Coronary artery disease and myocardial infarction

Coronary heart disease has numerous causes, both genetic and environmental. It is rarely cited as a cause for concern in terms of risk to offspring. However, familial hypercholesterolemia is an autosomal dominant disorder that is considered to account for about 10–20% of early coronary heart disease and, if this has been diagnosed in a parent, it is worth considering testing the children, so that early preventive measures can be introduced. Although the risk of inheriting the gene is 50% in such families, the risk of heart disease is considerably less than this, as a result of multiple confounding factors. The basic defect in familial hypercholesterolemia is a low-density lipoprotein receptor deficiency, and the gene is located on chromosome 19. Mutations have been identified in many cases, and provide an accurate means of screening in some families.[30]

References

1 Kelly TE. *Clinical Genetics and Genetic Counseling*. Chicago: Year Book, 1986.
2 Holt M, Oram S. Familial heart disease with skeletal malformations. *Br Heart J* 1960;**22**:236–42.
3 Hurst JA, Hall CM, Baraitser M. Syndrome of the month: the Holt–Oram syndrome. *J Med Genet* 1991;**28**:406–10.
4 Li QY, Newbury-Ecob RA, Terrett JA et al. Holt–Oram syndrome is caused by mutations in TBX5—a member of the Brachyury (T) gene family. *Nat Genet* 1997;**15**: 21–9.
5 Tartaglia M, Mehler EL, Goldberg R et al. Mutations in the protein tyrosine phosphatase gene PTPN11 cause Noonan syndrome. *Nat Genet* 2001;**29**:465–8.
6 Sharland M, Burch M, McKenna WM, Patton MA. A clinical study of Noonan syndrome. *Arch Dis Child* 1992;**67**:178–83.

7 Sarkozy A, Conti E, Diglio MC et al. Clinical and molecular analysis of 30 patients with multiple lentignes LEOPARD syndrome. *J Med Genet* 2004;**41**;e68.

8 Milewicz DM, Pycritz R, Crawford ES, Byers PH. Marfan syndrome: defective secretion, synthesis and extracellular matrix formation of fibrillin by cultured dermal fibroblasts. *J Clin Invest* 1992;**89**:79–86.

9 Ward OC. A new familial cardiac syndrome in children. *J Irish Med Assoc* 1964; **54**:103–6.

10 Splawski I, Shen J, Timothy KW et al. Spectrum of mutations in long QT syndrome genes KVLQT1, HERG, SCN5A, KCNE1 and KCNE2. *Circulation* 2000;**102**:1178–85.

11 Jervell A, Lange-Nielsen F. Congenital deaf-mutism, functional heart disease and prolongation of Q–T interval and sudden death. *Am Heart J* 1957;**54**:59–68.

12 Schmidt MA, Ensing GJ, Michels VV, Carter GA, Hagler DJ, Feldt RH. Autosomal dominant supravalvular aortic stenosis: large three-generation family. *Am J Med Genet* 1989;**32**:384–9.

13 Nickerson E, Greenberg F, Keating MT, McCaskill C, Shaffer LG. Deletions of the elastin gene at 7g11.23 occur in 90% of patients with Williams syndrome. *Am J Hum Genet* 1995;**56**:1156–61.

14 Ellis RWB, Van Creveld S. A syndrome characterised by ectodermal dysplasia, polydactyly, chondro-dysplasia and congenital morbus cordis. *Arch Dis Child* 1940; **15**:65–84.

15 Ruiz-Perez VL, Tompson SW, Blair HJ et al. Mutations in two non-homologous genes in a head-to-head configuration cause Ellis–van Creveld syndrome. *Am J Hum Genet* 2003;**72**:728–32.

16 Kartagener M, Stucki P. Bronchiectasis with situs inversus. *Arch Pediatr* 1962; **79**:193–207.

17 Guichard C, Harricane M-C, Lafitte J-J et al. Axonemal dynein intermediate chain (DNAI1) mutations result in situs inversus and primary ciliary dyskinesia (Kartagener syndrome). *Am J Hum Genet* 2001;**68**;1030–5.

18 Ryan AK, Goodship JA, Wilson DI et al. Spectrum of clinical features associated with interstitial chromosome 22q11 deletions: a European collaborative study. *J Med Genet* 1997;**34**:798–804.

19 Dennis NR, Warren J. Risks to the offspring of patients with some common congenital heart defects. *J Med Genet* 1981;**18**:8–16.

20 Emanuel R, Somerville J, Inns A, Withers R. Evidence of congenital heart disease in the offspring of parents with atrioventricular defects. *Br Heart J* 1983;**49**:144–7.

21 Zellers TM, Driscoll DJ, Michels VV. Prevalence of significant congenital heart defects in children of parents with Fallot's tetralogy. *Am J Cardiol* 1990;**65**:523–6.

22 Harper PS. *Practical Genetic Counselling*, 6th edn. Oxford: Butterworth-Heinemann, 2004.

23 Nora JJ, Berg K, Nora AH. *Cardiovascular Diseases. Genetics, epidemiology and prevention.* Oxford: Oxford University Press, 1991.

24 Thompson P, McRae C. Familial pulmonary hypertension: evidence of autosomal dominant inheritance. *Br Heart J* 1970;**32**:758–60.

25 Lane KB, Machado RD, Pauciolo MW et al. Heterozygous germline mutations in BMPR2 encoding TGF-beta receptor cause familial primary pulmonary hypertension. *Nat Genet* 1998;**26**:81–4.

26 Geisterfer-Laurence AAT, Kass S, Tanigawa G et al. A molecular basis for familial hypertrophic cardiomyopathy. *Cell* 1990;**62**:999–1006.

27 Elliott P, McKenna WJ. Hypertrophic cardiomyopathy (review). *Lancet* 2004;**363**: 1881–91.

28 Berko BA, Swift M. X-linked dilated cardiomyopathy. *N Engl J Med* 1987;**316**: 1186–91.

29 Muntoni F, Cau M, Ganau A et al. Deletion of muscle promotor region associated with X linked dilated cardiomyopathy. *N Engl J Med* 1993;**329**:921–5.

30 Goldstein JL, Hobbs HH, Brown MS. Familial hypercholesterolemia. In: Scriver CR, Beaudet AL, Sly WS et al. (eds), *The Metabolic and Molecular Bases of Inherited Disease*, 8th edn. London: McGraw-Hill, 2000.

CHAPTER 23

Contraception for the cardiac patient

Philip J Steer

The perfect contraceptive has not yet been invented; all methods have advantages and disadvantages. For many women with cardiac disease, the choices open to them are similar to those for women without cardiac disease, and will depend more on their personal characteristics (e.g. how good they are at remembering to take pills) and general life situation (e.g. whether they have a monogamous, stable and long-term sexual partnership with a man who is willing to take on the responsibility of contraception) than on their heart condition. For some women there will be additional risks, e.g. thrombosis from the combined oral contraceptive if they have cyanotic congenital heart disease, or subacute bacterial endocarditis if they use the intrauterine contraceptive device (IUCD). For those who are advised to avoid pregnancy, the risk of contraceptive failure looms large. It would be inappropriate to give a fully comprehensive and detailed account of contraceptive methods in a book on cardiac disease (for those who need more detail, I recommend John Guillebaud's recent text[1]). Accordingly, the account that follows gives only broad outlines of the methods available, and concentrates on those aspects particularly relevant to women with cardiac disease.

When should contraceptive advice be given?

Arguably, all women should have access to appropriate contraceptive advice before they choose to become sexually active. This is especially true of women who have a medical condition (in this case, cardiac disease) in which pregnancy represents a particular risk. Improved nutrition and the liberalization of many societies have led to a dislocation of the age at which women become sexually mature and able to conceive (which can be as early as 11 or 12 years of age), the age at which they can legally become sexually active (commonly 16 years of age) and the age at which their parents would expect them to become sexually active (which may be some years later). Thus, it can be difficult for the cardiologist to know when to start introducing the idea of contraception into their consultations. The appropriate time will vary according to the individual needs of the woman, and the society in which she lives.

My personal view is that basic sex education, including knowledge of contraception, should have been given by the time a woman is able to become pregnant. This is not to encourage her to undertake sexual activity earlier (indeed, there are many advantages to delaying sexual activity until the woman is psychologically mature enough to cope with long-term relationships, not the least of which includes reducing the risk of sexually transmitted infection and infertility), but to empower young women in situations in which she may be coerced by a partner or even her family into an early sexual relationship. Ideally, information about contraception should be embedded in a broader education about personal relationships and responsibilities. In the personal view of the author, all cardiologists providing pediatric cardiology services should arrange to assess and plan the contraceptive education needs of their patients when they reach about 12 years of age, and either provide information themselves, or arrange for an appropriate professional with a knowledge both of contraception and heart disease to provide it instead. Ideally, the family of the very young woman with heart disease should be involved in this process, especially her mother. However, the rights of the patient herself take precedence over the family view if these are at odds.

Contraceptive advice can profitably be given at the same time as a discussion with the woman about the long-term impact of her cardiac condition on her longevity, lifestyle and child-bearing potential. I have personally come across many women who have been given inadequate or misleading advice about the long-term prognosis for their condition (often in an understandable attempt to protect a young and optimistic woman from the sobering appreciation of the implications of her condition) or the risk to them of becoming pregnant. Some have happily embarked on a pregnancy, only to be faced with a substantial risk of death if they continue to term, or the emotionally traumatic alternative of termination of pregnancy.

The normal female desire to have children is not generally lessened by having heart disease and, for some women, this may lead them to choose surgical repair of their condition earlier than is otherwise necessary, so as to reduce the risk of pregnancy. Alternately, she may choose to delay child bearing until after surgery becomes necessary on medical grounds. In other women, their condition will deteriorate as they get older, and they may need to be advised to have their children as early as relationships allow.

Discussing these difficult issues in a sensitive and supportive manner requires skill, patience and understanding. It is vital that the patient's values are considered paramount, not those of physicians or her family. All too often the woman is presented by one or both of these groups with views that either minimize potential hazards or exaggerate them. The excuse is that this is 'in the patient's best interests'. There is only one attitude that is in the best interests of the woman concerned, and that is to tell her the truth. She has a right to be presented with as accurate a prognosis as possible for both mother and baby when pregnancy is discussed, and to be given an account of any potential hazards of procedures for contraception and sterilization. The woman who is aware that she may die within a few years may, at the extremes, have one of two diametrically opposed attitudes. One is that, if she is going to die, she would not want to leave a young child on his or her own, in the care of others. The other is that she would have done a good job in producing a healthy baby, who, if the mother dies, will live on, develop and be a credit to her memory. Many women will find it very hard to make a choice between these two alternatives and, for them, extensive counseling may be necessary.

The effectiveness of contraceptive methods

The failure rate of any particular method of contraception is expressed using the 'pearl index', which is the number of pregnancies that occur per 100 women-years of use. It should be borne in mind that there is a 'typical' failure rate based on the experience of the average user, and a 'best use' failure rate based on the optimal use of the technique. For some methods, these will be very different (e.g. the effectiveness of the use of condoms is very dependent on how well they are used) whereas for others, such as the IUCD, there is essentially no user-dependent component and therefore no difference in the failure rates. Typical failure rates for the various methods are shown in Table 23.1.

Table 23.1 Typical failure rates (Pearl index) of contraceptive methods (pregnancies per 100 women-years of use)

Method	'Typical' failure rate	'Best use' failure rate
No contraception used by normally fertile couple	85	85
Withdrawal	19	4
Male condoms	14	3
Female condom	21	5
Vaginal diaphragm	20	6
Cervical cap	18	6
Spermicides	26	6
Combined oral contraceptive pill	5	<1
Daily low-dose oral progestogen	5	2
Depot Provera (intramuscular injection of a progestogen)	<1	<1
Progestogen implants (e.g. Norplant)	<1	<1
Vaginal hormonal ring (e.g. Nuvaring)	Not yet established	<1
Plastic IUCD	3	3
Copper IUCD	<1	<1
Progestogen IUCD (e.g. Mirena)	<1	<1
Lactational amenorrhea	<2	<2

IUCD, intrauterine contraceptive device.

Methods available that have no direct influence on heart disease in the woman

'Natural' methods

There are a variety of techniques that use our understanding of how conception occurs to try to prevent pregnancy. Although often called 'natural', many seem far from natural in practice, e.g. abstinence is completely effective but for many defeats the purpose of having a relationship! The so-called 'safe period' relies on the assumption that the average woman ovulates 14 days from the beginning of her last menstrual period. Conception usually occurs only if intercourse takes place around the time of ovulation (sperm can remain viable for up to 72 hours and the egg for about 24 hours before fertilization occurs). Unfortunately, many women have irregular cycles and so they cannot rely on timing alone. There are various devices measuring temperature (the woman's temperature rises by about 0.5°C after ovulation as a result of secretion of progesterone from the ovary) or the viscosity of the cervical mucus. These methods can usually detect when ovulation has occurred, and intercourse more than 48 hours after ovulation is unlikely to result in a pregnancy until after the next period.

The likelihood of conception for each act of intercourse before the next menstrual period is only about 1%. Unfortunately, ovulation does not always occur reliably 14 days after the beginning of the menstrual period, and sometimes occurs even as early as day 5 (occasionally, even before the menstrual flow has completely stopped). Thus, the likelihood of conception between the end of the period and day 12 is about 4% for each act of intercourse. This means that penetrative intercourse is relatively safe for only about 10 days a month, and many couples find this irksome (it is sometimes known as the 'rhythm and blues' method). The temperature method is prone to disruption if the woman becomes pyrexial, e.g. from a cold, and many women find obtaining a good sample of cervical mucus difficult.

Barrier contraception

Male withdrawal before each ejaculation is often emotionally unsatisfactory for both partners. It is also often difficult for the male partner to time withdrawal accurately so that ejaculation occurs before he has withdrawn. In addition, a small number of sperm are often released into the vagina before orgasm and full ejaculation, and pregnancy can occur if even a single sperm reaches the egg. For all these reasons, the failure rate of this technique is usually unacceptable for women for whom pregnancy presents serious risks.

Male and female condoms have the advantage that they protect against sexually transmitted infections (STIs). However, they require considerable skill to use correctly, and many couples fail to acquire adequate instruction. Many couples find that male condoms interfere with the spontaneity of sexual intercourse. Both female condoms and diaphragms can be inserted well in advance of intercourse, but require premeditation. Female condoms are made of polyurethane rather than latex or rubber, and make rustling noises in use,

(a)   **(b)**   **(c)**

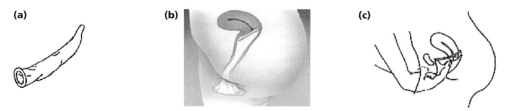

Figure 23.1 Contraceptive methods: (a) male condom; (b) female condom; (c) female diaphragm.

which some people find offputting! All of these methods should be used to-gether with a spermicide (most of which contain nonoxynol-9) if optimum success in preventing pregnancy is to be obtained. However, all of them have relatively high failure rates. Whether they are suitable for use by couples where the woman has heart disease therefore depends critically on how impor-tant it is to avoid pregnancy. If effectiveness is a priority, then clearly these tech-niques are not appropriate.

Cervical caps have to be individually fitted for each woman and cover only the cervix, rather than sitting between the posterior fornix and the retropubic vagina as shown for the diaphragm in Figure 23.1. They are difficult to use cor-rectly and are no longer widely available.

Lactational amenorrhea
In technologically undeveloped communities, prolonged breast-feeding is a traditional method of spacing pregnancies. The optimum time interval between pregnancies, in terms of minimizing the risk of ectopic pregnancy, miscarriage and placenta praevia, is 2 years. This probably relates to changes in the vascular supply to the uterus. Pregnancy increases blood flow to all parts of the uterus, and therefore early conception after pregnancy tends to result in abnormal im-plantation sites; once pregnancy changes have resolved, the major blood supply to the uterus is at the fundus, where implantation is optimal. In communities where breast-feeding is almost continuous throughout a woman's life, the average interpregnancy interval is about 2 years. Unfortunately, the absence of menstruation associated with breast-feeding is not a guarantee that ovulation has not occurred, because a menstrual period happens only after release of an ovum that is not fertilized or that does not implant successfully. Therefore, the first sign a woman may have that she has conceived again can be the swelling of her abdomen, or morning sickness. Thus, lactation is not a reliable contracep-tive method. However, together with a barrier method of contraception, or the progestogen-only pill (see later) the failure rate is probably acceptable unless another pregnancy is completely contraindicated.

Oral contraceptives
Combined estrogen–progestogen oral preparations are among the most effec-tive and convenient, readily available contraceptive methods available, and are

very widely used. Claims have been made for 'method failures' of less than 0.1/100 woman-years, but everyday clinical experience is that the overall failure rate is of the order of 1–5/100 woman-years. The combined pill works by suppressing ovulation. Most of the pregnancies are probably the result of 'patient failures', with the woman forgetting to take her pill. A missed pill is unlikely to result in conception during most of the pill-taking cycle, but ovarian suppression is at its lowest during the pill-free week, during which endometrial withdrawal bleeding occurs (usually interpreted by the woman as a 'period'), and thus missed pills just before or just after the pill-free week have the highest risk of allowing an unwanted conception. Some failures may be the result of gastrointestinal upsets with intestinal hurry and decreased absorption, and coincident administration of drugs such as rifampicin, phenytoin, phenobarbital, phenylbutazone and antibiotics, which speed metabolism or reduce absorption of the synthetic sex hormones. Women with heart disease are a well-motivated group, who generally read the instructions or are well instructed, and their failures with the pill should be at the lower end of the range. Recovery of fertility after ceasing to take an oral contraceptive is a bit slower than after other methods of contraception, but 80% of previously fertile women have had a baby within 18 months and 95% within 3 years.

Risks of oral contraceptives in patients with heart disease

The main concern is the risk of thromboembolic problems, including pulmonary embolism, biochemical changes predisposing to deterioration of atherosclerosis, hypertension, myocardial infarction in older women and hemodynamic changes consequent on fluid and electrolyte retention. These hazards have perhaps been overestimated in the past, because of overemphasis on isolated cases and the fact that when they were first introduced the amounts of synthetic sex hormones in contraceptive pills were substantially higher than they are today. Moreover, the content of combined pills has evolved and three generations of progestogens have been introduced, for example.

Thrombosis and embolism

The propensity of estrogen to increase the risk of venous thromboembolism has been appreciated since the first report of this effect in 1961. This resulted in a progressive decrease in the dose of estrogen used, so that currently most employ a dose of 30 μg or even less. However, multiple studies in the 1990s have shown that even this low dose is associated with a three- to sixfold increased relative risk of venous thromboembolism.[2] The risk is highest during the first year of use, but persists even with prolonged use. However, because the baseline risk of venous thromboembolism (VTE) is low in young healthy women (estimated as 1 VTE/10 000 women per year), the absolute risk remains low (3–6 VTE/10 000 women per year using oral contraception). These figures relate to combined oral contraceptives using norethisterone (first-generation progestogen) or levonorgestrel (second-generation progestogen). Third-generation progestogens such as gestodene and desogestrel, introduced because of their more favorable effect on metabolic profiles, have since been shown to double the risk of the VTE further and formulations using them are therefore particularly unsuitable for women at risk of VTE.[3,4] All these risks are substantially increased in women with thrombophilias such as factor V Leiden or protein C deficiency. Other risk factors include maternal obesity.

Provided that women with either a personal or family history of VTE are excluded, the risk of either a thrombosis or an embolism in the average woman taking a modern estrogen–progestogen oral contraceptive is low, of the order of 1 in 3300/year, even though it is three times higher than in women not taking these preparations. On the other hand, the comparable risk of thrombosis or embolism in a pregnancy that the contraceptive would have prevented is 10 per 10 000 pregnancies, twice as high as in women taking a contraceptive pill. Thus, the risk of VTE is probably acceptable when the need to avoid pregnancy is as high as it is in women with significant heart disease. Nevertheless, these issues must be brought to the patient's notice and ultimately the choice must be left to her.

The position with patients taking oral anticoagulants remains unclear. On the one hand, they are protected against the risk of thrombosis, but, on the other, they are by definition a high-risk group. If a patient on prophylactic anticoagulants strongly desires oral contraception and has a strong case for really effective contraception, such as previous failures with other procedures, then the unknown nature of the risk must be explained before acceding to her wishes. Many doctors would deny oral contraceptives to a patient on full anticoagulation for an artificial heart valve, but information to support such a stance is not available.

Biochemical changes and atherosclerosis

In the past, the balance of evidence was that the estrogen components of a combined pill tended to increase high-density lipoprotein (HDL)-cholesterol, which should reduce the risk of atherosclerosis, whereas progestogens appear to lower HDL-cholesterol and counterbalance the estrogen effect. Some progestogens also raise low-density lipoprotein (LDL)-cholesterol, which might have a deleterious effect. However, overall the general effect on cardiovascular risk was thought either to be neutral[5] or possibly even positive. The perception of neutrality has been supported by the Women's Health Initiative trial of hormone replacement therapy,[6] which reported a hazard risk for breast cancer of 1.26, for stroke 1.41 and no effect overall on the risk of cardiovascular disease. If a patient considered to be at risk for atherosclerosis requests oral contraception, it may well be prudent to estimate plasma lipids before starting the combined oral contraceptive pill. If the levels are normal, the risk is unlikely to be substantial; however, probably the estimation of plasma lipids should be repeated after 2 months of taking the pill and every 3 months thereafter.

Hypertension

The combined oral contraceptives can cause hypertension in a small number of normotensive women, but with careful monitoring of blood pressure (BP) this is not a major prospective contraindication to their use. However, there is some evidence that the combined oral contraceptive is contraindicated in women who are already hypertensive, and should be discontinued if hypertension is detected.[7]

It is therefore wise to be cautious in this respect in women with heart disease. Those who are normotensive and wish to take an oral contraceptive should have their BP checked 1 month after starting, again at 2 months and thereafter when the prescription is renewed. Women with heart disease who are already hypertensive are best advised of the risk, albeit small, of their hypertension deteriorating. If they feel that their reasons for taking an oral contraceptive outweigh this risk, then monthly checks on BP are desirable.

Myocardial infarction

Soon after oral contraceptives were first marketed in the 1960s, case reports linked their use to the occurrence of myocardial infarction. Over the past few decades, numerous studies have examined the cardiovascular complications associated with oral contraceptive use, and have reached conflicting conclusions. However, a recent meta-analysis of 19 case–control studies and four cohort studies[8] has found that current users of the oral contraceptive pill have an overall adjusted odds ratio of myocardial infarction of 2.48 compared with never users. Use of the oral contraceptive pill interacted with other risk factors such as smoking, hypertension, hypercholesterolemia and mutation in the prothrombin gene, resulting in odds ratios as high as 9. Interestingly, the overall odds ratio for past users was not significantly different from never users, being 1.15 (with confidence interval, $CI = 0.98–1.35$). As a result, women with predisposing factors for ischemic heart disease should be strongly advised not to take the combined estrogen–progestogen oral contraceptive pill. Patients known to have coronary artery disease should be told that these preparations are absolutely contraindicated.

Use of the oral contraceptive pill in other cardiac conditions

The World Health Organization (WHO) has classified contraindications into four grades, the first being no contraindication, the second where the advantages of the method generally outweigh the theoretical or proven risks, the third where the theoretical or proven risks usually outweigh the advantages (so that another method would be preferable, but a woman may still choose the method for personal reasons), and the fourth an unacceptable health risk. Table 23.2 indicates the varieties of heart disease in the various categories of contraindication.

Progestogen-only oral contraceptives

Not only do these contraceptives not contain estrogen, the dose of progestogen is also much lower than in the combined pill. They do not usually prevent

Table 23.2 Cardiac contraindications to use of the combined oral contraceptive pill

WHO grade 2 (advantages outweigh risks)	WHO grade 3 (risks outweigh advantages)	WHO grade 4 (contraindicated)
Dysrhythmias other than atrial fibrillation or flutter		Atrial fibrillation or flutter
Uncomplicated valve lesions including mitral and bicuspid aortic valve prolapse		Pulmonary hypertension or pulmonary vascular disease Pulmonary arteriovenous malformation
Prosthetic or tissue heart valves	Bileaflet mechanical valve in mitral or aortic position on warfarin	Björk–Shiley or Starr–Edwards valves, even on warfarin
Fully surgically corrected congenital heart disease	Heart disease or thrombosis well controlled on warfarin with careful supervision of INR	Poor left ventricular function (left ventricle ejection fraction <30%)
Non-reversible trivial left-to-right shunts, e.g. small VSD or trivial patent ductus arteriosus	All known interatrial communications – risk of paradoxical embolism	Dilated left atrium (>4 cm) Cyanotic heart disease
Repaired coarctation without aneurysm or hypertension	Repaired coarctation with aneurysm or hypertension	
Uncomplicated Marfan syndrome	Marfan syndrome with aortic dilatation, unoperated	
Uncomplicated pulmonary stenosis		Post-surgery Fontan heart, even on warfarin
Hypertrophic obstructive cardiomyopathy, pregnancy related or other cardiomyopathy, fully recovered with normal heart on echocardiography		Dilated cardiomyopathy or previous cardiomyopathy with residual left ventricular dysfunction
		Any past venous or arterial thromboembolic event, not on warfarin

INR, international normalized ratio; IUCD, intrauterine contraceptive device; VSD, ventricular septal defect; WHO, World Health Organization.

After Guillebaud.[9]

ovulation, but rely on preventing the midcycle increases in cervical mucus permeability, thus preventing sperm penetration into the female genital tract. As they do not prevent ovulation, they are less reliable than combined estrogen–progestogen preparations, with failure rates of 2–5/100 woman-years, and missing a single pill can result in pregnancy. For this reason, they require a high degree of patient motivation and are not suitable for women who find it difficult to remember to take the pill every day. Problems with irregular bleeding and episodes of amenorrhea, leading to suspicions of pregnancy, are common. As a result, discontinuation rates with the method are high—many women request an alternative after 1–2 years. As a result of their relatively high failure rate, they are not suitable for women at very high cardiac risk, for whom a pregnancy would be disastrous, e.g. in women with significant pulmonary hypertension.

The main reason for the promotion of the progesterone-only pill has been the assumption that, because there is no estrogen, and the progestogen dose is low, the effects on thrombosis and the cardiovascular system must be much less than with the combined pill. Unfortunately, there is a paucity of well-conducted studies, and the data sheet, even for norethisterone, which has been in use for over 40 years, says that it is contraindicated in women with previous thromboembolism. However, there is no evidence to support this assertion and papers are now appearing that support the view that thrombosis is unlikely to be a serious risk with the progesterone-only pill.[2,10] Moreover, a recent review of published literature suggests that the progesterone-only pill does not induce hypertension and is probably not contraindicated in women with hypertension.[11] Nor is there any significant evidence of metabolic disturbance with their use. For these reasons, many authorities (including Guillebaud[9]) suggest that the progesterone-only pill is suitable for motivated women with structural heart disease who can cope with some irregularity in their menstrual pattern.

Contraception postpartum may be particularly important to the cardiac patient, who may wish to postpone or prevent another pregnancy. In about 20% of women, the combined oral contraceptive pill will reduce breast milk production, which appears to be unaffected using the progestogen-only oral contraceptive. As lactational amenorrhea is quite an effective contraceptive on its own, there seems to be a logic in combining the two. However, it must be emphasized that the body of literature supporting the use of the progesterone-only pill is much smaller than that for the combined preparation.

Recently, a new progestogen-only pill (Cerazette) has been introduced containing 75 µg desogestrel. This does suppress ovulation, and therefore has a failure rate similar to that of the combined oral contraceptive pill. Moreover, the increased effectiveness prolongs its efficacy if the woman forgets to take her pill, so increasing the time that the woman can remember to take her pill and restore contraceptive efficacy, up to 12 hours after the missed dose. This improved efficacy makes it more suitable for women with high-risk cardiac lesions. Cerazette is metabolized after ingestion into etonorgestrel, which is used in the progestogen implant system Implanon. It can therefore be used to test a woman's tolerance of this hormone before the implant is inserted surgically.

Other forms of progestogen contraception

Vaginal rings
Vaginal rings releasing a progestogen (desogestrel) are already available in the USA and in some European countries. They have proved very popular in studies, with excellent cycle control and very few contraceptive failures. The ring is removed for 1 week out of 4, to allow a withdrawal bleed. It is too early to say whether they will be suitable for women with heart disease.

Injectable depot progestogens
Injectable progestogens, such as depot medroxyprogesterone acetate, are one solution to poor patient compliance, because they are administered by a nurse or similar professional, and relieve the patient of the responsibility for remembering to take pills. Medroxyprogesterone injections need to be given only once every 12 weeks to be effective. They have been repeatedly endorsed by the WHO and the International Planned Parenthood Federation, and are currently available for long-term contraceptive use in more than 130 countries. Despite this, they are used by fewer than 2% of women in the UK, because of concerns from women and professionals about the irregular uterine bleeding that they can provoke, especially when being discontinued. Nevertheless, women who find it difficult to take pills regularly may find it a preferable alternative to IUCDs or sterilization. The cardiovascular contraindications are essentially the same as for the progesterone-only pill.

Implants
One of the early subcutaneous progestogen implants to be introduced, Norplant, turned out to be difficult to remove, resulting in legal action from some women. This naturally had an adverse effect on public and professional confidence. However, more recently, Implanon has been introduced successfully into the UK. It is a single 40 mm long tube, 2 mm in diameter, and is far easier to insert than Norplant. It contains etonorgestrel. A major advantage is an extremely low failure rate, with current reports of less than one failure per 1000 insertions.[12] It is inserted into the upper non-dominant arm under local anesthetic; training in insertion is necessary. Removal is easy but also needs training. The risks associated with its use are likely to be similar to those with the other progestogens. Twenty percent of women become amenorrheic with its use, but many women develop irregular periods instead, and this is the most common reason why its removal is requested. It currently needs to be removed and replaced every 3 years.

Emergency contraception

The 'morning-after' pill
The 'morning-after 'pill is intended to prevent implantation if taken within 3 days of unprotected intercourse. The most widely used regimen consists of a

total of 100 µg ethinylestradiol and 500 µg levonorgestrel repeated after 12 hours. It is unwise to give a cardiac patient such a large dose of estrogen even for a short time, and systemic upsets—nausea, vomiting, headaches and dizziness—are common. A single dose (1.5 mg) of levonorgestrel (Levonelle) is more effective (1% pregnancy rate if used within 72 hours), has fewer side effects and is less prothrombotic, but it interacts with warfarin, increasing the international normalized ratio (INR) up to four times. However, insertion of an IUCD is effective even up to 5 days after unprotected intercourse, and this is probably the preferred alternative in women who need on-going contraception.

Intrauterine contraceptive devices

These devices have been described as the best available contraceptive for a proportion of parous women at certain times in their reproductive lives. They relieve the couple of taking day-to-day responsibility for contraception, apart from verifying the presence of the device monthly, after menstruation, by palpating the strings in the cervix. Failure rates of modern copper-containing IUCDs are comparable with oral contraceptives. The original ICUDs were made entirely of plastic (e.g. the Lippes loop) but they had an unacceptable failure rate and have been completely superseded by copper and progestogen-bearing devices. Once inserted, they are licensed to be effective for 3 and 5 years respectively.

Complications of the insertion procedure

About 10% of women develop tachycardia during insertion of an IUCD, and 2% will develop a bradycardia or develop a transient arrhythmia. Vasovagal syncope caused by dilatation of the cervix without analgesia or anesthesia can occur during insertion of a device; this phenomenon has been witnessed personally by me. However, it is rare; a recent review of 545 IUCD insertions reported only one case.[13] A cardiac patient should therefore be prepared for insertion of a device with a premedication including atropine, and insertion conducted under hospital conditions rather than in a family planning clinic. Insertion should be done by an experienced practitioner, with a skilled anesthetist in attendance in case of complications. Perforation of the uterus when a device is inserted is rare, occurring in about 1 in 1000 insertions. A copper-bearing device that has perforated should be removed promptly to prevent bowel adhesions forming. The implications for a patient with heart disease are those of the laparoscopy or laparotomy that is likely to be necessary for removal. A basic rule for the prevention of perforation during insertion is to discontinue the attempt promptly if the patient is not fully relaxed or experiences significant pain.

The risk of infection

The vagina and cervix always contain micro-organisms. The cervical glands and mucus plug present an anti-bacterial barrier to their ascent into the uterus. When they are introduced into the upper genital tract, some of these organisms are potentially pathogenic. The hazard can be much reduced by antiseptic cleansing of the vagina and cervix, and by good aseptic technique, but these areas are impossible to sterilize completely. Insertion of an IUCD is probably always accompanied by the introduction of some micro-organisms into the uterine cavity. The insertion of a device nearly always causes some minor intrauterine trauma, and it is likely that a transient bacteremia can result, much as with a dental extraction. However, both these invasions are usually dealt with by natural defense mechanisms, and only a few cases of endocarditis secondary to the insertion of an IUCD have been reported.[14] Nevertheless, in women with structural heart lesions, antibiotic prophylaxis seems wise, either with amoxicillin and gentamicin, or vancomycin and gentamicin.

As a result of this small risk of infection, the use of a copper IUCD in women with structural heart disease is regarded as WHO grade 3 contraindicated. However, early indications of the use of the progestogen-loaded IUCD (levonorgestrel intrauterine system, LNG-IUS, Mirena) suggest that because it suppresses endometrial activity and thickens cervical mucus, it reduces the risk of infection and might therefore be safer in this context. The Mirena has an extremely low failure rate, possibly as low as 0.2/100 women-years, which is less than most methods of sterilization other than hysterectomy.[9] So far, side-effect rates appear to be very low and it approaches 100% reversibility. It is currently licensed to be left in place for up to 5 years before replacement. Unlike the copper-loaded IUCD, which increases the heaviness of the menstrual flow, in 80% of women periods either cease or become very light. As a result of the very low failure rate, women can be reassured that loss of periods does not indicate pregnancy. The main disadvantage currently is its substantial cost.

'Emergency' contraception with an IUCD

Inserted within 5 days of unprotected intercourse, a copper-bearing intrauterine contraceptive device has a high degree of reliability in preventing implantation of a fertilized ovum. Cardiac patients presenting with this problem should be screened for STIs and the same precautions taken (prophylactic antibiotics and, particularly if nulliparous, premedication in a hospital setting) as for routine insertions.

Termination of pregnancy

When termination of an unplanned pregnancy is considered by a cardiac patient, it is not uncommon for the risks of continuing pregnancy to be either exaggerated or minimized by her cardiologist. It is essential in these cases that the patient be given an accurate prognosis for herself and for the baby, and that she draws her own conclusions as to the desirability of termination. Equally important is that she is not put under pressure by relatives, and at least one interview should be conducted with the patient on her own.

First trimester termination in a cardiac patient has the same basic risks as any other surgical procedure and should be conducted in a fully equipped hospital rather than in an isolated clinic. The added risks in cardiac patients arise from general anesthesia and from hemorrhage or infection. It is important in the prevention of these that retained products of conception are avoided. This involves the use of an adequate size suction catheter, even if this means dilating the cervix, and an ultrasound scan the following day to verify completion of the evacuation of the uterus. Patients with any anatomic cardiovascular lesion should have prophylactic antibiotics. Mifepristone (a progesterone antagonist) can be used to induce miscarriage, but the risk of retained products is such that it should be followed by surgical evacuation of the uterus (rather than prostaglandins, which have cardiovascular effects), if the ultrasonographer is not confident that the uterus is empty.

Second trimester termination has greater risks of pelvic trauma, hemorrhage and infection, and these should be balanced against the risks of continuing the pregnancy. Although probably the safest way of terminating a midtrimester pregnancy is cervical dilatation and evacuation of the fetus by a skilled surgeon, the number of clinicians trained and experienced to do this procedure is declining, in both the USA and the UK. Unfortunately, the alternative is to use mifepristone and a potent prostaglandin such as vaginally administered gemeprost or misoprostol to induce labour (if the fetus is 20 weeks' gestation or more, it is recommended that fetocide be performed first). The side effects of these prostaglandins include nausea, vomiting, diarrhea, pyrexia, bradycardia or tachycardia, fall in BP and reduced cardiac contractility. The cardiac patient must therefore be closely monitored, as for term labour and delivery. If untoward effects occur, an experienced gynecologist will be needed to complete the delivery surgically.

Tubal sterilization

The advice often given to cardiac patients is 'have your family while you are young and then get your tubes tied'. It is sensible to encourage this (if relationships allow) and, with progressive conditions such as Marfan syndrome, it should be emphasized that delayed child bearing will substantially increase the risk to the mother of the pregnancy when it eventually occurs. However, even when pregnancy is relatively contraindicated, with all women the decision for sterilization must still be theirs, based on accurate information. With less relentlessly progressive heart conditions, and when there is a possibility of cardiac surgery improving prognosis, advice should be more circumspect, because it is not unusual for sterilization in young women to be followed by regret and sometimes depression. Sterilization counseling in cardiac patients must be well informed and thorough. Women can be reassured that sterilization is extremely common; about 45% of couples above the age of 40 in the UK rely for contraception on sterilization of one or other partner.

The most common methods for tubal sterilization currently are laparoscopic procedures in which various forms of clips are applied to the fallopian tubes (Falope rings are used less nowadays because they cause more pain and the failure rate is higher). The Pomeroy operation, in which a loop of each tube is ligated and excised through a small abdominal incision, is used only when laparoscopic equipment is not available. With clips, failure rates are commonly quoted at 1 in 200–500. Failure rates are significantly higher if the operation is performed at the time of cesarean section or termination of pregnancy, because the fallopian tubes during pregnancy are too large for the commercially available clips and the Pomeroy procedure has to be used. Unfortunately, recanalization is more common when this procedure is done during pregnancy. On the other hand, this higher failure rate has to be balanced by the inconvenience of re-admission to hospital and further anesthesia, for 'interval' sterilization.

Cases of cardiac arrhythmia and cardiac arrest, and even isolated fatalities, have been reported during laparoscopy. It is not clear if these are due to the distension of the abdomen required alone or to the fact that it is distended with carbon dioxide. Full monitoring is required, and laparoscopy is regarded by some anesthetists as contraindicated in patients with organic heart disease. Under these circumstances, a 'mini-laparotomy' with application of clips to the fallopian tubes under direct vision may be preferable. Most gynecologists feel that they can operate more efficiently and avoid emotional and physical reactions from a cardiac patient with general rather than local anesthesia, but some anesthetists may prefer spinal anesthesia.

Vasectomy

In general this should be offered as an alternative to tubal sterilization. Even if it is suggested and has already been considered by the couple concerned, the procedure and its consequences must be explained thoroughly, and the couple given time to consider their options. Their conclusion can be motivated in a variety of ways, which they may be reluctant to reveal to a doctor. Their thoughts may range from a deep-seated fear on the man's side of a threat to virility or an increased risk of testicular or prostate cancer (both unfounded), or plans for a second marriage in the future (especially if his wife dies), to the woman's fear that it may provide her partner with the opportunity for unlimited promiscuity. Tact is particularly required in raising these issues when the woman has significant heart disease. Care must be taken to avoid the husband feeling any sort of pressure to have the operation for his partner's benefit. The potential for marital stress and break-up is obvious, particularly if the woman's life expectancy is limited. The couple may have already considered vasectomy If not, the possibility should be mentioned and it should be left to them to discuss it and the implications, and perhaps make a joint request for the man to have a vasectomy. The man should at some stage be seen alone before the operation, to ensure that he has considered all the implications and it is what *he* wants!

Acknowledgements

The contribution of the author of the equivalent chapter in the previous edition, on which this chapter draws in part, is gratefully acknowledged.

References

1 Guillebaud J. *Contraception — Your Questions Answered*. Edinburgh: Churchill Living-stone, 2004.

2 Kujovich JL. Hormones and pregnancy: thromboembolic risks for women. *Br J Haematol* 2004;**126**:443–54.

3 Gomes MP, Deitcher SR. Risk of venous thromboembolic disease associated with hormonal contraceptives and hormone replacement therapy: a clinical review. *Arch Intern Med* 2004;**164**:1965–76.

4 Pill research results in new guidance from CSM. *Fam Plan Today* 1995;**1**:1.

5 Burkman R, Schlesselman JJ, Zieman M. Safety concerns and health benefits associated with oral contraception. *Am J Obstet Gynecol* 2004;**190**:S5–22.

6 Rossouw JE, Anderson GL, Prentice RL et al. Risks and benefits of estrogen plus progestin in healthy postmenopausal women: principal results from the Women's Health Initiative randomized controlled trial. *JAMA* 2002;**288**:321–33.

7 Lubianca JN, Faccin CS, Fuchs FD. Oral contraceptives: a risk factor for uncontrolled blood pressure among hypertensive women. *Contraception* 2003;**67**:19–24.

8 Khader YS, Rice J, John L, Abueita O. Oral contraceptives use and the risk of myocardial infarction: a meta-analysis. *Contraception* 2003;**68**:11–17.

9 Guillebaud J. The levonorgestrel intrauterine system: a clinical perspective from the UK. *Ann NY Acad Sci* 2003;**997**:185–93.

10 Conard J, Plu-Bureau, Bahi N, Horellou MH, Pelissier C, Thalabard JC. Progestogen-only contraception in women at high risk of venous thromboembolism. *Contraception* 2004;**70**:437–41.

11 Hussain SF. Progestogen-only pills and high blood pressure: is there an association? A literature review. *Contraception* 2004;**69**:89–97.

12 Harrison-Woolrych M, Hill R. Unintended pregnancies with the etonogestrel implant (Implanon): a case series from postmarketing experience in Australia. *Contraception* 2005;**71**:306–8.

13 Farmer M, Webb A. Intrauterine device insertion-related complications: can they be predicted? *J Fam Plan Reprod Health Care* 2003;**29**:227–31.

14 Seaworth BJ, Durack DT. Infective endocarditis in obstetric and gynecologic practice. *Am J Obstet Gynecol* 1986;**154**:180–8.

Index